ANIMAL CLINICAL CHEMISTRY

A PRACTICAL GUIDE FOR TOXICOLOGISTS AND BIOMEDICAL RESEARCHERS

SECOND EDITION

ANIMAL CLINICAL CHEMISTRY

A PRACTICAL GUIDE FOR TOXICOLOGISTS AND BIOMEDICAL RESEARCHERS

SECOND EDITION

Edited by

G. O. EVANS

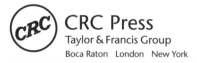

CRC Press
Taylor & Francis Group
Boca Raton   London   New York

CRC Press is an imprint of the
Taylor & Francis Group, an **informa** business

CRC Press
Taylor & Francis Group
6000 Broken Sound Parkway NW, Suite 300
Boca Raton, FL 33487-2742

© 2009 by Taylor & Francis Group, LLC
CRC Press is an imprint of Taylor & Francis Group, an Informa business

International Standard Book Number-13: 978-1-4200-8011-7 (Hardcover)

Library of Congress Cataloging-in-Publication Data
Animal clinical chemistry : a practical handbook for toxicologists and biomedical researchers / [edited by] G.O. Evans. -- 2nd ed.
p. ; cm.
"A CRC title."
Includes bibliographical references and index.
ISBN 978-1-4200-8011-7 (hardcover : alk. paper)
1. Toxicology--Animal models--Handbooks, manuals, etc. 2. Veterinary clinical chemistry--Handbooks, manuals, etc. I. Evans, G. O. II. Title.
[DNLM: 1. Animals, Laboratory. 2. Toxicity Tests--methods. QY 90 A5981 2009]
RA1199.4.A54A515 2009
615.9'020724--dc22   2009002683

Visit the Taylor & Francis Web site at
http://www.taylorandfrancis.com

and the CRC Press Web site at
http://www.crcpress.com

Contents

The Editor

After holding several senior positions and spending 13 years in health service laboratories, G. O. Evans left the post of principal clinical chemist at Birmingham Children's Hospital, England, to enter the field of laboratory animal toxicology and clinical pathology. He was head of clinical pathology at Wellcome Research Laboratories, Beckenham, England. He then joined Astra Charnwood and, later, the two AstraZeneca sites in the United Kingdom as director of clinical pathology. He is now a director of A. George Owen and Company (e-mail: agoco.melton@fsmail.net).

Evans was the editor of and a contributor to a number of chapters of the book *Animal Clinical Chemistry: A Primer for Toxicologists.* In addition to lecturing at various universities in the United Kingdom, he has published more than 40 papers on animal clinical pathology and toxicology. Other activities have included membership on the editorial board of the journal *Laboratory Animals* for more than 15 years and serving as scientific secretary and chairman of the Animal Clinical Chemistry Association in the United Kingdom. He recently authored *Animal Hematotoxicology: A Practical Guide for Toxicologists and Biomedical Researchers,* which was published by CRC Press.

Contributors

P. J. O'Brien
Clinical Pathology Laboratory
Veterinary Sciences Center
University College Dublin
Belfield, Dublin, Ireland

Claire L. Watterson
Clinical Pathology Department
Safety Assessment U.K. AstraZeneca
Macclesfield, Cheshire, England

Preface

This book is designed to help new entrants in the fields of laboratory animal clinical chemistry and toxicology, where the challenges are stimulating and the "rules" for human clinical chemistry do not always apply. There are many good general textbooks on human clinical chemistry/biochemistry and toxicology, and each organization has its favorites. This book aims to bridge the gap between these two mainstream sciences.

It has been more than 10 years since the book *Animal Clinical Chemistry: A Primer for Toxicologists* was published by Taylor & Francis, and that book evolved from the contributors to training courses held in the United Kingdom. This book has similar objectives and designs. Information has been collated from published papers, textbooks, and unpublished data, with references provided at the end of each chapter or in Appendix A, where readers are provided with some key references on published reference ranges for laboratory animals. Two chapters are devoted to preanalytical and analytical variables. These variables play a far more important part when data from animal studies are interpreted compared to data obtained for humans, where many of the variables can be well controlled or have less physiological effect.

Biological organisms cannot be understood solely by reducing them to the component parts and numbers. Toxicological science requires people with the knowledge and experience to interpret and place the clinical chemistry findings obtained from animal studies into an overall picture of toxicity; they must relate these findings to the same measurements made in early clinical trials and following adverse toxic events. The potential development of novel biomarkers that can be utilized and translated between animal and human clinical chemistry should make for scientific progress and excitement in the future.

1 Introduction

1.1 INTRODUCTION

We encounter a wide range of xenobiotics (foreign chemicals) during our lives, including drugs, manufactured consumer products, food additives, environmental pollutants, pesticides, industrial chemicals, and naturally occurring substances. These xenobiotics may be organic or inorganic chemicals of both synthetic and natural origin, and they also include those substances now loosely referred to as "biologicals" (e.g., vaccines and monoclonal antibodies). As we develop and use these novel compounds, there is a requirement to assess the risk to humans, animals, and the environment, and this is where toxicology plays its role as the gatekeeper for safety. In the last few decades, there has been a significant growth in the international activity of safety testing to meet the increasing requirement for consumer safety and to deal with the number and wide range of compounds. In summary, toxicology integrates scientific information to help preserve and protect health and the environment from the hazards presented by chemical and physical agents (Miya et al. 1988), and clinical pathology has a contribution to make by bridging the gap between preclinical studies and risk assessment to health and the environment.

In vivo studies enable toxicologists to make predictions for the safety of xenobiotics in man and other species; in this book, we will be concentrating on clinical chemistry tests used in safety evaluation studies with animals. To predict risk factors associated with the test compounds from laboratory data requires interpretation and integration with the other data obtained from toxicological studies. In our discussions, we will not be including clinical toxicology, which may be defined as the analysis of drugs, heavy metals, and chemical agents in body fluids and tissues (relating to the management of human or animal medicine), nor shall we be dealing with aspects of forensic toxicology and the related subject of analytical toxicology. Neither will we be discussing many of the in vitro techniques being developed as alternatives to in vivo studies for toxicological work that may replace the use of animals, although these techniques have already made a significant impact in dermal and ocular irritancy testing.

Many of the procedures used in conventional toxicity testing with animals have arisen by an apparently empirical process (e.g., period of exposure and selection of dose levels). Safety studies are performed with a variety of experimental animals, including rodents, rabbits, nonhuman primates, and farm animals, before progressing to studies with human volunteers, and other animals in the case of veterinary medicines. The individual study designs vary with the chosen animal species, route of administration, duration (dependent on the proposed or estimated exposure in man), and dosages, which may represent multiples of the proposed therapeutic dosage or different estimates of environmental exposure.

Test compounds can cause both local and systemic adverse effects; local effects occur at the sites of initial contact (e.g., injection sites), while systemic effects are observed in organs remote from the site of initial exposure. The degree of toxicity is dependent on the number of exposures or the duration. Effects can be classified as acute (i.e., short term following a single dose); repeated or multiple exposure effects can be referred to as short term (not more than 5% of life span), subchronic (5–20% of life span), and chronic (the entire or a major part of life span).

Often the distribution and metabolism of compounds vary between different animal species, and equal concentrations of xenobiotics (or metabolites) in different species do not necessarily mean equal pharmacological or toxic effects. Strain and sex differences in the metabolism of xenobiotics are also well recognized (Timbrell 1999). The selective applications for insecticides and pesticides make use of these variations between species. Toxic effects may be caused not by the parent compound but rather by one or more metabolites, and sometimes the identity of these metabolites in different species is not known at the time of animal toxicology studies. Biotransformations of xenobiotics occur primarily in the liver and kidney, and they are more commonly associated with reductions in potential toxicity, although the reverse is sometimes the case, resulting in increased toxicity. Phase 1 biotransformations of xenobiotics and/or metabolites involve the P450 cytochrome mono-oxygenase enzyme family. These enzymes hydroxylate lipophilic compounds, increasing their polarity solubility and then facilitating their excretion. In phase II, xenobiotics and/or their metabolites are biotransformed with polar compounds, which increases their solubility and urinary excretions.

Several other factors can contribute to toxicities. A relatively low toxicological profile with a racemic mixture may allow further development, but the problems encountered with thalidomide highlighted that the toxicities of the S and R enantiomers may differ markedly. Therefore, it is sometimes essential to determine the toxicology of the individual enantiomers even though the racemic mixture appears to cause little or no toxic changes because toxicity may be caused by an isomer-specific metabolite. When the toxicity of chemical mixtures is under examination, the interpretation becomes more difficult (Mumtaz et al. 1993). A mixture of two or more chemicals may result in a different qualitative or quantitative response relative to that predicted from the toxicities observed with separate exposure to the mixture constituents. These effects may be additive or ameliorate the collective toxicity findings. Thus, polypharmacy may complicate toxic changes as well as pharmacological actions.

The development of pro-drugs, designed to overcome pharmaceutical or pharmacokinetic limitations associated with the parent drug molecule, presents a different challenge because although the pro-drug may be pharmacologically inactive, it can show reduced or increased toxicity compared with the active parent compound (Bungaard 1991; Rooney et al. 2004). Adverse effects may be associated with supposedly "inactive" ingredients in drug formulations (Golightly et al. 1988), and vehicles used for compound delivery can markedly affect both exposure and

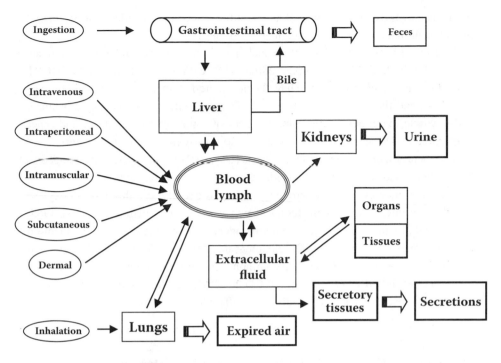

FIGURE 1.1 Ellipses on the left indicate routes of administration and absorption: ⇨ broad arrows indicate routes of elimination.

toxicity—for example, oily vehicles (Condie et al. 1986) and cyclodextrin (Frank, Gray, and Weaver 1976).

For xenobiotics and/or metabolites, the blood and urine are key elements in the metabolism, distribution, and elimination of compounds and their metabolites (see Figure 1.1, where various routes of exposure are indicated). A variety of biochemical measurements can be used to evaluate a broad range of physiological and metabolic functions, identifying possible target organs, measuring impaired function, and assessing the persistence and severity of tissue injury.

1.2 REGULATORY REQUIREMENTS

There have been several published recommendations and suggestions for tests that should be included in toxicology studies (reviewed by Davies 1996). In 1995, an International Committee for Harmonization of Clinical Pathology Testing (IHCPT) in toxicity and safety studies (Weingand et al. 1996) suggested a list of the minimum or core tests that should be included in safety studies. This included a choice of plasma/serum tests for detecting hepatotoxicity (see Chapter 3), but these recommendations have not been entirely adopted into regulatory documents. Several of these common tests are interrelated, and, when combined, these tests can provide better information by pattern recognition (e.g., urea and creatinine for glomerular function and several plasma enzymes for hepatotoxicity). The selection of tests should be influenced by the expected mode of action of the test compound, data obtained from previous animal studies, and the regulatory guidelines.

In Table 1.1, tests that have been included in regulatory guideline documents (MHW 1990; OECD 1995b, 2002a, 2002b; U.S. EPA 1997, 2008) and the IHCPT guidelines are listed. These tests have been selected as measures of metabolic perturbations and tissue injury, and they include measurements of electrolyte balance, carbohydrate metabolism, and some markers of injury to liver, kidney, and other major organs. These tests will be discussed more fully in subsequent chapters.

The inclusion of ornithine decarboxylase (U.S. EPA 2008) has been questioned as to whether it was confused with ornithine carbamoyl transferase (OCT), which is a far more common enzyme measurement for hepatotoxicity; ornithine decarboxylase (ODC) is of interest mainly in studies of polyamine metabolism (Carakostas 1988; Evans 1989; Evans 1993). Succinate dehydrogenase is included in one Organization of Economic Cooperation and Development document (OECD 2002a), designated SDH; this abbreviation is used more commonly for sorbitol dehydrogenase, which is given in a second OECD document (OECD 2002b), and where both documents refer to published data for sorbitol dehydrogenase (Travlos et al. 1996).

TABLE 1.1
Plasma/Serum Chemistry Tests Cited in Recent Regulatory and Nonregulatory Documents[a]

Glucose[b]	Alanine amino transferase[b]
Urea (urea nitrogen)[b]	Alkaline phosphatase[b]
Creatinine[b]	Aspartate aminotransferase[b]
Total protein[b]	Gamma glutamyl transferase[b]
Albumin[b]	Ornithine carbamoyl transferase
Calculated globulin[b]	Ornithine decarboxylase[c]
Total calcium[b]	Sorbitol dehydrogenase[b]
Sodium[b]	Glutamate dehydrogenase[b]
Potassium[b]	Total bilirubin[b]
Chloride[b]	Total bile acids[b]
Total cholesterol[b]	Succinate dehydrogenase[c]
Triglycerides	5´-Nucleotidase[b]
Magnesium	Lactate dehydrogenase
Protein electrophoresis	Creatine kinase
Inorganic phosphate/cholinesterase	
Phosphorus	

Note: In addition, methemoglobin, acid-base balance, various unspecified lipids, and hormones are suggested by the U.S. EPA (2008).

[a] OECD 1998a, 1998b, 2002a, 2002b, 2006; U.S. EPA 1997, 2008; and IHCPT, Weingand et al. 1996.
[b] Tests contained in the IHCPT (1996).
[c] Tests questioned in the text.

Cholinesterase measurements in erythrocytes and plasma/serum are required if there is evidence that the xenobiotic could affect this enzyme (e.g., organophosphate and carbamate pesticides). Triglycerides are included in the guidelines for testing of pharmaceuticals by the Japanese Ministry of Health and Welfare and for industrial chemicals by the Japanese Ministry of International Trade and Industry. Many laboratories choose to include triglycerides as another measure of lipid metabolism.

In an OECD interlaboratory collaborative study to validate the updated guideline 407 for repeat 28-day oral toxicity study in rats (OECD 2006), the 13 participating laboratories all measured glucose; urea; creatinine; total protein; albumin, globulin, or albumin-to-globulin ratio; total calcium; sodium; potassium; chloride; total cholesterol; aspartate aminotransferase; alanine aminotransferase; and alkaline phosphatase. Of the 13 participating laboratories, some laboratories did not measure inorganic phosphate ($n = 2$), triglycerides ($n = 2$), total bilirubin ($n = 2$), and gamma glutamyl transferase ($n = 3$). Thus, this study gives a limited "snapshot" of current practices and perhaps reflects in part some opinions that these latter measurements have little value in rat safety studies, although these were measured by the majority of laboratories.

1.3 URINALYSIS

Table 1.2 lists the measurements suggested for urinalysis, although some guidelines have no requirement for the inclusion of these tests in rodent studies (e.g., U.S. EPA 2008). The core recommended tests include assessment of urine appearance (color

TABLE 1.2

Urinalysis Tests Cited in Recent Regulatory and Nonregulatory Documents[a,b]

Appearance
Volume
Specific gravity
pH
Sediment (microscopic)
Protein
Glucose
Ketones
Bilirubin
Blood
Nitrate (nitrite; see text)
Urobilinogen

[a] OECD 2002a, 2002b, 2006; U.S. EPA 2008; and IHCPT,1996.
[b] Not required for carcinogenicity studies based on U.S. EPA OPPTS or OECD test guidelines.

and turbidity), volume, specific gravity or osmolality, pH, and either the quantitative or semiquantitative determination of total protein and glucose.

Many of these listed qualitative tests are performed using dry reagent test strips/ dipsticks that are designed for use with human urine, so there are some limitations when they are used with rodent urine samples (see Chapter 13). There are some advantages in using these test strips at an early stage: because these same test strips are widely used for urinalysis in human and veterinary medicine, any misleading results due to the xenobiotic or its metabolites are identified at early stages of toxicity testing. Urinalysis is performed primarily to monitor renal function and is also a simple indicator of fluid balance. More detailed discussions of urine measurements are contained in Chapter 4. In the published regulatory list, nitrate should be interpreted as nitrite; urinary nitrates derived from dietary metabolites are converted by bacterial action to nitrites, which are increased in urinary infections. This excess production is detected by the test strip and indicates the presence of bacteria.

It is recommended in some guidelines that urinalysis should be conducted at least once during a study, with an overnight collection (approximately 16 h). For carcinogenicity studies, some guidelines do not specify the inclusion of urinalysis. Various methods for urine collection have been reviewed by Kurien, Everds, and Scofield (2004) and are discussed further in Chapter 4.

1.4   NEUROTOXICITY, SAFETY PHARMACOLOGY, AND IMMUNOTOXICOLOGY

Some laboratories may also support one or several of these disciplines for regulatory studies and there are some specific regulatory requirements. The requirement for cholinesterase measurements when dealing with pesticides has already been mentioned; this is discussed later in Chapter 11.

In safety pharmacology, a number of renal functional tests, such as creatinine and electrolyte measurements, can be supported by most clinical chemistry laboratories (Kinter, Gossett, and Kerns 1994; Seuter 1996; ICH 2000). In some of the later chapters discussing assessments of hepatotoxicity and renal toxicity, a few functional tests are mentioned. Although it may be desirable to include function tests in repeated-dose toxicity studies, given the additional and sometimes invasive procedures, these tests may be better performed by incorporation into single-dose toxicity studies or separate additional studies (Matsuzawa et al. 1997).

In an immunotoxicity guideline (FDA 2006), plasma total globulin measurements and ratios of albumin to globulin are listed, with the suggestion that alterations of total globulin concentrations could be followed by measurement of plasma immunoglobulins (see Chapter 8).

1.5   FREQUENCY OF MEASUREMENTS

The frequency and timing of clinical pathology testing are dependent upon study duration, study objectives, the biological activity of the test material, and the species tested. For repeated-dose studies in nonrodent species, clinical pathology testing is recommended at or very close to study termination, and at least once at an earlier interval because of the small number of animals per group and intra- and interindividual animal variability. For rodent repeated-dose studies, clinical pathology testing is essential at or very close to study termination. For 13-week studies, blood samples can be taken at approximately 4 and 13 weeks; in the longer-term chronic studies, additional blood samples should be considered at 26 and 52 weeks. For studies of 2- to 6-week duration, testing is also appropriate within 7 days of initiation of dosing.

Interim blood sampling of rats may not be necessary when the dose levels are similar in the short- and longer-duration studies. The sample timings in the guidelines refer to the core tests, but some specialized tests require samples to be collected at times in relation to the toxic injury in acute studies (e.g., cardiac biomarkers) or to expected peaks in the circadian or reproductive cycle rhythms. Additional times for blood sampling should be avoided if the procedures could compromise the health of the animals. In all procedures, consideration should be given to the possible stress effects of the sample collection procedures and the amount of blood collected in relation to the total blood volume.

The timing of the urine collections is a critical factor in detecting renal injury. Tubular necrosis is an event more likely to occur early in a study, and therefore urine samples are best taken during this early period, whereas renal papillary necrosis is more likely to occur in a later part of a study (Heywood 1981). In some acute cardiac toxic events, the cardiac biomarkers increase within a few hours of injury, so sampling needs to be timed within this window because later samples may not show elevations of these biomarkers.

Some other considerations not included in the regulatory guidelines are discussed in this and the following paragraphs. For both rodents and nonrodents, clinical pathology testing should be performed on the same animals as those examined for morphologic pathology findings, and it is also recommended that blood samples from "recovery" or "withdrawal" satellite groups should be analyzed at study termination. Many investigators generally apply the same core tests for studies in all species, but some may select tests for one but not all species. For mice, the number of tests may be reduced due to smaller available blood volumes.

In designing a study in which several additional tests cannot be obtained from a single blood collection and may require more carefully timed collections (e.g., plasma hormones), it may be necessary to include additional animals in the study. Although, ideally, both hematology and plasma chemistry sample collections should be taken from the same animals, subgroups should sometimes be used for mice and these two collections allocated to the subgroups. If the volume of collected sample is smaller than the total volume required for analysis, the tests should be prioritized in order of importance (e.g., enzyme tests for hepatic injury may be analyzed first). In some laboratories, it is the practice to repeat collections from some animals when the first collection has not been sufficient for all tests.

Although in many cases the values for plasma and serum are similar for core analytes, each laboratory has its preference for plasma or serum; plasma will be used to describe measurements rather than serum in most instances in this book. Current biochemical analyzers require small volumes of plasma for each test (typically 2–30 μL); in addition, there is "dead" volume within the sample cup that the sample probe cannot reach (this may be equivalent to a sample volume of >20 μL). Immunoassays often require larger test volumes in some part due to the relative concentrations of the several analytes being in the picomolar rather than the millimolar range. Some of the limitations, frequency, and stress effects associated with sample collections are discussed later in Chapter 12.

The practice of pooling samples for groups of animals from the same group or cage for analysis should be avoided because it can lead to difficulties when interpreting the results. For example, samples from three healthy animals mixed with one sick animal could affect the mean result; gross hemolysis found in one sample would affect the potassium results when mixed with nonhemolyzed samples. Another example is where three animals produce large amounts of urine, which are then mixed with a very small volumes obtained from another animal within the group. The practice of placing several smaller animals within one metabolism cage for urine collections also should be avoided.

1.6 BIOMARKERS

Since laboratory measurements commenced, we have used biomarkers; however, in the last decade there has been a great deal of discussion and debate about the term *biomarker,* its definition, and its usage (Colburn 1997; Biomarkers Definitions Working Group 2001; Frank and Hargreaves 2003). The term biomarker is often used to encompass relatively new indices—for example, plasma and urine profiles obtained with nuclear magnetic resonance spectroscopy (NMR), metabonomics, proteomics, etc. (Grandjean et al. 1994; Timbrell, Draper, and Waterfield 1994). However, the term is equally applicable to the traditional core tests.

A biomarker is a characteristic that is objectively measured and can be evaluated as an indicator of normal biological, pathogenic, or pharmacologic processes. It can be a physiological or a biochemical measurement, so not all biomarkers are laboratory measurements (e.g., blood pressure and electrocardiography). Biomarkers may indicate (1) exposure, (2) response, or (3) susceptibility. Exposure biomarkers indicate that there is or has been exposure to a xenobiotic, its metabolites, or its adducts. Biomarkers of response indicate biochemical changes in the animal as a result of exposure to a xenobiotic or its metabolites (e.g., hepatic enzyme induction). Biomarkers of susceptibility indicate that an animal may be more or less susceptible to exposure to a xenobiotic (e.g., cholinesterase polymorphisms in man and the Ah receptors in animals). These markers of susceptibility are of special interest in the emerging sciences of pharmacogenomics and pharmacogenetics.

An alternative view of clinical biomarkers is expressed as three types: 0, I, and II. Type 0 are markers of the natural history of the disease and correlate longitudinally with know clinical indices. Type I markers capture the effect of an intervention in accordance with the mechanism of action (MOA) of the xenobiotic or drug even though the MOA might not be known to be associated with the clinical outcome. Type II markers are considered to be surrogate endpoints where a change of the biomarker predicts clinical benefit. Again, all of these biomarker types may be biochemical or physiological measurements.

Biomarkers in clinical pathology can be established on evidence that supports the performance characteristics of the test—analytical accuracy and reproducibility—and in which the use of the test is supported by toxicological, pharmacological, or physiological in vivo evidence. Some biomarkers are designed to confirm either the theoretical principle or the mechanism of action of a drug. Ideally, a biomarker should apply to all laboratory animal species, have similar diagnostic value, and be predictive for human safety; the biomarker should be specific, sensitive, and minimally invasive. Unfortunately, many biochemical markers in current use are not ideal in these respects.

It is sometimes suggested that the current choice of biochemical tests in regulatory animal studies has been governed by investigators more familiar with human medicine, even though several of the tests were originally evaluated in animal studies before their introduction to human medicine. There is now perhaps a greater enthusiasm for developing new biomarkers that will bridge the gaps between animal studies and subsequent improved diagnostic accuracy in humans and animals.

In the past decade, some newer tests have emerged that should be considered for inclusion in some studies, and several of these tests are mentioned in subsequent chapters. For example, troponin measurements have proved to be useful in acute cardiac toxicity, and the range of immunoassays suitable for endocrinological measurements in rodents has expanded. However, many of the newer tests require much wider validation to demonstrate their usage in toxicology testing.

1.7 GOOD LABORATORY PRACTICE (GLP)

Laboratories performing regulatory studies must ensure that the studies comply with the principles of good laboratory practice (GLP) as interpreted by national and international regulatory authorities and their inspectorates (Paget 1979; FDA 1979, 2007a; Weinberg 1995; OECD 1997). The GLP principles include requirements for job descriptions for personnel, their responsibilities, and management responsibilities. Other aspects of GLP include training, general laboratory facilities, calibration and maintenance of equipment, reagent preparation and quality control procedures for assays, and the characterization of other experimental variables. There is an emphasis on adequate documentation; authorized and documented standard operating procedures (SOPs); a definition of the "raw" data and linking these to the metadata of time, analyst etc.; detailing amendments to the data; and the authorization of these amendments. Adherence to the principles of GLP is essential for those laboratories that perform regulatory studies, and it provides a good framework for laboratories that do not.

In many laboratories, the laboratory data are transmitted from the analyzers and stored electronically. The processes for direct or indirect capture of data, data reporting, and data storage need to validated, operated, and maintained in accordance with GLP (OECD 1995a; FDA 2007b). Guidance on electronic data and electronic signatures was provided by the FDA in 1997, but this guidance proved difficult to interpret and implement, thus leading to a reconsideration by the regulatory authority (FDA 2007b). Given the large volume of data and long-term storage requirements, electronic data must be readable, and it must be possible to re-create accurate and complete representations of the data, even though data may have been obtained from an obsolete and discarded analyzer.

1.8 USE OF ANIMALS

The four principles of reduction, refinement, replacement, and responsibility for the use of animals must be of concern to all investigators (Rowan 1990). Public opinion and pressure to reduce the number of animals in experiments by the use of alternatives such as in vitro studies still appears to be a long-term rather than a short-term goal in most animal studies; currently, significant growth has taken place in the numbers of genetically modified animals being studied. Most transgenic animals are developed for research purposes and have yet to be commonly studied in toxicology (Dunn 2005). The physiological and stress effects of the removal of blood from smaller laboratory animals and the possible effects on test values must be considered; some of these effects are discussed in Chapter 12.

Typically, for general toxicology studies, animals are divided into four groups: a control group and three different dose groups—low, medium, and high; the medium- and high-dose groups are at several ascending multiples of the low dose, using both sexes. Where the vehicle is novel or for inhalation studies, a fifth group acting as an additional control for a vehicle may be included. For subchronic rodent studies, 10–15 animals per sex per group are appropriate, with twice as many animals in chronic studies; additional animals may be in the group where there is a recovery or off-dose period at the end of the study. For nonrodent studies with dogs or with nonhuman primates, there are commonly five animals per sex per group; two of the five are retained during recovery or off-dose period studies. These numbers are constrained by animal welfare issues, but they represent small numbers—particularly for the large animals—when examining the analytical results (Mann, Crouse, and Prentice 1991). Too severe a reduction in the numbers of animals studied may lead to interpretative problems due to the often wider intra- and interanimal variations observed in laboratory animals, even though we currently study fairly homogeneous populations. The challenge for clinical chemists and toxicologists is to extract more valuable information from the studies we perform in order to improve risk–benefit assessment.

1.9 BIOLOGICAL AND CHEMICAL SAFETY IN THE LABORATORY

It would be remiss of analysts to ignore the safety risks associated with their own work when toxicology studies help to define these risks. Ballantyne (1993) has reviewed some of the additional hazards associated with work in toxicology laboratories. In general, precautions taken for handling human samples can be equally applied to animal samples, and extended further where the risks appear to be greater—for example, working with samples containing carcinogens or highly toxic compounds, from immunocompromised animals, or where the animal model has been deliberately infected with parasite, virus, or bacteria.

Biological samples including blood and urine may present health risks to the personnel collecting and analyzing the samples. When diverse blood samples are transported, received, or analyzed, every effort should be made to reduce the biohazards for laboratory staff (Truchaud et al. 1994; WHO 2003). Suitable containers or bags should be used to transport samples from the animal care buildings to the laboratory. Allergies to laboratory animals and their samples remain a risk for laboratory workers, and efforts should be made to minimize exposure to animal dander, etc. (Venables et al. 1988; Hunskaar and Fosse 1990; Cullinan et al. 1994; Wood and Smith 1999).

Although most laboratories use purpose-bred animals, occasionally bacteria, parasites, and yeasts may be found in blood (Owen 1992). When immunosuppressants or immunostimulants are being tested, this may increase the risks of viral infections and potential viral transmission. When wild-caught animals are being studied, for example, in underdeveloped countries, the risks from viral infections must be considered (Veillet 1998). Guidance for periodic cleaning and disinfection of analyzers is usually provided by manufacturers, but more frequent measures are required following analysis of highly infectious materials.

Warnings are usually provided by manufacturers on electrical and reagent chemical hazards. These risks are increased by exposure to laboratory chemicals and test compounds where the toxicological risks are unknown; additional consideration must be given when staff handles mutagenic materials. Sodium azide is a simple example of a common additive often used in small quantities in laboratory reagents that has a known toxicological profile, which should be considered when it is used (Chang and Lamm 2003). Samples from some studies may contain radioactivity and these should be treated according to local rules pertaining to radiation safety. Sometimes the laboratory may be asked to analyze samples containing small amounts of radioactivity; this requires a risk assessment in terms of analysts and contamination of equipment (Astill and Nuttall 1997).

1.10   GENERAL CONSIDERATIONS OF TOXICITY

For in vivo safety evaluation studies, Zbinden (1993) proposed three principal goals:

*   spectrum of toxicity: detection of adverse effects in selected laboratory animal species and description of the dose–effect relationship over a broad range of doses;
*   extrapolation: prediction of adverse effects in other species, particularly man; and
*   safety: prediction of safe levels of exposure in other species, particularly man.

The term *adverse* defines a biochemical, morphological, or physiological change that occurs in response to a stimulus either singly or in combination with other stimuli. These changes adversely affect the performance of the whole organism or reduce its ability to respond to an additional environmental challenge (Lewis et al. 2002). Using this definition of adverse—the highest level of exposure at which no adverse effect or no adverse effects are observed in the animal population—we can define the no observed effect level (NOEL) and the no observed adverse effect level (NOAEL).

For food additives that often have low biological activity, the onus on the toxicologist is to demonstrate a NOAEL (i.e., a nontoxic level) and to identify separately any changes in data that may be the result of an adaptive response to repeated overdose. This is in contrast to the situation with drugs, where it is important both to demonstrate potential toxic response and to define a NOEL. Here, the difficulties are in distinguishing among nonadverse pharmacological responses, desired pharmacological actions, adaptive responses, and apparent toxic effects (James 1993). It remains debatable whether safety evaluation should be based on demonstrating the absence of toxic signs rather than target organ toxicity (Heywood 1981). Toxicology studies are generally designed to characterize the adverse effects of a xenobiotic by identifying its effects on target organs and on key metabolic functions, as well as to determine if these effects are reversible.

Therefore, biochemical measurements can help in

identifying target organ toxicity;
confirming other observations, particularly changes found by histopathological examination;
defining NOEL or NOAEL levels;
compound selection—screening of analogues;
elucidating toxic mechanisms; and
elucidating interspecies differences in toxicity studies.

The prediction of toxic risk can be defined as the probability that an adverse event may occur or result from a particular challenge. However, it must be remembered that, if the incidence rate of an adverse reaction is less than 0.01%, the adverse event that is apparent when a drug is administered to one million people may be undetected in toxicology studies in which the total number of animals may be less than one thousand. Animal toxicity studies may sometimes lead to the erroneous elimination of promising drugs for man and occasionally fail to predict toxicity that may occur in man.

In several retrospective studies of new drugs, it has been shown that some animal studies have been predictive for adverse events in humans while others have failed to detect adverse effects and predict toxicity in man (see Chapter 14). What these published studies often fail to show is the very large number of unpublished studies that have prevented compounds from being given to humans because of the results obtained from animal toxicity studies. Alternatively, the presence of adverse signals from animal studies has not prevented the administration of compounds to humans; this has led to questioning how these data are reviewed.

It remains a major public concern that drugs are removed during the marketing phase due to adverse drug reactions (ADRs). Data from the United States suggest an estimated 5% mortality rate for drug-induced liver injury; drugs caused 15–30% of fulminant liver failure cases and 2–5% of the patients hospitalized with jaundice (Sturgill and Lambert 1997). In the last 10 years in Britain, the number of adverse drug reactions has increased by more than 40% and accounts for 1 in 16 admissions to hospitals.

Clinical pathology must meet future challenges and broaden its practice. We need to extend the repertoire of tests—not for the sake of the exercise, but rather to maximize the predictive values of the tests we offer for human and animal safety. We need to seek and provide further evidence for the correlation of biochemical changes with histological findings, and to gain a better understanding of the small but statistically significant changes that we detect. Other future challenges include the need to support studies designed to reduce preanalytical variables, as well as more involvement with animal welfare issues and nutritional studies where concern is focused on reducing obesity in the aged rat with little reference to alterations of biochemical values.

REFERENCES

Astill, M. E., and K. L. Nuttall. 1997. Undisclosed radioactivity in specimens: How much of a problem? *Clinical Chemistry* 43:1097.

Ballantyne, B. 1993. Hazards in the toxicology laboratory. In *General and applied toxicology,* ed. B. Ballantyne, T. Marrs, and P. Turner, pp. 359–667. Basingstoke, England: Macmillan Press.

Biomarkers Definitions Working Group. 2001. Biomarkers and surrogate endpoints: Preferred definitions and conceptual framework. *Clinical Pharmacology and Therapeutics* 69:89–96.

Bungaard, H. 1991. Novel approaches to prodrug design. *Drugs of the Future* 16:443–458.

Carakostas, M. C. 1988. What is ornithine decarboxylase? *Clinical Chemistry* 34: 2606–2607.

Chang, S., and S. H. Lamm. 2003. Human health effects of sodium azide exposure: A literature review and analysis. *International Journal of Toxicology* 22:175–186.

Colburn, W. A. 1997. Selecting and validating biological markers for drug development. *Journal of Clinical Pharmacology* 37:355–362.

Condie, L. W., R. D. Laurie, T. Mills, M. Robinson, and J. P. Bercz. 1986. Effect of gavage vehicle on hepatotoxicity of carbon tetrachloride in CD-1 mice: Corn oil versus Tween-60 aqueous emulsion. *Fundamental and Applied Toxicology* 7:199–206.

Cullinan, P., D. Lowson, M. J. Nieuwenhuijsen, S. Gordon, R. D. Tee, K. M. Venables, J. C. McDonald, and A. J. Newman Taylor. 1994. Work-related symptoms sensitization and estimated exposure in workers not previously exposed to laboratory rats. *Occupational and Environmental Medicine* 51:589–592.

Davies, D. T. 1996. Study design and regulatory requirements. In *Animal clinical chemistry: A primer for toxicologists,* ed. G. O. Evans, pp.11–19. London: Taylor & Francis.

Dunn, D. A., C. A. Pinkert, and D. L. Kooyman. 2005. Foundation review: Transgenic animals and their impact on the drug discovery industry. *Drug Discovery Today* 10:757–767.

Evans, G. O. 1989. More on ornithine decarboxylase. *Clinical Chemistry* 35:897–898.

———. 1993. Clinical pathology testing recommendations for nonclinical toxicity and safety studies. *Toxicologic Pathology* 21:463–464.

Frank, D. W., J. E. Gray, and R. N. Weaver. 1976. Cyclodextrin nephrosis in the rat. *American Journal of Pathology* 83:367–382.

Frank, R., and R. Hargreaves. 2003. Clinical biomarkers in drug discovery and development. *Nature Reviews Drug Discovery* 2:566–580.

Golightly, L. K., S. S. Smolinske, M. L. Bennett, E. W. Sutherland, and B. H. Rumack. 1988. Pharmaceutical excipients. Adverse effects associated with "inactive" ingredients in drug products (part II). *Medical Toxicology and Adverse Drug Experience* 3:209–240.

Grandjean, P., S. S. Brown, P. Reavey, and D. S. Young. 1994. Biomarkers of chemical expo-
    sure: State of the art. *Clinical Chemistry* 40:1360–1362.
Heywood, R. 1981. Target organ toxicity. *Toxicology Letters* 8:349–858.
Hunskaar, S., and R. T. Fosse. 1990. Allergy to laboratory mice and rats: A review of the
    pathophysiology, epidemiology and clinical aspects. *Laboratory Animals* 24:358–374.
James, R. W. 1993. The relevance of clinical pathology to toxicology studies. *Comparative
    Hematology International* 13:190–195.
Kinter, L. B., K. A. Gossett, and W. D. Kerns. 1994. Status of safety pharmacology in the
    pharmaceutical industry. *Drug Development Research* 32:208–216.
Kurien, B. T., N. E. Everds, and R. H. Scofield. 2004. Experimental animal urine collection: A
    review. *Laboratory Animals* 38:333–361.
Lewis, R. W., R. Billington, E. Debryune, A. Gamer, B. Lang, and F. Carpanini. 2002.
    Recognition of adverse and nonadverse effects in toxicology studies. *Toxicologic
    Pathology* 30:66–74.
Mann, D., D. A. Crouse, and E. D. Prentice. 1991. Appropriate animal numbers in biomedi-
    cal research in light of animal welfare considerations. *Laboratory Animal Science*
    41:6–14.
Matsuzawa, T., M. Hashimoto, H. Nara, M. Yoshida, S. Tamura, and T. Igarashi. 1997. Current
    status of conducting function tests in repeated dose toxicity studies in Japan. *Journal of
    Toxicological Sciences* 22:375–382.
Miya, T. S., J. E. Gibson, J. B. Hook, and R. O. McClellan. 1988. Contemporary issues in
    toxicology. Preparing for the twenty-first century: Report of the Tox-90s commission.
    Toxicology and Applied Pharmacology 96:1–6.
Mumtaz, M. M., I. G. Sipes, H. J. Clewell, and R. S. Yang. 1993. Risk assessment of chemi-
    cal mixtures; biologic and toxicologic issues. *Fundamental and Applied Toxicology*
    21:258–269.
Owen, D. G. 1992. *Parasites of laboratory animals. Laboratory animal handbook,* vol. 12.
    London: Royal Society of Medicine Press.
Paget, G. E. 1979. *Good laboratory practice.* Lancaster, England: MTP Press Ltd.
Rooney, P. H., C. Telfer, M. C. McFayden, W. T. Melvin, and G. I. Murray. 2004. The role
    of cytochrome P450 in cytotoxic bioactivation: Future therapeutic directions. *Current
    Cancer Drug Targets* 4:257–265.
Rowan, A. N. 1990. Refinement of animal research technique and validity of research data.
    Fundamental and Applied Toxicology 15:25–32.
Seuter, F. 1996. Safety pharmacology studies. *Scandinavian Journal of Laboratory Animal
    Science* 23:297–304.
Sturgill, M. G., and G. H. Lambert. 1997. Xenobiotic-induced hepatotoxicity: Mechanisms
    of liver injury and methods of monitoring hepatic function. *Clinical Chemistry*
    43:1512–1526.
Timbrell, J. 1999. *Principles of biochemical toxicology,* 3rd ed. London: Taylor & Francis.
Timbrell, J. A., R. Draper, and C. J. Waterfield. 1994. Biomarkers in toxicology. New uses for
    old molecules? *Toxicology and Ecotoxicology News* 1:4–14.
Travlos, G. S., R. W. Morris, M. R. Elwell, A. Duke, S. Rosenblum, and M. B. Thompson.
    1996. Frequency and relationship of clinical chemistry and liver and kidney histopathol-
    ogy findings in 13-week toxicity studies in rats. *Toxicology* 107:17–29.
Truchaud, A., P. Schnipelsky, H. L. Pardue, J. Place, and K. Ozawa. 1994. Increasing the bio-
    safety of analytical systems in the clinical laboratory. *Clinica Chimica Acta* 226:S5–13.
Veillet, F. 1998. Les agents infectieux d'actualité et leur déspitage chez les rongeurs de labo-
    ratoire. *Science Technical Animal Laboratory* 23:115–121.
Venables, K. M., R. D. Tee, E. R. Hawkins, D. J. Gordon, C. J. Wale, N. M. Farrer, T. H. Lam,
    P. J. Baxter, and A. J. Newman Taylor. 1988. Laboratory animal allergy in a pharmaceu-
    tical company. *British Journal of Industrial Medicine* 45:660–666.

Weinberg, S., ed. 1995. *Good laboratory practice regulations*. New York: Marcel Dekker Inc.

Weingand, K. et al. 1996. Harmonization of animal clinical pathology testing in toxicity and safety studies. The Joint Scientific Committee for harmonization of clinical pathology testing. *Fundamental and Applied Toxicology* 29:198–201.

Wood, M., and M. W. Smith. 1999. *Health and safety in laboratory animal facilities. Laboratory animal handbook,* no. 13. London: Royal Society of Medicine Press.

WHO (World Health Organization). 2003. *WHO laboratory biosafety guidelines,* 2nd ed. Geneva: World Health Organization.

Zbinden, G. 1993. The concept of multispecies testing in industrial toxicology. *Regulatory Toxicology and Pharmacology* 17:85–94.

GENERAL REFERENCES FOR TOXICOLOGY

Derelanko, M. J., and M. A. Hollinger. 2001. *Handbook of toxicology,* 2nd ed. Boca Raton, FL: CRC Press.

Hayes, A. W., ed. 2007. *Principles and methods of toxicology,* 5th ed. Boca Raton, FL: CRC Press.

Niesink, R., M. A. Hollinger, and J. de Vries. 1996. *Toxicology principles and applications.* Boca Raton, FL: CRC Press.

Timbrell, J. 2001. *Introduction to Toxicology,* 3rd ed. London: Taylor & Francis.

REGULATORY DOCUMENTS

FDA (U.S. Food and Drug Administration). 1979. Nonclinical laboratory studies: Good laboratory practice regulations. *Federal Register* 43:59986–60025.

———. 2006. ICH guidance for industry. S8 Immunotoxicity studies for human pharmaceuticals. Washington, D.C.: Department of Health and Human Services, Food and Drug Administration.

———. 2007a. Title 21 CFR 58. Good laboratory practice for nonclinical laboratories. Washington, D.C.: Department of Health and Human Services Food and Drug Administration.

———. 2007b. Title 21 CFR Part 11. Electronic records: Electronic signatures. Washington, D.C.: Department of Health and Human Services, Food and Drug Administration.

ICH (International Conference for Harmonization). 2000. S7A Safety pharmacology studies for human pharmaceuticals. Geneva: International Conference for Harmonization.

MHW (Ministry of Health and Welfare, Japan). 1990. Guidelines for toxicity studies of drugs manual. Editorial supervision by new drugs division, Pharmaceutical Affairs Bureau, Tokyo.

OECD (Organization for Economic Cooperation and Development). 1995a. No. 10. The application of the principles of GLP to computerized systems. Organization for Economic Cooperation and Development, Paris.

———. 1995b. Test no. 407. Repeated-dose 28-day oral toxicity study in rodents. Organization for Economic Cooperation and Development, Paris.

———. 1997. Principles of good laboratory practice. Organization for Economic Cooperation and Development, Paris.

———. 1998a. Guidelines for the testing of chemicals. Test no. 408. Repeated-dose 90-day oral toxicity study in rodents. Organization for Economic Cooperation and Development, Paris.

———. 1998b. Guidelines for the testing of chemicals. Test no. 409. Repeated-dose 90-day oral toxicity study in nonrodents. Organization for Economic Cooperation and Development, Paris.

————. 2002a. Guidance notes for analysis and evaluation of repeat-dose toxicity studies. Series on Testing and Assessment, no. 32, and Series on Pesticides, no. 10. Organization for Economic Cooperation and Development, Paris.

————. 2002b. Guidance notes for analysis and evaluation of chronic toxicity and carcinogenicity studies. Series on Testing and Assessment, no. 35, and Series on Pesticides, no. 14. Organization for Economic Cooperation and Development, Paris.

————. 2006. Report of the validation of the updated guideline 407: Repeat-dose 28-day oral toxicity in laboratory rats. Series on Testing and Assessment, no. 59. Organization for Economic Cooperation and Development, Paris.

U.S. EPA (Environmental Protection Agency). 1997. Toxic Substances Control Act test guidelines: Final rule. 40 CFR. Part 799.

————. 2008. Health effects testing guidelines subpart D. Chronic exposure. No. 40 CFR Part 798. Washington, D.C.: Environmental Protection Agency.

2 General Enzymology

2.1 INTRODUCTION

Enzymes are proteins with catalytic properties that include the specific activation of their respective substrates; several enzymes are used in toxicological studies to measure cellular injury, enzyme induction, and activation or inhibition of the enzymes. The distribution of enzymes varies among the different body organs and tissues and may vary in the different cell types within an organ (Clampitt and Hart 1978; Keller 1981; Braun et al. 1983; Lindena et al. 1986; Milne and Doxey 1986; Davy et al. 1988). The tissue distributions vary between species and an enzyme can also be affected by age and sex (e.g., alkaline phosphatase). Caution must be exercised when interpreting data on tissue enzyme distribution when a single extraction and assay system has been used because this does not allow for the variable requirements for optimizing the extraction of the enzyme and for the measurement of the enzyme. Not all enzymes will be extracted with the same efficiency if the extraction procedure is carried out with one pH buffer.

The intracellular distribution of enzymes varies and the proportions may be such that an enzyme can be regarded as relatively specific to a particular type of organelle. Several enzymes are cytosolic (e.g., lactate dehydrogenase), while others are located in organelles, such as glutamate dehydrogenase in mitochondria or acid phosphatase in lysosomes. Some enzymes, such as aspartate aminotransferase, occur in mitochondria and in the cytosol, whereas other enzymes may be largely membrane bound (e.g., gamma glutamyl transferase).

Many enzymes show molecular heterogeneity, and the different forms are termed isoenzymes (or isozymes). These isoenzymes catalyzing the same reaction differ in physical and chemical properties and can therefore be differentiated by several techniques, such as electrophoresis, chromatography, immunological separation, selective inhibition, or modified substrate methods. Currently, the term *isoenzyme* should be restricted to the enzyme forms that originate at the genomic level that encode the structure of a particular enzyme. The isoenzyme patterns in different tissues vary, and their measurement may help in identifying the source of changes in total enzyme activity. There are also some nongenetic causes of multiple forms of enzymes (see CK isoforms in Chapter 7).

Given the tissue and cellular variations, it is not surprising to find marked differences in plasma enzymes between species (Lindena and Trautschold 1986). For example, plasma alkaline phosphatase (ALP) and lactate dehydrogenase (LDH) activities show greater variability in rats and monkeys when compared to man; therefore, they have a poorer predictive or diagnostic value in these species. In young animals, the osseous ALP isoenzyme is the dominant plasma form in most species, but the proportion of intestinal ALP in plasma is far greater in the adult rat than in other laboratory species. Plasma gamma glutamyl transferase (GGT) activities are lower in most rodent species compared with the enzyme levels found in man.

Although in some instances the contribution to a plasma enzyme can be related to the tissue with the highest enzyme concentration, this is not always the case (e.g., in the rat where the renal tissue GGT and alkaline phosphatase are higher in renal tissue than in hepatic tissue but where these plasma enzymes rarely change following renal injury because any increased amounts of the enzyme are released into the urine rather than the plasma). Enzymes located on biliary epithelial cells are released primarily into the bile. The plasma activity of an enzyme depends on several factors, including the enzyme concentrations in different tissues, the intracellular location of the enzyme, the rate of synthesis of the enzyme, the severity of tissue and cellular damage, the molecular mass of the enzyme, and the rate of clearance of the enzyme from plasma.

In the earlier stages of tissue damage, cytoplasmic enzymes may leak from cells when membrane permeability has altered (Keil 1990). As the severity of tissue damage progresses, enzymes normally present in subcellular organelles will be released into the circulation (Schmidt and Schmidt 1987; Bouma and Smit 1988). The molecular mass of the enzyme also governs its cellular and renal clearances. There are considerable variations in the published data for plasma half-lives (or clearance rates from plasma), and these variations are partly due to the different methodologies used for these measurements and the lack of suitable enzyme preparations.

Table 2.1 shows some of the estimated elimination half-lives for some of the common enzymes; it is important to consider these clearance rates when enzyme changes occur. In acute injury such as myocardial infarction, enzyme changes may be detected by ensuring that the sample collection times make due allowance for the enzyme half-life; otherwise, changes may not be detected. Enzymes with longer half-lives (i.e., days rather than minutes) can be more useful in the detection of low-grade or chronic tissue injury because the increased half-life provides a wider time window for sampling.

Plasma enzymes may be classified as (1) plasma-specific enzymes, (2) other secreted enzymes (e.g., amylase), and (3) intracellular enzymes. The plasma-specific enzymes include those that are secreted by some organs and have a direct action in

TABLE 2.1
Range of Estimates of Half-Lives (h) of Some Plasma Enzymes in Three Species

	Rat	Dog	Human
Alkaline phosphatase (liver isoenzyme)	28–72	140	40–180
Alanine aminotransferase	3–10	3–50	32–52
Aspartate aminotransferase	3–10	10–12	4–46
Creatine kinase	0.5–4	1–10	3–35

the plasma (e.g., pseudo- or nonspecific cholinesterase and coagulation enzymes). Within this class of enzyme, organ damage often correlates with reduced plasma enzyme activities (i.e., reduced pseudocholinesterase levels following some forms of hepatic injury). More than 2000 enzymes have now been described and many were identified using the substrate and by adding the suffix *ase* (e.g., phosphat*ase*). Although the singular term *alkaline phosphatase* is commonly used, there is a group of phosphatases that are optimally active at an alkaline pH.

The International Union of Biochemistry uses a four-group Enzyme Commission (EC) number to define the enzyme by its function; the enzymes are assigned to one of six classes:

oxidoreductases;
transferases;
hydrolases;
lyases;
isomerases; and
ligases.

Table 2.2 shows some of the enzymes used in toxicology studies. Although many enzymes have been and continue to be evaluated as markers of tissue injury, the number of enzymes commonly used remains a relatively small proportion of the total number of enzymes.

Attention in toxicology studies is focused mainly on increased plasma activities following cellular injury. In some studies, the plasma enzymes may show good correlation with the extent of tissue injury, but this is not always the case. For example, tissue regeneration may also be accompanied by changes in plasma enzymes following enzyme leakage from the cell, with plasma enzyme activities falling but at different rates, depending on the rates of clearance of each enzyme from the circulation. It should not be assumed that enzymes applied in human clinical practice show the same diagnostic value in the various animal species (Woodman 1981). The plasma enzymes commonly measured are used mainly to assess hepatotoxicity, cardio- and myotoxicity, pancreatic toxicity, and neurotoxicity, whereas in the assessment of nephrotoxicity, we use urinary enzyme measurements (please see later chapters). In some cases, the focus is on the reduction of enzyme activity (e.g., cholinesterase) and there are a few examples where reductions of the aminotransferases occur.

Several of the common enzyme measurements aimed at detecting hepatotoxicity are not specific to the liver, show a widespread tissue distribution, and are therefore affected by damage to extrahepatic tissue (e.g., alanine aminotransferase, aspartate aminotransferase, and lactate dehydrogenase following injury to cardiac or skeletal muscles). The development of troponin assays has provided an alternative to enzyme measurements as indicators of cardiotoxicity, but not for myotoxicity; here, the timing and the methods of sample collection are particularly critical for the detection of cardiac or muscle damage (see Chapter 7).

TABLE 2.2

Some Enzymes, Their Abbreviations, and Enzyme Commission (EC) Numbers

Enzyme	Abbreviation	EC Number
ALD	Aldolase	4.1.2.13
ALT (GPT)	Alanine aminotransferase	2.6.1.2
AAP	Alanine aminopeptidase	3.4.1.2
ALP	Alkaline phosphatase	3.1.3.1
AMY	Amylase	3.2.1.1
AST (GOT)	Aspartate aminotransferase	2.6.1.1
AChE	Acetyl cholinesterase	3.1.1.7
ARG	Arginase	3.5.3.1
BChE	Butyryl cholinesterase	3.1.1.8
CK (CPK)	Creatine kinase	2.7.3.2
GGT	Gamma glutamyl transferase	2.3.2.2
GLDH	Glutamate dehydrogenase	1.4.1.3
GST	Glutamyl S-transferase	2.5.1.18
HBD	Hydroxybutyrate dehydrogenase	—
ICDH	Isocitrate dehydrogenase	1.1.1.42
LDH	Lactate dehydrogenase	1.1.1.27
LAAP	Leucine arylamidase	3.4.11.2
LAP	Leucine aminopeptidase	3.4.11.1
LIP	Lipase	3.1.1.3
NAG	N-acetylglucosaminidase	3.2.1.30
5´-NT	5´-Nucleotidase	3.1.3.5
OCT	Ornithine carbamoyl transferase	2.1.3.3
SDH	Sorbitol dehydrogenase	1.1.1.14

2.2 ENZYME MEASUREMENTS

Enzyme activities are expressed generally as international units: one unit is the amount of enzyme that will catalyze under optimum conditions the transformation of 1 pmol of substrate per minute. The activities are expressed as IU/L or mLU/mL. The katal (kat; nanokatal = nKat) has been proposed as an alternative unit; it is defined as the catalytic activity that, under defined conditions, converts 1 mol of substrate per second. Thus, the units are moles per second (mol/s). One IU/L corresponds to 16.67 nKat/L. Unfortunately, these definitions of enzyme units do not include other major variables that affect their measurement, such as the composition and pH of buffer, identity and concentration of the substrate, temperature, and the presence of activators. This has led to a variety of national and international recommendations for the common enzyme measurements, which confuse comparisons between published data. Calibration of enzyme methodologies—particularly for less common enzymes—remains a laboratory issue (Jansen et al. 2006).

Enzymes may be measured by monitoring a reduction in substrate concentration or an increase of reaction product. The majority of the common enzymes can be measured using a kinetic approach in which the velocity of the enzyme reaction is monitored by serial measurements over a short time period. For some enzymes, the measurement reactions are linked to the enzyme cofactors nicotinamide adenine dinucleotide (NAD) or nicotinamide dinucleotide phosphate (NADP), and changes in these cofactors are measured in the ultraviolet spectrum. Reactions can be linked through second- or third-step reactions where these cofactors are involved (e.g., for AST and ALT). Other enzymes may be measured colorimetrically (e.g., ALP and GGT). Very few enzymes have been measured as enzyme mass, although proteomic methods may lead to greater utilization of enzyme mass measurements.

Enzyme reactions accelerate with increased temperature and the Q10 for the majority of enzyme reactions varies from 1.7 to 2.5 (i.e., the reaction approximately doubles for every 10°C rise); most laboratories measure enzyme activities at 37°C. Similarly, several enzymes are thermally inactivated (e.g., at temperatures of 56°C and above, the activity of some ALP isoenzymes is reduced). Conversely, urinary GGT is deactivated when frozen. Although plasma CK is inactivated rapidly in storage, incubation with high redox potential thiols such as N-acetyl cysteine or glutathione will overcome this problem. Dooley (1979) reported that substrate concentrations required for measurements of AST differed substantially among rat, dog, monkey, and humans. Reagents described as having optimal or optimized reagent concentrations for human plasma are not optimal for laboratory animal samples. Nevertheless, most laboratories routinely use reagents formulated for use with human samples—primarily for convenience in reagent preparation and in the absence of data showing that that these reagents are totally inappropriate for use with the differing species used in toxicology.

Variations between species using different enzyme substrates have been shown for cholinesterase (Myers 1953; Evans 1990) and other enzymes (e.g., angiotensin converting enzyme; Evans 1989). For alkaline phosphatase, the majority of methods employ 4-nitrophenylphosphate as the substrate, but there are two main alternative buffers—diethanolamine and 2-aminopropanol—that can cause interspecies differences (Masson and Holmgren 1992). For isoenzymes, the majority of laboratories currently use a variety of electrophoretic separation methods; although selective inhibition of isoenzymes with antibodies is being used increasingly, there are problems associated with protein specificity and relative isoenzyme concentrations in animal samples.

2.3 COMMON ENZYME MEASUREMENTS IN REGULATORY GUIDELINES

2.3.1 ALANINE AMINOTRANSFERASE (ALT)

ALT (also known as glutamic pyruvic transaminase, GPT) catalyzes the reaction

$$l\text{-alanine} + alpha\text{-oxoglutarate} \leftrightarrow pyruvate + glutamate$$

In many species, the proportion of ALT in hepatic tissue is greater than in any other organs (e.g., rat and dog); in other species, the proportions of ALT in hepatic and cardiac tissue are similar (e.g., rabbit) (Clampitt and Hart 1978; Lindena et al. 1986). General texts often state that ALT is a cytosolic enzyme, although mitochondrial ALT is present in many tissues of some species including the rat (DeRosa and Swick 1975; Ruŝĉák et al. 1982). It is the relative proportions of cytosolic to mitochondrial forms and the variations between major organs that lead to such statements and, although these ALT isoenzymes exist, they are not widely measured in diagnostic enzymology at present. Again, in some texts, it is suggested that plasma ALT is specific for liver injury in the dog and, although the majority of observations of increased ALT are associated with liver changes in the dog, there are some examples where plasma ALT is increased in muscle necrosis (Valentine et al. 1990) or as a consequence of acute intestinal enteropathies in dogs (Dodurka and Kraft 1995) and other causes (Balazs, Farber, and Feuer 1978; Swenson and Graves 1997). In some species, such as the common marmoset, plasma ALT activity is low and may be less useful as a marker of hepatotoxicity (Davy, Jackson, and Walker 1984; Cowie and Evans, 1985).

In rodents, preanalytical factors such as food intake and restraint may alter plasma ALT (see Chapter 12 also). A 50% food restriction over 210 days in rats resulted in elevated ALT values compared to controls (Schwartz, Tornaben, and Boxhill 1973), while reduced levels of ALT were observed in a study of fasting effects on the oral toxicity of several xenobiotics (Kast and Nishikawa 1981). Changes of ALT related to diet may reflect perturbations of gluconeogenesis (Toropila et al. 1996). There are now several examples where plasma ALT falls after the administration of xenobiotics due to effects on pyridoxal phosphate, which is a cofactor necessary for action of the aminotransferases AST and ALT (Dhami et al. 1979; Rhodes et al. 1987; Waner et al. 1990; Waner and Nyska 1991). Such effects may confuse the interpretation of data when hepatotoxicity occurs and tends to increase ALT, but where there is an opposing effect due to reductions in pyridoxal phosphate. Further complications with ALT have been described by Wells and To (1986) in covalent binding studies with acetaminophen.

2.3.2   Aspartate Aminotransferase (AST)

AST (also known as glutamic oxaloacetate transaminase, GOT) catalyzes the reaction

$$\text{aspartate} + \text{2-oxoglutarate} \leftrightarrow \text{l-glutamate} + \text{oxaloacetate}$$

Similarly to ALT, this enzyme is widely distributed in the tissues, including cardiac, skeletal, hepatic, and renal tissues. It is commonly used in conjunction with ALT to identify the site of tissue damage. Some published texts emphasize its use for nonhepatic tissues, but plasma levels of this enzyme do change following the administration of various hepatotoxins. Mitochondrial and cytosolic forms of AST exist; the proportion of mitochondrial to cytosolic form is generally greater than for ALT and thus may indicate the extent of cellular damage. Simple methodology for measuring the mitochondrial AST is not readily available and this remains a research technique (Rej 1980; Sada, Tashiro, and Morino 1990; Watazu et al. 1990).

Some investigators have expressed the activities of the two aminotransferases as a ratio (AST:ALT) to assist with interpretation. However, it is necessary for each laboratory to establish its own discriminating ratios because the use of different methods and animal species affects the values obtained for these ratios. From the factors affecting these measurements in different species, it can be seen that ratios established for one species cannot be used for another species.

Pyridoxal phosphate is a cofactor for both of these enzymes and is often supplied as a separate component of reagent kits. The addition of pyridoxal phosphate can increase the measured activities of both aminotransferases' activity by a small percentage (Stokol and Erb 1998) and can alter statistical differences observed between treatment groups in rat studies (Evans and Whitehorn 1995). Given the potential for some compounds to cause pyridoxal deficiencies mentioned earlier, the omission of pyridoxal phosphate from the reagents may be a preferred practice. Both ALT and AST are found in urine, but the concentrations are relatively low and these urinary enzymes do not have a significant role in the assessment of renal injury.

2.3.3 ALKALINE PHOSPHATASE

This group of relatively nonspecific enzymes hydrolyzes a variety of ester orthophosphates under alkaline conditions and exhibits optimal activity between pH 9 and 10. The group may act as hydrolases, liberating inorganic phosphate, or as phosphotransferases to an acceptor molecule such as a sugar. It is common practice to refer to the measurement as though it is a single enzyme, but the common analytical methods cover a variety of alkaline phosphatases. Several plasma isoenzymes of alkaline phosphatase are recognized, including hepatic, osseous, intestinal, and placental forms; the relative proportions of these isoenzymes in plasma vary with species. ALP is widely distributed in tissues—notably on the border membranes of the bile canaliculi and on the sinusoidal surfaces of the liver, the intestinal mucosa, the osteoblasts of bone, the renal proximal tubules, the placenta, and the mammary glands. In most species, age-related changes of osseous ALP are observed, reflecting bone growth in the neonatal and juvenile periods (Syakalima et al. 1997a). Although the diagnostic emphasis is mainly on increases of plasma ALP and hepatotoxicity, the enzyme may be reduced in hypothyroidism and pernicious anemia and may change in several nonhepatic-related conditions (Fernandez and Kidney 2007).

ALP may be measured using 4-nitrophenol phosphate as the substrate and one of three buffering systems—2-amino-2-methyl-1-propanol (AMP), diethanolamine (DEA), and N-methyl-D-glucamine (Matsushita et al. 2002); the first two systems are the most popular. Higher values are observed with DEA buffered methods compared to AMP methods. In the fasting rat and in rats dosed with alpha-naphthyl isothiocyanate, the optimum pH was reported to move from 9.4 to 10 (Yabe and Kast 1988). Many methods have been described for the separation and quantification of ALP isoenzymes because an increase of total ALP activity can be difficult to interpret given the widespread distribution of these enzymes These separation methods include electrophoresis (Pickering and Pickering 1978a; Milne and Doxey 1986); heat stability; wheat germ lectin affinity (Calderón de la Barca, Lundorff Jensen, and Bøg-Hansen 1993; Hoffman et al. 1994); use of enzyme selective inhibitors such as urea, phenylalanine, and levamisole (van Belle 1972, 1976; Moss 1982; Wellman et al. 1982a); immunochemical (Saini et al. 1978; Wellman et al. 1982b; Farley et al. 1992); treatment with neuraminidase (Eckersall et al. 1986); and high-performance liquid chromatography (Dziedziejko et al. 2005).

The hepatic isoenzyme is the dominant isoenzyme in plasma of most laboratory animals, but in the rat the intestinal and osseous isoenzymes are the dominant forms in plasma. Food intake has a marked effect on plasma ALP values in the rat, reflecting the intestinal component, with postprandial plasma ALP increase (Madsen and Tuba 1952; Sukumaran and Bloom 1953; Pickering and Pickering 1978b). When rats are fasted or food consumption is reduced secondarily due to toxicity, plasma ALP values are lower; however, this observation does not occur with other laboratory animals to the same extent and protein-deficient diets over 12 weeks increased serum ALP in beagles (Davenport et al. 1994). The intestinal ALP isoenzymes have very short half-lives of less than 10–60 minutes in most species. In the dog, the administration of glucocorticoids induces ALP activity, the so-called steroid- or corticosteroid-induced ALP (CALP) (Dorner, Hoffmann, and Long 1974; Eckersall 1986; Teske et al. 1989; Solter et al. 1993; Rutgers et al. 1995; Syakalima et al. 1997b; Thuroczy et al. 1998; Wiedmeyer, Solter, and Hoffmann 2003). This is associated with hepatopathies, which affect the plasma membrane and subcellular organelles; this plasma enzyme is increased in hypercorticism and during acute phase responses.

2.3.4 Amylase (AMY) and Lipase (LIP)

These enzymes are considered together because they are used primarily to evaluate changes in the pancreas (see Chapter 5). These two low molecular weight enzymes (42–45 kDa) are found mainly in the pancreas, although amylase is also found in salivary glands and liver. The origin of plasma amylase may therefore be described as pancreatic (P) or from the salivary glands (S). Plasma amylase can be useful in monitoring sialoadenitis in the salivary glands of rats, although not in the dog and rabbit, where the enzyme is less likely to be increased in this condition.

2.3.5 Creatine Kinase (CK) or Creatine Phosphokinase (CPK)

This enzyme is used primarily in studies of cardiotoxicity and myotoxicity and will be discussed in Chapter 7. The enzyme is primarily cytoplasmic and dimeric with subunits B (brain) and muscle (M) and they are glycoproteins (McBride, Rodgerson, and Hilborne 1990). There are three cytosolic enzymes: the muscle type dimer (CK-MM), the brain type dimer (CK-BB), and the myocardial type dimer (CK-MB) (Lang 1981). Mitochondrial isoenzymes and isoforms of CK also exist. The isoenzyme distribution varies between tissues; for example, in the dog and baboon, the dominant isoenzyme in the myocardium is CK-MM, while CK-BB is the dominant isoenzyme in the tissues of the gastrointestinal tract (Yasmineh et al. 1976; Kikuta and Onishi 1986; Aktas et al. 1993). The plasma CK enzyme levels are increased following myocardial damage, muscle injury including the effects of intramuscular injections, and surgically induced mesenteric infarction in dogs (Graeber et al. 1981; Roth, Jaquet, and Rohner 1989).

2.3.6 Gamma Glutamyl Transferase (GGT)

This enzyme, also called gamma glutamyl transpeptidase, catalyzes the transfer of gamma glutamyl groups from glutamyl peptides to an acceptor peptide or l-amino acid; it is one of six membrane-bound enzymes that act in the gamma glutamyl cycle, playing a major role in the regulation of reduced glutathione. The highest concentrations of GGT are found in the kidney and pancreas and then the liver. The enzyme is located on the brush border cells of the renal proximal convoluted tubules and on the canicular surfaces of the hepatic parenchymal cells (Ratanasavanh et al. 1979; Taniguchi and Ikeda 1998; Whitfield 2001). In the rat kidney, the level of GGT is approximately 200 times higher than the level found in hepatic tissue. However, despite its relatively high renal tissue concentrations plasma, GGT does not appear to alter following renal injury, although urinary GGT measurements are helpful in monitoring renal tubular damage.

In hepatic studies, plasma GGT can be used as an indicator of cholestasis, even in rats where plasma GGT levels are normally very low (often less than 2 IU/L). The use of GGT as a marker of enzyme induction and in the presence of hepatic tumors is less predictive in laboratory animals compared with data from human studies (Braun et al. 1987; Batt et al. 1992). GGT synthesis is induced in the liver by some xenobiotics (e.g., barbiturate) and by compounds that act via the thyroid on the liver (e.g., propylthiouracil and some glucocorticoids) (Sulakhe, Tran, and Pulga 1990).

2.3.7 Glutamate Dehydrogenase (GLDH or GDH)

This enzyme catalyzes the conversion of glutamate to 2-oxoglutarate. It is essentially a mitochondrial enzyme occurring in liver and kidney tissues; the highest concentrations are present in the liver. Plasma levels are generally low in most species; it has been recommended for detecting hepatotoxicity when there is cellular necrosis (O'Brien et al. 2002), although it loses diagnostic sensitivity in older rats, where the plasma values are more variable.

2.3.8 Ornithine Carbamoyl Transferase (OCT)

This enzyme, also called ornithine carbamyl transferase, catalyzes the reaction

$$\text{carbamoyl phosphate} + \text{ornithine} \leftrightarrow \text{citrulline} + \text{phosphate}$$

The high concentration of OCT is in hepatic tissue relative to other tissues; this leads to this enzyme being regarded as a liver-specific enzyme. OCT is localized in the periportal mitochondria and is the second of the five enzymes in the urea cycle. The enzyme measurement should not be confused with ornithine decarboxylase (ODC), which is of interest in studies of polyamine metabolism. The use of the method has been limited by some of technical requirements for the older assays, but newer enzymatic methods may increase its use (Peltenburg et al. 1991; Isobe, Matsuzawa, and Nagamura 1993; Ishikawa et al. 2002). In a number of rat studies, ALT was found to be more predictive of hepatotoxicity than OCT (Bondy et al. 2000).

2.3.9 Sorbitol Dehydrogenase (SDH)

Also known as iditol dehydrogenase, this enzyme catalyzes the interconversion of sorbitol to fructose in the presence of the coenzyme nicotinamide adenine dinucleotide. The enzyme is cytosolic, with the highest tissue concentration in the liver and a short half-life of less than a few hours. The plasma enzyme is relatively unstable and activity can be rapidly lost when serum is stored at room temperature; storage at lower temperatures reduces the deactivation of the enzyme. The enzyme measurement can be useful in canine, nonhuman primate, and rat studies as a confirmatory test for hepatotoxicity (Dooley, Turnquist, and Racich 1979; Pakuts, Whitehouse, and Paul 1988; Blazka et al. 1996; Travlos et al. 1996). However, the changes in liver injury are often relatively small compared to baseline values.

2.4 LESS COMMON ENZYME MEASUREMENTS

2.4.1 Alcohol Dehydrogenase (EC.1.1.1.1)

This enzyme is a cytoplasmic enzyme located mainly in the centrilobular region of the liver; it catalyzes the oxidation of ethanol to acetaldehyde with nicotinamide adenine dinucleotide as coenzyme. The enzyme is present in relatively low levels in plasma, and it has been used as a marker of hepatotoxicity by some investigators (Moser, Papenberg, and von Wartburg 1968; Khayrollah et al. 1982; Zimatkin, Pronko, and Grinevich 1997).

2.4.2 Aldolase (ALD: EC. 4.1.2.13: Fructose-1,6-Diphosphate Aldolase)

This enzyme converts fructose 1,6-diphosphate to glyceraldehyde-3-phosphate and dihydroxyacetone phosphate. It is used as a marker of muscle or liver injury (Sibley and Lehninger 1949).

2.4.3 Aminopeptidases and Arylamidases

These enzymes have been linked here because they have some common applications in diagnostic enzymology. Alanine aminopeptidase (AAP) and leucyl arylamidase (LAAP) hydrolyze the N-terminal amino acids and some amino amides; the enzymes respectively hydrolyze leucyl- and alanyl-4-nitroanilide substrates. These enzymes occur in microsomes and are also membrane bound; they have been used in studies of both hepatotoxicity and nephrotoxicity. They should not be confused with cytosolic leucine aminopeptidase (LAP); this enzyme is an aminopeptidase that hydrolyzes N-amino acid residues of proteins, in particular those with an N-terminal l-leucine, where l-leucyl-β-napthylamide is commonly used as substrate. Urinary alanine aminopeptidase is a useful marker of nephrotoxicity (Jung and Scholz 1980).

2.4.4 ARGINASE (EC 3.5.3.1)

This enzyme acts in the urea cycle, catalyzing the conversion of arginine to urea and ornithine. Arginase 1 is a cytoplasmic enzyme found mainly in the liver, but it is also found in erythrocytes and other tissues. In mouse tissue, arginase I is more widespread than arginase II (Yu et al. 2003). Given that arginase shares a common substrate with nitric oxide synthase, there is increasing interest in this enzyme in hepatology, nephrology (Waddington 2002), cancer, and other areas of high interest to those investigating nitric oxide pathways; the specificity of this enzyme for hepatic injury remains to be tested in a wider context. Analytical methods using sandwich ELISA and colorimetric and fluorometric techniques have been described. Increases of plasma/serum arginase have been demonstrated in various animal models of induced hepatotoxicity (Aminlari et al. 1994; Ikemoto et al. 2001).

2.4.5 GLUTATHIONE S-TRANSFERASES (GST)

These are a family of mainly cytosolic enzymes involved in the detoxification of xenobiotics by reactions between reduced glutathione and electrophilic compounds in phase II biotransformations. Some forms are also known as ligandin (EC 2.5.1.1.18). GSTs also sequester and transport endogenous hydrophobic compounds such steroids, bilirubin, bile acids, heme, and other metabolites in addition to xenobiotics. These enzymes are widely distributed in the body tissues, with the highest concentrations occurring in the liver and the testes and then the kidneys of the rat. There is a small amount of microsomal GST. The enzymes are dimeric, with several isoenzymes formed either as homo- or heterodimers from a number of subunits The enzyme nomenclature has led to some historic confusion, but essentially GSTs can be grouped structurally into alpha (A), mu (M), pi (P), theta (T), and zeta (Z) classes based on these subunits (Mannervik and Danielson 1988; Van der Aar Eaton and Bammler 1999; Salinas and Wong 1999; Awasthi 2006).

These GSTs can also be described according to the species: Using rat as an example, a GST may be described as rGSTA1-1, where r indicates rat (h = human) and A is the alpha unit; this enzyme is a homodimer 1-1. Within a class, the GSTs show approximately 40% homology and <30% homology between classes; sex differences have been observed (Igarashi et al. 1985). The proteins are globular with molecular masses of between 23 and 29 kDa and short half-lives of less than 60 minutes. Some of these enzymes may be measured by radioimmunoassay, immunofluorimetry, or enzyme immunoassays. Plasma GSTs have been used as markers of hepatotoxicity and in nephrotoxicity (De Simplicio 1982; Beckett and Hayes 1993; Kilty et al. 1998).

2.4.6 LACTATE DEHYDROGENASE (LDH OR LD)

This enzyme catalyzes the reversible oxidation of lactate to pyruvate; it is a cytosolic tetrameric enzyme with five major isoenzymes in plasma consisting of H (heart) and M (muscle) subunits. Five isoenzymes are numbered according to decreasing anodic mobility during electrophoretic separation: LDH 1 has four H subunits, LDH5 has four M subunits, and LDH2, LDH3, and LDH4 are hybrid combinations containing HHHM,

HHMM, and HMMM, respectively (Markert, Shaklee, and Whitt 1975). The wide-spread tissue distribution of LDH differs with the various species (Garbus et al. 1967; Cornish, Barth, and Dodson 1970; Karlsson and Larsson 1971; Schultze et al. 1994). Some additional isoenzymes of LDH have been described, and some LDH isoenzymes may complex with drugs—for example, streptokinase (Podlasek and McPherson 1989). Because LD is a cytoplasmic enzyme, it is increased in serum during hepatocyte or myocyte necrosis and conditions that are toxic to hepatocytes or myocytes. However, it lacks specificity and sensitivity when compared to other enzymes for detection of specific organ injury. In laboratory animals, the primary use for LD has been the detection of experimentally induced myocardial injury (see Chapter 7).

There is a marked difference in the half-lives of the five isoenzymes; a progressive decrease in half-life occurs as the M subunit becomes the dominant form. The isoenzymes are not stable in storage, and there are phylogenic differences for plasma and tissue LDH isoenzymes (Yoshikuni et al. 2001). Mice infected with the Riley strain of the lactate dehydrogenase virus have a five- to tenfold increase of LDH that is maintained throughout life. This virus is presumed to destroy or block a population of macrophages that remove LD from circulation, resulting in a marked reduction in clearance of either endogenous or exogenously administered LD (Hayashi et al. 1988, 1992).

2.4.7   5′-NUCLEOTIDASE (5′-NT)

This enzyme is an alkaline phosphomonoesterase that catalyzes the hydrolysis of nucleoside 5′-monophosphates (e.g., adenosine-5′-monophosphate and inosine-5′-monophosphate). It appears to be distributed widely in the body tissues and to be mainly a membrane-bound enzyme, but it is also found in the cytoplasm, lysosomes, and other subcellular organelles. In the liver, the enzyme is located on the bile canicular membrane and on other cells, including the sinusoidal cells, leading to its use for the detection of hepatobiliary injury (Goldberg 1973; Dooley and Racich 1980; Carakostas, Power, and Banerjee 1990; Sunderman 1990). The enzyme measurement has largely been discarded in clinical medicine; however, more recently, the 5′-NT enzymes have been implicated in the inhibition of antiviral nucleosides, so interest may be revived (Hunsucker, Mitchell, and Spychala 2005).

2.4.8   PARAOXANASE (PON1; EC.3.1.1.2)

This enzyme may be measured in studies of organophosphate-induced neurotoxicities. More recently, its cardioprotective role in association with high-density lipoprotein has received some attention. Paraoxanase has also been used as marker of hepatotoxicity (Gil et al. 1994; Hernandez et al. 1997; Ferre et al. 2002).

2.5   OTHER ENZYME MEASUREMENTS

2.5.1   TISSUE CYTOCHROMES P450

The P450 enzyme family is a group of mono-oxygenases found mainly in hepatocytes, but also in the small intestine, kidneys, lungs, and brain. More than 30 P450 isoforms have been described, although only a few appear to play a major part in the metabolism of xenobiotics; some of these reactions involve biotransformations of lipophilic drugs to more polar compounds, which are then renally excreted. The enzymes are recognized as being an important key to individual differences in drug metabolism, some of which result in the separation of recipients into responders and nonresponders to treatments (Batt et al. 1994; Spatzenegger and Jaeger 1995; Horsmans 1997; Lewis 2001; Lee, Obach, and Fisher 2003; Wilkinson 2005). Hepatic enzyme induction is associated with alterations of drug metabolism and systemic exposure; it can cause hepatotoxicity with hypertrophy and necrosis and may lead to hepatic tumors. In addition, there may be effects on the thyroid via TSH and testicular toxicities following perturbations of steroid metabolism. Some of the important P450 enzymes can be measured in liver tissue extracts.

2.5.2 OTHER DRUG-METABOLIZING ENZYMES IN PLASMA

Plasma esterases such as cholinesterase and arylesterases are involved in the hydrolysis of some xenobiotics and may affect the elimination of some compounds. Carboxylesterases appear to be absent from some laboratory animals, but are present in rats and guinea pigs and may also play a part in the hydrolysis of xenobiotics (Williams 1987).

2.6 SUMMARY

In summary, very few of the many enzymes in the body are measured routinely in toxicology studies, and even fewer of these are organ-specific markers. Most of the common enzymes—ALT, ALP, AST, GGT, OCT, and SDH—are aimed at detecting hepatic injury. Other enzymes—such as alcohol dehydrogenase, arginase, malate dehydrogenase (MDH), isocitrate dehydrogenase (ICDH), glucose-6-phosphate dehydrogenase (G6PDH), and lactate dehydrogenase—are among many of the enzymes evaluated in studies of hepatotoxicity that have been discarded as having limited or no additional value. Of these, perhaps arginase is worthy of reevaluation as improved methods are available, but it remains to be seen if this enzyme has any advantages over the other urea cycle enzymes that have already been tried.

Several urinary enzymes are useful in the assessment of nephrotoxicity, and these are discussed separately in Chapter 4. Although there is some application of cholinesterases in studying hepatotoxicity, these enzymes are important markers in pesticide-induced toxicities and are discussed in Chapter 11. Creatine kinase (CK) remains a useful marker for myotoxicity, but it is rapidly losing its place to troponins in the detection of cardiotoxicity (see Chapter 7). Amylase and lipase remain the enzyme markers of pancreatic toxicity.

After evaluation in toxicology studies, several enzymes have been discarded as having little or no additional diagnostic value, or perhaps due to the lack of suitable automated methods and available reagents. These findings are not dissimilar to those in human and veterinary medicine. Enzyme patterns obtained by proteomic techniques may lead to more sensitive assays based on mass rather than activity, and this may lead to biochip technology to further develop novel assays.

REFERENCES

Aktas, M., D. Auguste, H. P. Lefebvre, P. L. Toutain, and J. P. Braun. 1993. Creatine kinase in the dog: A review. *Veterinary Research Communications* 17:353–369.

Aminlari, M., T. Vaseghi, M. J. Sajdianfard, and M. Samsami. 1994. Changes in arginase, aminotransferases and rhodanes in sera of domestic animals with experimentally induced liver necrosis. *Journal of Comparative Pathology* 110:1–9.

Awasthi, Y. C. 2006. *Toxicology of glutathione transferases.* Boca Raton, FL: CRC Press.

Balazs, T., T. M. Farber, and G. Feuer. 1978. Drug induced serum alkaline phosphatase and alanine aminotransferase activities not related to hepatic injuries. *Archives of Toxicology* 1 (Suppl.): 159–163.

Batt, A. M., J. Magdalou, M. Vincent-Viry, M. Ouzzine, S. Fournel-Gigleux, M. M. Galteau, and G. Siest. 1994. Drug metabolizing enzymes related to laboratory medicine: Cytochromes P-450 and UDP-glucuronosyltransferases. *Clinica Chimica Acta* 226:171–190.

Batt, A. M., G. Siest, J. Magdalou, and M-M. Galteau. 1992. Enzyme induction by drugs and toxins. *Clinica Chimica Acta* 209:109–121.

Beckett, G. J., and J. D. Hayes. 1993. Glutathione S-transferases: Biomedical applications. *Advances in Clinical Chemistry* 30:281–380.

Blazka, M. E., M. R. Elwell, S. D. Holladay, R. E. Wilson, and M. I. Luster. 1996. Histopathology of acetaminophen-induced liver changes: Role of interleukin 1 alpha and tumor necrosis factor alpha. *Toxicologic Pathology* 24:181–189.

Bondy, G. S., C. L. Armstrong, I. H. Curran, M. G. Barker, and R. Mehta. 2000. Retrospective evaluation of serum ornithine carbamyl transferase as an index of hepatotoxicity in toxicological studies with rats. *Toxicology Letters* 114:163–171.

Bouma, J. M. W., and M. J. Smit. 1988. Elimination of enzymes from plasma in the rat. In *Enzymes—Tools and targets, advances in clinical enzymology,* vol. 6, ed. D. M. Goldberg, D. W. Moss, E. Schmidt, and F. W. Schmidt, pp. 111–119. Basel, Switzerland: Karger.

Braun, J. P., P. Bernard, V. Burgat, and A. G. Rico. 1983. Tissue basis for use of enzymes in toxicology. *Veterinary Research Communications* 7:331–335.

Braun, J. P., G. Siest, and A. G. Rico. 1987. Uses of gamma-glutamyltransferase in experimental toxicology. *Advances in Veterinary Science and Comparative Medicine* 31:151–172.

Calderón de la Barca, A. M., A. Lundorff Jensen, and T. C. Bøg-Hansen. 1993. Affinity methods with lectins: A tool to identify canine alkaline phosphatase isoenzymes. *Journal of Biochemical and Biophysical Methods* 27:169–180.

Carakostas, M. C., R. J. Power, and A. K. Banerjee.1990. Serum 5′-nucleotidase activity in rats: A method for automated analysis and criteria for interpretation. *Veterinary Clinical Pathology* 19:109–113.

Clampitt, R. B., and R. J. Hart. 1978. The tissue activities of some diagnostic enzymes in ten mammalian species. *Journal of Comparative Pathology* 88:607–621.

Cornish, H. H., M. L. Barth, and V. N. Dodson. 1970. Isozyme profiles and protein patterns in specific organ damage. *Toxicology and Applied Pharmacology* 16:411–423.

Cowie, J. R., and G. O. Evans. 1985. Plasma aminotransferase measurements in the marmoset (*Callithrix jacchus*). *Laboratory Animals* 19:48–50.

Davenport, D. J., R. A. Mostardi, D. C. Richardson, K. L. Gross, K. A. Greene, and K. Blair. 1994. Protein-deficient diet alters alkaline phosphatase, bile aids, proteins and urea-nitrogen in dogs. *Journal of Nutrition* 124:2677S.

Davy, C. W., A. Brock, J. M. Walker, and D. A. Eichler. 1988. Tissue activities of enzymes of diagnostic interest in the marmoset and rat. *Journal of Comparative Pathology* 99:41–53.

Davy, C. W., M. R. Jackson, and J. M. Walker. 1984. Reference intervals for some clinical chemistry parameters in the marmoset (*Callithrix jacchus*): Effect of age and sex. *Laboratory Animals* 18:135–142.

DeRosa, G., and R. W. Swick. 1975. Metabolic implications of the distribution of alanine aminotransferase isoenzymes. *Journal of Biological Chemistry* 250:7961–7967.

De Simplicio, P. 1982. Glutathione and glutathione S-transferase in rat liver and plasma after carbon tetrachloride and thioacetamide intoxication. *Pharmacology Research Communications* 14:909–920.

Dhami, M. S. I., R. Drangova, R. Farkas, T. Balazs, and G. Feuer. 1979. Decreased aminotransferase activity of serum and various tissue in the rat after cefazolin treatment. *Clinical Chemistry* 25:1263–1266.

Dodurka, T., and W. Kraft. 1995. Alanine aminotransferase (ALT) aspartate aminotransferase (AST) glutamate dehydrogenase (GLDH), alkaline phosphatase (AP) and gammaglutamyltransferase (GGP) in intestinal diseases of dogs. *Berliner und Munchener Tierarzliche Wochenschrift* 108:244–248.

Dooley, J. F. 1979. The role of clinical chemistry in chemical and drug safety evaluation by use of laboratory animals. *Clinical Chemistry* 25:345–347.

Dooley, J. F., and L. Racich. 1980. A new kinetic determination of serum 5´-nucleotidase activity with modifications for a centrifugal analyzer. *Clinical Chemistry* 26:1291–1297.

Dooley, J. F., L. J. Turnquist, and L. Racich. 1979. Kinetic determination of serum sorbitol dehydrogenase activity with a centrifugal analyzer. *Clinical Chemistry* 25:2026–2029.

Dorner, J. L., W. E. Hoffmann, and G. B. Long. 1974. Corticosteroid induction of an isoenzyme of alkaline phosphatase in the dog. *American Journal of Veterinary Research* 35:1457–1458.

Dziedziejko, V., K. Safranow., D. Sowik-Zyka, A. Machoy-Mokrzynska, B. Millo, Z. Machoy, and D. Chlubek. 2005. Comparison of rat and human alkaline phosphatase isoenzymes and isoforms using HPLC and electrophoresis. *Biochimica et Biophysica Acta* 1752:26–33.

Eaton, D. L., and T. K. Bammler. 1999. Concise review of the glutathione S-transferases and their significance to toxicology. *Toxicological Science* 49:156–164.

Eckersall, P. D. 1986. Steroid induced alkaline phosphatase in the dog. *Israeli Journal of Veterinary Medicine* 42:253–259.

Eckersall, P. D., A. Thomas, G. M.Marshall, and T. A. Douglas. 1986. The effect of neuraminidase on the molecular weight and the isoelectric point of the steroid induced alkaline phosphatase of dogs. *Journal of Comparative Pathology* 96:587–591.

Evans, G. O. 1989. Species relationships for plasma angiotensin converting enzyme activity using a furanacryloyl tripeptide substrate. *Experimental Animals* 38:897–898.

———. 1990. Species relationships for plasma acylcholine-acyl hydrolase using three different substrates. In *Fourth Congress, International Society for Animal Clinical Biochemistry,* p. 270. Davis: University of California.

Evans, G. O., and L. C. Whitehorn. 1995. Effects of pyridoxal 5´-phosphate on plasma alanine aminotransferase determinations in toxicological studies. *Toxicology Letters* 80:34–37.

Farley, J. R., S. L. Hall, C. Richie, S. Herring, C. Orcutt, and B. E. Miller. 1992. Quantitation of skeletal alkaline phosphatase activity in canine serum. *Journal of Bone and Mineral Research* 7:779–792.

Fernandez, N. J., and B. Kidney. 2007. Alkaline phosphatase beyond the liver. *Veterinary Clinical Pathology* 36:223–232.

Ferre, N., J. Camps, E. Prats, E. Vilella, A. Paul, L. Figuera, and J. Joven. 2002. Serum paraoxonase activity: A new additional test for the improved evaluation of chronic liver disease. *Clinical Chemistry* 48:261–268.

Garbus, G. B., B. Highman, and P. D. Altland. 1967. Alterations in serum enzymes and isoenzymes in various species induced by epinephrine. *Comparative Biochemistry and Physiology* 22:507–516.

Gil, F., M. C. Gonzalvo, A. F. Hernandez, E. Vilanueva, and A. Pla. 1994. Differences in the kinetic properties, effect of calcium and sensitivity in inhibitors of paraoxon hydrolase activity in rat plasma and microsomal fraction of the liver. *Biochemical Pharmacology* 48:1559–1568.

Goldberg, D. M. 1973. 5′-Nucleotidase: Recent advances in cell biology, methodology and clinical significance. *Digestion* 8:87–99.

Graeber, G. M., P. J. Cafferty, M. J. Reardon, C. P. Curley, N. B. Ackerman, and J. W. Harmon. 1981. Changes in serum total creatine phosphokinase in experimental mesenteric infarction. *Annals of Surgery* 193:499–505.

Hayashi, T., M. Ozaki, I. Mori, M. Saito, T. Mitoh, and H. Yamamoto. 1992. Enhanced clearance of lactic dehydrogenase-5 in severe combined immunodeficiency (SCID) mice: Effect of lactic dehydrogenase on enzyme clearance. *International Journal of Experimental Pathology* 73:173–181.

Hayashi, T., K. Salata, A. Kingman, and A. L. Notkins. 1988. Regulation of enzyme levels in the blood; influence of environmental and genetic factors on enzyme clearance. *American Journal of Pathology* 132:503–511.

Hernandez, A. F., M. C. Gonzalvo, F. Gil, E. Villanueva, and A. Pla. 1997. Divergent effects of classical inducers on rat plasma and microsomal fraction paraoxonase and arylesterase. *Environmental Toxicology and Pharmacology* 3:83–86.

Hoffman, W. E., N. Everds, M. Pignatello, and P. F. Solter. 1994. Automated and semiautomated analysis of rat alkaline phosphatase isoenzymes. *Toxicological Pathology* 22:633–638.

Horsmans, Y. 1997. Major cytochrome P450 families: Implications in health and liver diseases. *Acta Gastroenterologica Belgique* 60:2–10.

Hunsucker, S. A., B. S. Mitchell, and J. Spychala. 2005. The 5′-nucleotidases as regulators of nucleotide and drug metabolism. *Pharmacology and Therapeutics* 107:1–30.

Igarashi, T., T. Satoh, K. Iwashita, S. Ono, K. Uneo, and H. Kitagawa. 1985. Sex difference in subunit composition of hepatic glutathione S-transferase. *Journal of Biochemistry* 98:117–123.

Ikemoto, M., S. Tsunekawa, Y. Toda, and M. Totani. 2001. Liver-type arginase is a highly sensitive marker for hepatocellular damage in rats. *Clinical Chemistry* 47:946–948.

Ishikawa, H., T. Matsuzawa, K. Ohashi, and Y. Nagamura. 2003. A novel method of measuring serum ornithine carbamoyltransferase. *Annals of Clinical Biochemistry* 40:264–268.

Isobe, K., T. Matsuzawa, and Y. Nagamura. 1993. A new enzymatic method of ornithine carbamoyltransferase activity. *Analytical Letters* 26:465–486.

Jansen, R., G. Schumann, H. Baadenhuijsen, P. Franck, C. Franzini, R. Kruse, A. Kuypers, C. Weykamp, and M. Panteghini. 2006. Trueness verification and traceability assessment results from commercial systems for measurement of six enzyme activities in serum. An international study in the EC4 framework of the Calibration 2000 project. *Clinica Chimica Acta* 368:160–167.

Jung, K., and D. Scholz. 1980. An optimized assay of alanine aminopeptidase activity in urine. *Clinical Chemistry* 26:1251–1254.

Karlsson, B. W., and G. B. Larsson. 1971. Lactic and malic dehydrogenases and their multiple molecular forms in the Mongolian gerbil as compared with the rat, mouse and rabbit. *Comparative Biochemistry and Physiology* 40B:93–108.

Kast, A., and J. Nishikawa. 1981. The effects of fasting on oral acute toxicity of drugs in rats and mice. *Laboratory Animals* 15:359–364.

Keil, E. 1990. Determination of enzyme activities in serum for the detection of xenobiotics effects on the liver. *Experimental Pathology* 39:157–164.

Keller, P. 1981. Enzyme activities in the dog: Tissue analyses, plasma values, and intracellular distribution. *American Journal of Veterinary Research* 42:575–582.

Khayrollah, A. A., Y. Y. Al-Tamer, M. Taka, and L. Skursky. 1982. Serum alcohol dehydrogenase in liver diseases. *Annals of Clinical Biochemistry* 19:35–42.

Kikuta, Y., and T. Onishi. 1986. The contribution of intestinal creatine kinase activity and its isoenzymes in dogs. *Nippon Juigaku Zasshi.* 48:547–551.

Kilty, C., S. Doyle, B. Hassett, and F. Manning. 1998. Glutathione S-transferases as biomarkers of organ damage: Applications of rodent and canine GST enzyme immunoassays. *Chemico–Biological Interactions* 111–112:123–135.

Lang, H. 1981. *Creatine kinase isoenzymes.* Berlin: Springer–Verlag.

Lee, J. S., S. Obach, and M. B. Fisher. 2003. *Drug metabolizing enzymes: Cytochrome P450 and other enzymes in drug discovery and development.* Boca Raton, FL: CRC Press.

Lewis, D. F.V. 2001. *Guide to cytochromes P450. Structure and function.* Boca Raton, FL: CRC Press.

Lindena, J., U. Sommerfeld, C. Hopfel, and I. Trautschold. 1986. Catalytic enzyme activity concentration in tissues of man, dog, rabbit, guinea pig, rat and mouse. *Journal of Clinical Chemistry and Clinical Biochemistry* 24:35–47.

Lindena, J., and I. Trautschold. 1986. Catalytic enzyme activity concentration in plasma of man, sheep, dog, cat, rabbit, guinea pig, rat and mouse. Approach to a quantitative diagnostic enzymology. *Journal of Clinical Chemistry and Clinical Biochemistry* 24: 11–18.

Madsen, N. B., and J. Tuba. 1952. On the source of alkaline phosphatase in rat serum. *Journal of Biological Chemistry* 195:741–750.

Mannervik, B., and U. H. Danielson. 1988. Glutathione transferases—Structure and catalytic activity. *CRC Critical Reviews in Biochemistry* 23:283–337.

Markert, C. L., J. B. Shaklee, and G. S. Whitt. 1975. Evolution of a new gene. Multiple genes for LDH isoenzymes provide a model of the evolution of gene structure function and regulation. *Science* 189:102–114.

Masson, P., and J. Holmgren. 1992. Comparative study of alkaline phosphatase in human and animal samples using methods based on AMP and DEA buffers: Effect on quality control. *Scandinavian Journal of Clinical and Laboratory Investigation* 52:773–775.

Matsushita, M., T. Irino, T. Kawaguchi, and T. Komoda. 2002. The effect of different buffers and amounts of intestinal alkaline phosphatase on total alkaline phosphatase activity. *Clinica Chimica Acta* 319:49–55.

McBride, J. H., D. O. Rodgerson, and L. H. Hilborne. 1990. Human, rabbit, bovine and porcine creatine kinase isoenzymes are glycoproteins. *Journal of Clinical and Laboratory Analysis* 4:196–198.

Milne, E. M., and D. L. Doxey. 1986. Alkaline phosphatase and its isoenzymes in the tissues and sera of normal dogs. *Veterinary Research Communications* 10:229–236.

Moser, K., J. Papenberg, and J. P. von Wartburg. 1968. Heterogenität und organverteilung der alkohodehydrogenase bei verschiedenen spezies. *Enzymologia Biologica et Clinica* 9:447–450.

Moss, D. W. 1982. Alkaline phosphatase isoenzymes. *Clinical Chemistry* 28:2007–2016.

Myers, D. K. 1953. Studies on cholinesterase: 9. Species variation in the specificity pattern of the pseudocholinesterases. *Biochemistry Journal* 55:67–79.

O'Brien, P. J., M. R. Slaughter, S. R. Polley, and K. Kramer. 2002. Advantages of glutamate dehydrogenase as blood biomarker of acute hepatic injury in rats. *Laboratory Animals* 36:313–321.

Pakuts, A. P., L. W. Whitehouse, and C. J. Paul. 1988. Plasma sorbitol dehydrogenase determination in experimental hepatotoxicity using the Abbott bichromatic analyzer. *Journal of Clinical Chemistry and Clinical Biochemistry* 26:693–695.

Peltenburg, H. G., M. A. Janssen, P. B. Soeters, J. G. Flendrig, and W. T. Hermens. 1991. Measurement of ornithine carbamyl transferase (OCT) in plasma by means of enzymatic determination of ammonia. *Clinica Chimica Acta* 203:395–402.

Pickering, C. E., and R. G. Pickering. 1978a. Studies of rat alkaline phosphatase. 1. Development of methods for detecting isoenzymes. *Archives of Toxicology* 39:249–266.

———. 1978b. Studies of rat alkaline phosphatase. 2. Some applications of the methods for detecting the isoenzymes of plasma alkaline phosphatase in rats. *Archives of Toxicology* 39:267–287.

Podlasek, S. J., and R. A. McPherson. 1989. Streptokinase binds to lactate dehydrogenase subunit-M which shares an epitope with plasminogen. *Clinical Chemistry* 35:67–73.

Ratanasavanh, D., A. Tazi, M. M. Galteau, and G. Siest. 1979. Localization of gamma-glutamyltranferase in subcellular fractions of rat and rabbit liver: Effect of phenobarbital. *Biochemical Pharmacology* 28:1363–1365.

Rej, R. 1980. An immunochemical procedure for determination of mitochondrial aspartate aminotransferase in human serum. *Clinical Chemistry* 26:1694–1700.

Rhodes, D. C., H. N. Dring, S. A. Blackmer, and H. B. Lewis. 1987. Drug-induced decreases in serum alanine aminotransferase (ALT). *Veterinary Clinical Pathology* 16:12.

Roth, M., P. Y. Jaquet, and A. Rohner. 1989. Increase of creatine kinase and lactate dehydrogenase in the serum of rats submitted to experimental intestinal infarction. *Clinica Chimica Acta* 183:65–69.

Ruščák, M., J. Orlický, and V. Žubor. 1982. Isoelectric focusing of the alanine aminotransferase isoenzymes from the brain, liver and kidney. *Comparative Biochemistry and Physiology* 71B:141–144.

Rutgers, H. C., R. M. Batt, C. Vaillant, and E. Riley. 1995. Subcellular pathologic features of glucocorticoid-induced hepatopathy in dogs. *American Journal of Veterinary Research* 56:898–907.

Sada, E., S. Tashiro, and Y. Morino. 1990. The significance of serum mitochondrial aspartate aminotransferase activity in obstructive jaundice: Experimental and clinical studies. *Japanese Journal of Surgery* 20:392–405.

Saini, P. K., G. M. Peavy, D. E. Hauser, and S. K. Saini. 1978. Diagnostic evaluation of canine serum alkaline phosphatase by immunochemical means and interpretation of results. *American Journal of Veterinary Research* 39:1514–1518.

Salinas, A. E., and M. G. Wong.1999. Glutathione S-transferases—A review. *Current Medicinal Chemistry* 6:279–309.

Schmidt, E., and F. W. Schmidt. 1987. Enzyme release. *Journal of Clinical Chemistry and Clinical Biochemistry* 25:525–540.

Schultz, A. E., K. P. Gungaga, J. G. Wagner, C. M. Hoorn, W. R. Moorhead, and R. A. Roth. 1994. Lactate dehydrogenase activity and isozyme patterns in tissues and bronchoalveolar lavage fluid from rats treated with monocrotaline pyrrole. *Toxicology and Applied Pharmacology* 126:301–310.

Schwartz, E., J. A. Tornaben, and G. C. Boxhill. 1973. The effects of food restriction on hematology, clinical chemistry and pathology in the albino rat. *Toxicology and Applied Pharmacology* 25:515–524.

Sibley, J. A., and A. L. Lehninger. 1949. Determination of aldolase in animal tissues. *Journal of Biological Chemistry* 177:859–861.

Solter, P. F., W. E. Hoffman, L. L. Hungerford, M. E. Peterson, and J. L. Dorner. 1993. Assessment of corticosteroid-induced alkaline phosphatase isoenzymes as a screening test for hyperadrenocorticism in the dog. *Journal of the American Veterinary Medical Association* 203:534–538.

Spatzenegger, M., and W. Jaeger. 1995. Clinical importance of hepatic cytochrome P450 in drug metabolism. *Drug Metabolism Reviews* 27:397–417.

Stokol, T., and H. Erb. 1998. The apo-enzyme content of aminotransferases in healthy and diseased domestic animals. *Veterinary Clinical Pathology* 27:71–78.

Sukumaran, M., and W. L. Bloom. 1953. Influence of diet on serum alkaline phosphatase in rats and men. *Proceedings of the Society for Experimental Biology and Medicine* 6:631–634.

Sulakhe, S. J., S. T. Tran, and V. B. Pulga. 1990. Modulation of gamma-glutamyltranspeptidase activity in rat liver membranes by thyroid hormones. *International Journal of Biochemistry* 22:997–1004.

Sunderman, F. W. 1990. The clinical biochemistry of 5´-nucleotidase. *Annals of Clinical and Laboratory Science* 20:123–139.

Swenson, C. L., and T. K. Graves. 1997. Absence of liver specificity for canine alanine aminotransferase (ALT). *Veterinary Clinical Pathology* 26:26–28.

Syakalima, M., M. Takiguchi, J. Yasuda, and A. Hashimoto. 1997a. The age dependent levels of serum ALP isoenzymes and the diagnostic significance of corticosteroid-induced ALP during long term glucocorticoid treatment. *Journal of Veterinary Medical Science* 59:905–909.

———. 1997b. Separation and quantification of corticosteroid-induced, bone and liver alkaline phosphatase isoenzymes in canine serum. *Zentralblatt für Veterinarmedizin A* 44:603–610.

Taniguchi, N., and Y. Ikeda. 1998. Gamma-glutamyl transpeptidase: Catalytic mechanisms and gene expression. *Advances in Enzymology and Related Areas of Molecular Biology* 72:239–278.

Teske, E., J. J. Rothuizen, J. J. de Bruijne, and A. Rijnberk. 1989. Corticosteroid induced alkaline phosphatase isoenzyme in the diagnosis of hypercorticism. *Veterinary Record* 1989:12–14.

Thuroczy, J., L. Balogh, G. Huszenicza, G. A. Janoki, and M. Kulcsar. 1998. Diagnosis of hyperadrenocorticism in dogs as compared to human diagnostic methods: A review. *Acta Veterinaria Hungarica* 46:157–173.

Toropila, M., I. Ahlers, E. Ahlersova, M. Ondrasovic, and K. Benova. 1996. The effect of prolonged starvation on changes in the activity of selected adaptive enzymes in rat liver. *Veterinary Medicine (Praha)* 41:41–44.

Travlos, G. S., R. W. Morris, M. R. Elwell, A. Duke, S. Rosenblum, and M. B. Thomson. 1996. Frequency and relationship of clinical chemistry and liver and kidney histopathology findings in 13-week toxicity studies in rats. *Toxicology* 107:17–29.

Valentine, B. A., J. T. Blue, S. M. Shelley, and B. J. Cooper. 1990. Increased alanine aminotransferase activity associated with muscle necrosis in the dog. *Journal of Veterinary Internal Medicine* 4:140–143.

van Belle, H. 1972. Kinetics and inhibition of alkaline phosphatases from canine tissues. *Biochimica et Biophysica Acta* 289:158–168.

———. 1976. Kinetics and inhibition of rat and avian alkaline phosphatases. *General Pharmacology* 7:53–58.

van der Aar, E. M., K. T. Tan, J. N. Commandeur, and N. P. Vermeulen. 1998. Strategies to characterize the mechanisms of action and active sites of glutathione S-transferases: A review. *Drug Metabolism Reviews* 30:569–643.

Waddington, S. N. 2002. Arginase in glomerulonephritis. *Kidney International* 61:876–881.

Waner, T., and A. Nyska. 1991. The toxicological significance of decreased activities of blood alanine and aspartate aminotransferase. *Veterinary Research Communications* 15:73–78.

Waner, T., A. Nyska, E. Bogin, R. Levy, and A. Galiano. 1990. Drug-induced decrease of serum alanine and aspartate aminotransferase activity in the rat, as a result of treatment with oxodipine, a new calcium channel blocker. *Journal of Clinical Chemistry and Clinical Biochemistry* 28:25–30.

Watazu, Y., H. Okabe, H. Sugiuchi, Y. Uji, Y. Shirahase, and N. Kaneda. 1990. Proteolytic measurements of mitochondrial aspartate aminotransferases in human serum. *Clinical Biochemistry* 23:127–130.

Wellman, M. L., W. E. Hoffmann, J. L. Dorner, and R. E. Mock. 1982a. Comparison of the steroid-induced, intestinal and hepatic isoenzymes of alkaline phosphatase in the dog. *American Journal of Veterinary Research* 43:1204–1207.

———. 1982b. Immunoassay for the steroid-induced, intestinal and hepatic isoenzymes of alkaline phosphatase in the dog. *American Journal of Veterinary Research* 43:1200–1203.

Wells, P. G., and E. C. To. 1986. Murine acetaminophen hepatoxicity: Temporal interanimal variability in plasma glutamic-pyruvic transaminase profiles and relation in vivo chemical covalent binding. *Fundamental and Applied Toxicology* 7:17–25.

Whitfield, J. B. 2001. Gamma-glutarnyl transferase. *Critical Reviews in Clinical Laboratory Science* 38:263–355.

Wiedmeyer, C. E., P. E. Solter, and W. E. Hoffmann. 2003. Alkaline phosphatase expression in tissues from glucocorticoid-treated dogs. *American Journal of Veterinary Research* 63:1083–1088.

Wilkinson, G. R. 2005. Drug metabolism and variability among patients in drug response. *New England Journal of Medicine* 352:2211–2221.

Williams, F. M. 1987. Serum enzymes of drug metabolism. *Pharmacology and Therapeutics* 34:99–109.

Woodman, D. D. 1981. Plasma enzymes in drug toxicity. In *Aspects of drug toxicity testing methods*, ed. J. W. Gorrod, pp. 145–156. London: Taylor & Francis.

Yabe, T., and A. Kast. 1988. The optimum pH of serum alkaline phosphatase after induced cholestasis in the male rat, mouse and rabbit. *Journal of Toxicological Sciences* 13:179–191.

Yasmineh, W. G., R. B. Pyle, N. Q. Hanson, and B. K. Hultman. 1976. Creatine kinase iosenzymes in baboon tissues and organs. *Clinical Chemistry* 22:63–66.

Yoshikuni, K., T. Matsuda, J. Poracova, A. Sakai, K. Shimada, N. Tabuchi, and K. Tanishima. 2001. Phylogenic study of denaturation of lactate dehydrogenase isoenzymes from different species by high and low temperatures. *Annals of Clinical Biochemistry* 38:548–553.

Yu, H., P. K. Yoo, C. C. Aguirre, R. W. Tsoa, R. M. Kern, W. W. Grody, S. D. Cederbaum, and R. K. Iyer. 2003. Widespread expression of arginase I in mouse tissues. Biochemical and physiological interactions. *Journal of Histochemistry and Cytochemstry* 51:1151–1160.

Zimatkin, S. M., P. S. Pronko, and V. P. Grinevich. 1997. Alcohol action on liver: Dose dependence and morpho-biochemical correlations. *Casopis Lekaru Ceskych* 136:598–602.

3 Assessment of Hepatotoxicity

3.1 STRUCTURE, PHYSIOLOGY, AND BIOCHEMISTRY

Hepatocytes are the commonest cell type found in the liver, constituting about 70% of the total liver mass. The plasma membranes of these cells have three functional domains: the sinusoidal domain, an intercellular domain with gap junctions that is the contact area between hepatocytes, and the canalicular domain, where many of the hepatic secretory functions are performed. The hepatocytes are arranged in single cell layers around sinusoids, which are vascular capillary vessels connected to the hepatic portal vein and hepatic artery; the perisinusoidal space of Disse separates the endothelial cell from the hepatocytes. Fenestrations (or windows) in the cells lining the sinusoids allow the formation of hepatic lymph fluid and the movement of proteins into the space of Disse. The lymph leaves the liver through the lymphatic vessels, the lymph nodes, and the thoracic duct, although a small proportion leaves the liver through lymph vessels associated with the hepatic vein.

The hepatocytes are large nucleated cells with the Golgi apparatus lying between the cell nucleus and the bile canaliculi. Closely associated with the Golgi apparatus are the lysosomes; the mitochondria and peroxisomes are generally scattered through the cell cytoplasm. The abundant, rough endoplasmic reticulum of the hepatocyte is often near the mitochondria and the smooth endoplasmic reticulum is found centrally associated with glycogen granules. Within the hepatocyte is a cytoskeleton where microtubules transport materials between the sinusoidal surface of the cell and the areas near the Golgi apparatus. The mitochondria act as the cellular powerhouse, carrying out many diverse metabolic activities; protein synthesis is performed by the ribosomes; and the Golgi apparatus transports, secretes, and stores many metabolites.

The lobes of the liver are divided into smaller lobules with a roughly hexagonal arrangement of hepatocytes around a central vein. At the vertices of the lobules are bile ducts, terminal branches of the hepatic artery, and portal veins—termed the portal triad. Connective stromal tissues extend throughout the liver, providing support for cells and routes for blood vessels, lymphatic vessels, and bile ducts. The hepatocytes form groups of cells around small branches of the portal vein, hepatic arteriole, bile duct, lymph vessel, and nerves; this functional unit is called an acinus (plural: acini). The acini form part of a larger structure, which can be divided into three zones:

zone 1: the periportal hepatocytes closest to the portal triad receiving blood
    rich in nutrients and oxygen;
zone 2: the midzonal/centrilobular hepatocytes; and
zone 3: the perivenous zone.

The levels of oxygen and nutrients decrease from zone 1 to zone 3.

There is continual slow turnover of hepatic cells, with cells added through mitosis and removed by apoptosis. The liver has a large functional reserve, so hepatic failure does not become apparent until at least 70% of the functional capacity is lost. The liver is capable of marked regeneration following hepatocellular injury or hepatectomy; this regeneration is triggered by circulating mitogenic and growth factors (e.g., tumor necrosis factor [TNF]-alpha, interleukin 6, epidermal growth factor, and hepatic growth factors).

Partly related to an oxygen gradient and the flow of nutrients from the hepatic portal vein, the metabolic and enzymic processes vary within these three zones. For example, glycogen in the periportal zone is depleted and synthesized more rapidly during fasting and after feeding, although it appears to be evenly distributed in the acinar cells during steady state. In zone 1, the cells are larger and the mitochondria more numerous than in the other zones. Compared to zone 3, hepatocytes in zones 1 and 2 have higher concentrations of ammonia; urea and glutamine are mainly synthesized in the periportal zone and the enzymes of the urea cycle are situated in these two zones.

Kuppfer cells are macrophages residing in the sinusoids that remove bacteria, foreign proteins, particulate matter, and senescent erythrocytes. The Kuppfer cells form part of the mononuclear phagocyte system (the reticuloendothelial system); these cells originate from the bone marrow as peripheral blood monocytes before differentiation into Kuppfer cells. Activation of Kuppfer cells by xenobiotics causes the release of inflammatory mediators, growth factors, and reactive oxygen species. These activations appear to modulate hepatic injury and carcinogenesis (Roberts et al. 2007).

The hepatic stellate (or Ito) cells are fat-storing cells found in the perisinusoidal spaces between the hepatocytes and sinusoids: these cells can later become involved in hepatic fibrosis. When hepatic lipid is increased by greater than 5% by weight, the histological changes are described as steatosis, or fatty changes.

Approximately 20% of the blood flowing to the liver enters via the hepatic artery, with the larger remainder flowing through the hepatic portal veins from the small intestine, stomach, spleen, and pancreas. The terminal branches of the hepatic portal vein and artery empty into the liver sinusoids. Plasma from this blood supply is filtered into the space of Disse to provide a major fraction of the body's lymph. The blood flows from the sinusoids and empties into the lobular central vein, which then connects into hepatic veins that leave the liver to join the vena cava. Oxygenated blood is supplied to the liver via the hepatic artery and blood oxygenation gradually decreases as blood flows to the hepatic venules. The blood entering the liver via the hepatic artery carries nutrients, digested food particles, and orally absorbed xenobiotics or their metabolites.

The hepatocytes secrete bile into the canaliculi, which are intercellular spaces between the adjacent hepatocytes, and then into the bile ducts. The small bile ductules join to form larger ducts, and eventually the bile flows through the common bile duct into the intestine. In larger laboratory animals, a gall bladder where bile is stored and concentrated between feedings is attached to the upper part of the bile duct. There is no gall bladder in rats and the bile duct fuses with the pancreatic duct, unlike in larger animals where the ducts remain separate and the gall bladder exists. Where the bile duct joins the intestine, there is a sphincter known as the sphincter of Oddi. The liver produces bile continuously, even when the small intestine is not digesting food, and the bile flow is dependent on the rate of hepatic bile production and the actions of the enteric hormones cholecystokin and secretin.

Bile fluid performs two important functions: (1) the emulsification, solubilization, and transport of lipids and fat-soluble vitamins by the detergent effects of bile acids, and (2) the elimination of many waste products, including bilirubin and cholesterol secreted via the bile into the gastrointestinal tract. Bile acids and bile salts are the principal components of the bile fluid, acting as detergents in the digestion of fat in the intestinal tract.

The bile acids have a steroid nucleus with aliphatic side chains synthesized from cholesterol in the hepatocytes as either cholic or chenodeoxycholic acids. These two bile acids are conjugated with either glycine or taurine (Klaassen and Watkins 1984; Reichel and Sauerbruch 1995). The bile acids are both hydrophobic (lipid soluble, derived from cholesterol) and hydrophilic (polar)—properties that help in the lipid emulsification and solubilization. The transport of bile acids from the sinusoid to the hepatocytes involves various mechanisms, including a sodium taurocholate cotransporting polypeptide and organic anion transporting polypeptide (OATP). The bile acids then are secreted by export transport systems from the hepatocyte into the bile canaliculi to enter the enterohepatic circulation between the biliary system and the intestinal tract, where they can reenter the portal venous system after absorption and protein binding (Kuipers et al. 1985; Dobrinska 1989; Ferenci, Zollner, and Trauner 2002). Plasma bile acid levels are affected by food intake and the extrahepatic circulation.

Bilirubin is formed from the breakdown of hemoglobin; it is then conjugated prior to secretion in the bile. Erythrocytes are destroyed primarily in the spleen to release hemoglobin, which then is broken down to heme (part of the porphyrin structure of hemoglobin) and separated from the globin parts of the hemoglobin molecule. The heme is converted first to bilverdin by the reversible action of biliverdin reductase and then to unconjugated bilirubin (Figure 3.1). In the liver, the bilirubin undergoes conjugation with glucuronic acid, rendering it more soluble prior to excretion into the bile. Some of the conjugated bilirubin is metabolized by the gut flora to form stercobilinogen and then oxidized to stercobilin, while some of the conjugated bilirubin is reabsorbed and excreted as urobilinogen or the oxidized urobilin via the kidneys. When unconjugated bilirubin is markedly increased—for example, when there is excessive red cell breakdown—it sometime imparts a yellow color to the liver tissues because it is fat soluble and remains in the tissues.

Historically, the conjugated and unconjugated forms were known as direct and indirect bilirubin, respectively. The unconjugated bilirubin reacts more slowly in analytical methods and the plasma total bilirubin reflects the balance between production and excretion. In most laboratory animals, the plasma total bilirubin is lower

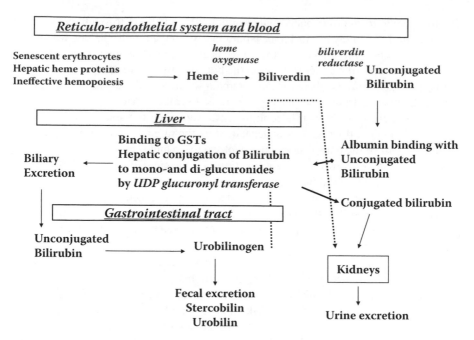

FIGURE 3.1 Formation and excretion of bilirubin.

than in humans due to the low renal threshold for circulating conjugated bilirubin. In some genetic rat strains (e.g., the Gunn rat), bilirubin cannot be converted to glucuronide due to an enzyme deficiency, and therefore plasma bilirubin is higher in these strains. In dogs where the renal threshold is low, conjugated bilirubin may be detected in urine prior to the detection of bilirubinemia.

The hepatocytes are the most active sites of protein synthesis, and albumin plays important roles in the transport of bilirubin, anions, fatty acids, several hormones, and xenobiotics. Albumin also is important in determining the colloidal osmotic pressure of plasma and other body fluids. Other proteins synthesized in the liver include the acute-phase response proteins, complement proteins, and the coagulation cascade proteins (see Chapter 8). The levels of plasma proteins reflect the balance between the rates of synthesis, utilization, and degradation. The liver also plays an important role in the metabolism of cholesterol and lipoproteins (see Chapter 9).

Glutathione (N-(N-L-gamma–glutamyl-L-cysteinyl) glycine) is a tripeptide thiol compound formed from cysteine, glycine, and glutamic acid, and it acts as an antioxidant. In the reduced state, the thiol group of cysteine donates an electron to reactive oxygen species, and this then binds with another reactive glutathione to form glutathione disulfide (GSSG). Glutathione (GSH) helps to maintain the ferrous state of iron in heme and also to remove toxic peroxides in metabolic reactions catalyzed by glutathione peroxidase. GSH is a substrate for several conjugation reactions catalyzed by glutathione S-transferases in the cytosol, mitochondria, and microsomes. Several of the glutamyl S-transferases are found in the cytosol. These enzymes catalyze the conjugation of glutathione with many electrophilic compounds, reducing organic hydroperoxides, and they participate in steroid isomerization reactions.

Reactive oxygen species (ROS) include free radicals, peroxides, and oxygen ions. They are formed in the normal metabolism of oxygen but can increase during cellular stress; this results in oxidative stress. Free radicals are produced in cellular organelles such as the mitochondria; enzymes such as superoxide dismutases and catalases, together with antioxidants such as ascorbate, urate, and glutathione, play important roles in the normal defense mechanisms against ROS damage. ROS are implicated in many mechanisms, including DNA damage, fatty acid oxidation, inactivation of some enzymes by cofactor oxidation, amino acid oxidation, inflammatory responses, and redox signaling in apoptosis and ischemic injury.

Gamma glutamyl transferase (GGT) catalyzes the transfer of amino acids across the cellular membrane and links with the glutamyl cycle pathways. Some of the interactions among glutathione, glutamyl S-transferase, aminotransferases, and taurine metabolism are shown in Figure 3.2. Cysteine and other thiols are important factors in the homeostatic mechanisms controlling oxidative stress and intracellular calcium concentrations.

Cytochrome P450 (abbreviated as CYP or P450) enzymes are a large and diverse group of heme proteins that act mainly as catalysts in mono-oxygenase reactions (Spatzenegger and Jaeger 1995). Their spectral characteristics of being colored cellular proteins lead to their name of cytochrome, and the CYPs are localized within the inner mitochondrial membranes or endoplasmic reticulum. The active site of the P450 cytochromes is a heme iron center linked to the protein by thiol groups of cysteine residues. The cytochrome P450 enzymes with oxidized ferric ions bind substrates and initiate oxygen binding and electron transport from donor proteins

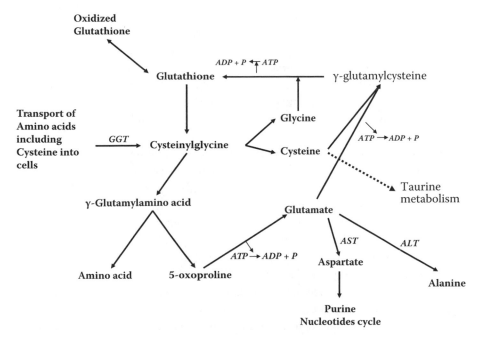

FIGURE 3.2   The gamma glutamyl cycle and its linkages with taurine metabolism, transamination, and oxidation of glutathione.

(e.g., cytochrome P450 reductase, cytochrome b5). Molecular oxygen is then bound and split by the reduced heme iron, one atom of oxygen is inserted into an organic molecule to form an alcohol or epoxide, and the remaining molecule is reduced to water.

The CYPs are present in the liver; the greatest concentration is in the smooth endoplasmic reticulum of the centrilobular hepatocytes. They are also present in many other tissues, including the gastrointestinal tract. CYPs are capable of reacting with multiple endogenous and exogenous compounds, and they are active in bilirubin metabolism, cholesterol synthesis, hormone synthesis and catabolism, and vitamin D metabolism. They are of particular interest because of their role in the oxidative metabolism of xenobiotics as part of phase I reactions and the biotransformation of lipophilic compounds to more polar compounds, which are readily excreted by the kidney into the urine.

Peroxisome proliferator-activated receptors (PPARs) are nuclear receptor proteins that play essential roles in the regulation of cell differentiation development and metabolism (McGuire and Lucas 1991; Gibson and Lake 1993; Berger and Moller 2002). Several types of PPARs have been identified, including alpha, gamma, and delta (or beta); these PPARs are molecular targets for several drug therapies (e.g., in diabetes) (Stumvoll and Haring 2002).

In summary, the liver plays a major role in the regulation of many blood constituents by metabolism, storage, or excretory mechanisms. Some of its functions include:

carbohydrate homeostasis with the production of glucose via glycolysis, gluco-neogenesis, and glycogen storage or mobilization;

regulation of amino acids for protein synthesis (protein catabolism by the liver leads to the production of urea, which is excreted by kidneys);

synthesis of cholesterol, triglycerides, lipoproteins, fatty acids, and more complex lipids required for lipid and steroid metabolism;

bile production and secretion to facilitate lipid absorption in the intestine and excretion of lipid soluble molecules;

storage of carbohydrates, fats, lipids, minerals, and vitamins;

production of coagulation proteins, factors, and heparin to prevent blood clotting and enable blood to flow under normal circumstances, but altering coagulation to prevent and accelerate blood coagulation following injury;

production of albumin and other proteins, including those involved in immunity and acute-phase responses;

synthesis of heme protein required for hemoglobin, the removal of hemoglobin from senescent erythrocytes, and reutilization of iron;

removal of bacteria, antigens, and (foreign) proteins and production of immune proteins, including complement;

contribution to the production of heat and maintenance of body temperature; and

synthesis of insulin-like growth hormones, therefore acting as an endocrine organ.

3.2   HEPATIC METABOLISM OF XENOBIOTICS

The major roles of special interest in toxicology are the detoxifying and excretory mechanisms used by the liver to remove toxic or unwanted xenobiotics and endogenous waste products (e.g., ammonia). Metabolic reactions affecting xenobiotics may be one of two types: phase I or phase II. Phase I reactions involve oxidation, reduction, or hydrolysis, where the solubility of a compound in water is increased by generating hydroxyl, carboxy, or epoxide functional groups on the parent compound. These reactions are generally followed by phase II reactions, which involve conjugations with glucuronate, sulfate, glutathione, or acetate moieties, and these conjugation reactions generally further increase the compound's solubility and renal excretion.

In phase II reactions, the resulting conjugates often are less likely to be biologically inactive, but disruption of phase II reactions can lead to accumulation of phase I metabolites. Hepatic elimination of xenobiotics occurs either by biotransformation or biliary excretion. Most of the compounds excreted in the bile have a small molecular mass of less than 500 Da, and there are separate excretory mechanisms (transporters) for acidic, basic, and neutral compounds. These compounds excreted in the bile may become available later for intestinal absorption into the blood (i.e., via the enterohepatic circulation) (Dobrinska 1989).

3.3   HEPATOTOXICITY

This is often due to metabolites of a xenobiotic formed by bioactivation or biotransformation in the liver and not the parent compounds, and reactive metabolites are more likely to cause damage at the sites of phase I bioactivation reactions. Many different mechanisms cause hepatotoxicity and affect different cellular locations (Figures 3.3 and 3.4). Liver injury can be broadly classified as those injuries that are predictable and show a dose- and time-dependent pattern (type 1 lesions or intrinsic toxicity) and that occur in animals and are predictive of hepatic effects in man. Type II lesions are unpredictable or idiosyncratic, often with a low incidence, and animal studies often fail to be predictive of adverse effects in humans (Buratti and Lavine 2002; Boelsterli 2003; Lee 2003). These idiosyncratic reactions may or may not show dose and time dependency. Idiosyncratic reactions are often characterized by a delay in onset after starting the drug therapy, although in some cases prior exposure to the drug may hasten the onset of hepatotoxicity on rechallenge. In addition to toxic changes, hepatic responses induced by xenobiotics may be adaptive, exaggerated physiological, or expected pharmacological responses.

Given the multiple metabolic functions performed by the liver, it should not be surprising that the hepatotoxic effects of xenobiotics are so different; several different morphological patterns of xenobiotic-induced hepatotoxicity can be observed (Plaa 1991; Batt and Ferrari 1995; Zimmerman 1999; Plaa and Charbonneau 2001; Kaplowitz 2002; Kaplowitz and DeLeve 2003; Lee 2003). For example, in acute toxicity, cell degeneration leads to necrosis (cell death), and this may or may not be accompanied by steatosis (an accumulation of lipids and "fatty" liver where hepatic lipid content is >5%). Necrosis may affect small groups of hepatocytes (i.e., focal

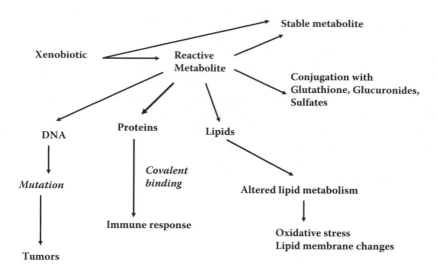

FIGURE 3.3 Potential effects of xenobiotics and reactive metabolites.

necrosis) or larger numbers of cells located in one or more of the zones—centrilobular, midzonal, or periportal necrosis.

Again, hepatotoxicity can be separated into two main categories: hepatotoxins that cause hepatocyte injury with necrosis and/or steatosis and those that alter cholestasis with reductions of bile flow and effects on the biliary system. Morphological descriptions for both of these broad categories can be varied and may include cholestatic effects (hepatocanalicular, canalicular, and cholangiolar) or cytotoxic effects (steatosis, necrosis, or apoptosis); there may be a mixture of these effects (Hardisty and Brix 2005; Greaves 2007). In some severe cases, the effects are overlapping, and it

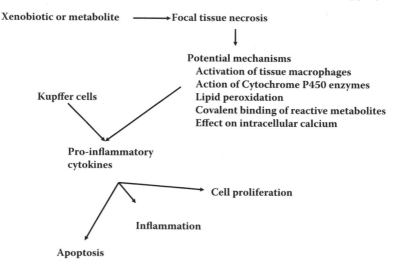

FIGURE 3.4 Potential cellular effects of xenobiotics or metabolites.

is important to distinguish between adaptive or exaggerated physiological responses and cellular injury.

Hepatitis describes infiltration of the hepatic tissue by mononuclear cells, which may or may not be associated with hepatocellular changes. There are also different patterns of cellular injury, such as those affecting the hepatocellular organelles—particularly, the microsomes, peroxisomes, and mitochondria. When hepatocellular injury occurs, the aminotransferases are probably the most useful markers, and they may be supplemented by measurements of other plasma enzymes—ALP, GLDH, and plasma bilirubin (see the following sections on laboratory investigations). Several markers of cellular function require tissues for the measurements of altered function (e.g., microsomal cytochrome P450 measurements).

Cholestatic effects are caused by impairment to the intrahepatic or extrahepatic bile flow; obstruction of the bile flow by stone formation is rare in laboratory animals. The more common causes of cholestasis result from alterations of bilirubin metabolism, which may or may not be a consequence of increased hemoglobin degradation, bile retention, or alterations to bile acid transporter systems. In these cases, plasma bilirubin, GGT, and alkaline phosphatase are increased in the absence of hepatic necrosis. Alpha-napthylisocyanate (ANIT) provides a well-tested animal model of induced cholestasis, but it does not replicate hepatotoxicities caused primarily by altered transporter systems. Plasma bilirubin may also be increased when a xenobiotic affects bilirubin transporter systems or uridine diphosphate glucuronosyl transferase reactions (Zucker et al. 2001). In severe hemolytic conditions, the capacity of plasma haptoglobins to bind hemoglobin is saturated, and the remaining unconjugated bilirubin, which is bound to albumin, remains in the plasma because it does not readily pass through the renal glomeruli. This results in hyperbilirubinemia and is accompanied by the evidence from altered erythrocytic measurements in the blood count.

A considerable number of hepatotoxins have been used to model noncholestatic hepatotoxicity; these compounds include carbon tetrachloride, aflatoxin B, allyl alcohol, tetracycline, thioacetamide, dimethylnitrosamine, nonsteroidal anti-inflammatory drugs (NSAIDs), Phenobarbital, peroxisome proliferators, and acetaminophen. However, many of these compounds are often given at high dosages that produce marked morphological changes, whereas the current challenges surely are to improve biomarkers for detecting minimal morphological changes and reducing the number of potential idiosyncratic effects.

Some of the causes of hepatotoxicity outlined by Lee (2003) include:
  covalent binding of xenobiotics mediated by cytochrome P450s;
  alterations of mitochondrial function affecting beta-oxidation of fatty acids;
  altered production of reactive oxygen species and metabolites;
  alteration of transporter proteins;
  alterations of actin fibrils and filaments;
  disruption of intracellular calcium homeostasis;
  T-lymphocyte activation and cytolysis; and
  alpha-tumor necrosis factor stimulation of apoptosis.

Effects on hepatic protein synthesis are caused by many hepatotoxins, but the changes may take some time to become apparent given the half-lives of the involved proteins. Reductions of plasma albumin and acid glycoprotein may affect the binding and exposures to xenobiotics and plasma bilirubin. Other effects on proteins may also be due to reduced food intake due to toxicity. The production of many plasma proteins, including those involved in complement and coagulation cascades, can be affected by reductions of hepatic protein synthesis.

The liver plays a major role in adaptive and innate immunity, and alterations of hepatic structure and function can result in major changes in either or both of these systems (Beaune and Lecoeur 1997; Luster et al. 2000; Parker and Picut 2005). There may be direct actions on the synthesis and utilization of proteins such as the complement proteins and immunoglobulins. With some xenobiotics, a metabolite is haptogenic or forms an antigen by binding with a macromolecule to form an antigen that acts as immunogens. Other xenobiotics may act as direct haptens requiring no biotransformation. Glucuronidation of some compounds produces reactive acyl glucuronides in phase II reactions, and these glucuronides also can induce a cell-mediated or humoral immune response. Immune mechanisms have been implicated in several idiosyncratic hepatotoxic reactions, but it is unlikely that all idiosyncratic reactions are mediated by these mechanisms (Pohl et al. 1988; Boelsterli 1993; Uetrecht 1999; Iverson and Uetrecht 2001).

Several xenobiotics can induce microsomal enzymes, particularly the P450 enzymes (Wang, Nakajima, and Honma 1999). These enzyme inducers increase the proliferation of the smooth endoplasmic reticulum and the concentrations of several fatty acids and phospholipids; they often cause a marked increase of liver weight. Xenobiotic induction of hepatic enzymes is the cause of several drug–drug interactions (DeLeve 1998). Enzyme induction also can alter the interactions of the liver and thyroid glands with enhanced production of thyroxine, leading to an increased trophic drive on the thyroid (Klaassen and Hood 2001; see Chapter 10). The CYPs can also alter some thiol-containing membrane proteins, which regulate calcium homeostasis, and these changes can lead to increased intracellular calcium concentrations and cell death and altered glutathione metabolism with an effect on oxidative processes.

There are known associations among P450 inducers, peroxisome proliferators, and hepatomegaly that sometimes lead to tumorgenesis in rodents. Proliferation of peroxisomes—particularly in the hepatic parenchyma of rodents—is caused by a diverse group of chemicals including some fibrates, phthalate esters, and halogenated solvents. The larger numbers of peroxisomes increase peroxisomal beta-oxidation of fatty acids, with hepatic hypertrophy and hyperplasia in rodents. Several peroxisome proliferators cause hypolipidemia, and several have been deliberately used as lipid-lowering agents (e.g., fibrates) (McGuire et al. 1991). This peroxisome proliferation can also be associated with metastatic hepatocellular carcinomas in rodents, but the causative agents do not appear to affect or damage DNA directly (Moody et al. 1991; Gibson and Lake 1993; Kluwe 1994; Berger and Moller 2002).

The hepatic mitochondria help to preserve cellular integrity by regulating oxidative phosphorylation and the redox potential. There are a number of toxic effects on mitochondria, including the inhibition of DNA synthesis production of reactive metabolites or inhibition of fatty acid beta-oxidation, alteration of mitochondrial permeability, and increased oxidative stress (McKenzie et al. 1995). Necrosis may follow severe changes in mitochondrial function after oxidative injury.

3.4 LABORATORY INVESTIGATIONS

The measurements suggested by various regulatory authorities and the International Committee for International Harmonization of Clinical Pathology Testing (IHCPT) were listed in Chapter 1 (Weingand et al. 1996). The IHCPT list of tests was again reviewed in 2005 by the American Society for Veterinary Clinical Pathology (Boone et al. 2005). The tests suggested by the IHCPT included:

hepatocellular tests (two from the following)
   alanine aminotransferase (ALT)
   aspartate aminotransferase (AST)
   sorbitol dehydrogenase (SDH)
   glutamate dehydrogenase (GLDH)
   total bile acids
hepatobiliary tests (two from the following)
   alkaline phosphatase (ALP)
   gamma glutamyl transferase (GGT)
   5′-nucleotidase
   total bilirubin
   total bile acids

The various recommendations also include supplementary tests for albumin, total protein, triglycerides, cholesterol glucose and coagulation measurements (prothrombin time and activated partial thromboplastin time), which can provide valuable information on the functioning of the liver. Functional products of hepatic metabolism that are commonly measured include total bilirubin, cholesterol, triglycerides, albumin, and prothrombin time (Zimmerman 1999). Using strict terminology, some measurements (e.g., ALT and GGT are indicators of hepatic injury rather than liver-function tests (LFTs), but they are commonly described as LFTs). This author suggests the use of the following plasma enzymes: ALT, AST, ALP, GGT, and GLDH—with OCT or SDH as optional additions, remembering that plasma ALP has a high intestinal component and plasma GGT is low in the rat.

The core tests should include those for hepatocellular and cholestatic injury because both or either may occur. Given that it is not always possible to predict whether a xenobiotic will cause either cellular or biliary injury, the choice of enzymes and bilirubin/bile salts needs to include markers for both of these types of toxicity and to take into consideration the intracellular locations of these enzymes. These common tests are far more effective when used in groups, and reliance should not be placed on any single test for the diagnosis of hepatotoxicity. The recognition of an increase in several of these test values and a pattern of changes offer more evidence of an adverse effect due to a xenobiotic.

There have been several additional discussion documents (Shah 1999; Zimmerman 1999; Dufour et al. 2000; FDA 2000; Amacher 2002) and evaluations using several hepatotoxicants (Carakostas et al. 1986; Travlos et al. 1996; Fujii 1997; Bondy et al. 2000), but there continue to be much discussion and effort expended on improving methods for the detection of hepatotoxicity because it remains an important safety issue. Several additional assays have been advocated (e.g., GST and bile acids), but because they are not widely used in human medicine, they fail to meet a criterion for biomarkers to bridge between animal and human studies. Many of the enzyme assays relate to the steps in the gamma-glutamyl and urea cycles, so perhaps it is time to focus on searching for markers of other hepatotoxic mechanisms. Proteomic and gene expression studies have identified some potential additional markers, but these remain to be evaluated and compared to the current available measurements (Amacher, Schomaker, and Burkhardt 2001; Waring et al. 2001). Some of the potential and emerging markers for hepatotoxicity are mentioned in later paragraphs.

3.4.1 ENZYMES

Given the important impact of hepatotoxicity for safety risk assessment, many enzyme tests have been evaluated, and the majority of plasma enzyme measurements reflect cellular disruption and organelle damage. These tests include ornithine carbamoyl transferase (OCT), glutamyl S-transferase (GST), arginase, cholinesterases, lactate dehydrogenase (LDH), leucine aminopeptidase, leucine arylaminidase, malate dehydrogenase (MDH), alcohol dehydrogenase, paraoxanase, and glucose-6-phosphate dehydrogenase (see Chapters 2 and 11). The enzymes AST, ALT, OCT, and GGT together with arginase and malate dehydrogenase catalyze reactions in the gamma-glutamyl cycle reactions and urea metabolism (Figures 3.2 and 3.5).

The use of some additional enzyme tests has been limited by the lack of available commercially prepared reagents or methodologies unsuitable for the current generation of automated biochemical analyzers. Older manual methods, which were less precise, have largely been discarded, and they are not commonly used in human medicine.

There are four broad effects on plasma enzymes in hepatotoxicity:

enzymes that reflect cholestasis rather than parenchymal damage (i.e., reduced bile flow—for example, ALP and GGT);
enzymes sensitive to cytotoxic effects and relatively specific for liver (e.g., ALT and SDH);
enzymes sensitive to cytotoxic effects but with relatively wide tissue distribution and therefore low specificity (e.g., lactate dehydrogenase, LDH); and
enzymes that exhibit a depressed plasma activity (e.g., cholinesterases and paraoxanase).

3.4.1.1 Aminotransferases

In animals (and humans), plasma ALT is an effective marker of liver damage and it should always be measured, although it is not entirely specific for liver (see

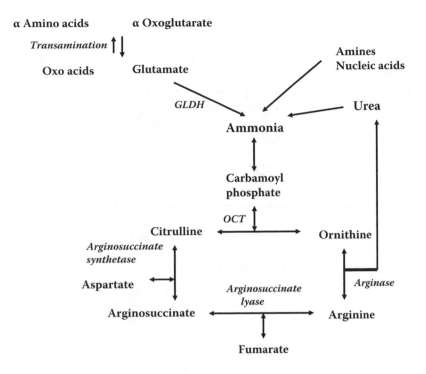

FIGURE 3.5 Urea cycle and its enzymes.

Chapter 2). Plasma ALT can increase or decrease following microsomal enzyme induction effects in the rat and the dog (Amacher, Schomaker, and Burkhardt 1998; Amacher et al. 2001) and when there is a heavy fatty infiltration of hepatic cells, where plasma enzymes may reflect the displacement of cytoplasm as the fat load increases. This enzyme may also be increased in biliary toxicity and following bile duct obstruction through the effects of bile salts on the neighboring hepatocyte cell membranes. ALT can be affected by food intake and stress (Chapter 11). Plasma ALT is the most useful enzyme for detecting hepatocellular injury in most laboratory animal species.

Plasma AST measurements are a useful adjunct to ALT, and increased AST can be an indication of mitochondrial and cytoplasmic injury, although this enzyme is less specific for hepatotoxicity compared to ALT. Sustained increases of the plasma aminotransferase levels can indicate a progressive injury, but the aminotransferases may not be elevated during acute necrosis if the timing of the sample collection has allowed the increased circulating plasma enzymes to be cleared. Plasma ALT and AST may be decreased when the enzyme cofactor pyridoxal phosphate is reduced in vivo (Dhami et al. 1979; also see Chapter 2).

The term *transaminitis* has been use in human medicine to describe mild elevations of the aminotransferases in the absence of other abnormal clinical laboratory findings in asymptomatic individuals, with apparently no supporting evidence from preclinical studies (Balazs, Farber, and Feuer 1978; Amacher 1998).

3.4.1.2 Alkaline Phosphatase (ALP)

Alkaline phosphatase (ALP) is present within biliary and canalicular membranes, kidney, intestine, and bone; therefore, ALP is not specific for the liver. Plasma alkaline phosphatase (ALP) can be used as a measure of cholestasis (Moss 1982; Schlaeger, Haux, and Katterman 1982), although the high intestinal proportion in the rat and the intra- and intervariability in nonhuman primates reduce its diagnostic value.

As with the aminotransferases, hepatic ALP production can be increased by some anticonvulsants and exogenous and endogenous corticosteroids. Glucocorticoid-induced increases of plasma ALP occur in the dog, associated with hepatopathy involving plasma membrane changes and subcellular organelles. Here, ALP isoenzyme measurements are useful in elucidating the nature of increased ALP and associated with a hepatopathy with progressive changes of the plasma membrane and other subcellular organelles (Solter et al. 1994; Rutgers et al. 1995; also see Chapter 2 for additional references on corticosteroid-induced ALP in dogs).

3.4.1.3 Gamma-Glutamyl Transferase (GGT)

Although the highest concentrations of this membrane-localized enzyme are in the kidney and pancreas, increases of plasma GGT have been reported following cholestasis in rats, where GGT changes are more specific than those observed for ALP, even though the basal plasma GGT levels are very low (Huseby and Torstein 1978; Leonard, Neptun, and Popp 1984; Evans 1986; also see Chapter 2). Plasma GGT activity is rarely altered by primary hepatocellular toxicity in laboratory animals.

3.4.1.4 Glutamate Dehydrogenase (GLDH)

Of the various dehydrogenases, glutamate dehydrogenase (GLDH) can be a good indicator for mitochondrial damage in juvenile rats. However, this measurement has less value in older rats, where there is greater inter- and intra-individual variability (O'Brien et al. 2002).

3.4.1.5 Sorbitol Dehydrogenase (SDH)

This is a cytosolic enzyme and indicator of hepatocellular damage in laboratory animals (Dooley, Turnquist, and Racich 1979; Abdelkader and Hauge 1986; Travlos et al. 1996).

3.4.1.6 Lactate Dehydrogenase (LDH) and Other Dehydrogenases

LDH is too widely distributed in the tissues to be of value in the diagnosis of hepatotoxicity. Other dehydrogenases, such as isocitrate dehydrogenase (Boyd 1962; Keller 1981), malate dehydrogenase, glucose-6 phosphatase dehydrogenase, and alcohol dehydrogenase, have not been widely evaluated in toxicology studies. None of these enzymes is widely used in clinical medicine (Zimmerman 1982).

3.4.1.7 Urea Cycle Enzymes

Two of the urea cycle enzymes (Figures 3.2.and 3.5), which are located in the hepatocytes and both ornithine carbamoyl transferase (OCT) and arginase can provide evidence of liver damage in animals, although more data are available for OCT (Cornelius et al. 1963; Carakostas et al. 1986; Bondy et al. 2000). However, their use has been limited by the available methodology. Liver arginase has been used in both the rat and the dog as a marker of hepatocellular injury, but it has not been widely evaluated (Noonan and Meyer 1979; Ikemoto et al. 2001). It remains to be seen whether this enzyme is more predictive of hepatotoxicity compared to other enzymes of the urea cycle.

3.4.1.8   5′-Nucleotidase (5′-NT)

This enzyme is associated with the canalicular and sinusoidal membranes. It is also found in the cytoplasm, lysosome, and other intracelluar organelles. 5′-NT can offer some diagnostic value when the measurements of ALP and GGT in cholestatic hepatotoxicity are equivocal, but it is not widely used (Kryszewski et al. 1973).

3.4.1.9   Leucine Aminopeptidase (LAP)

This enzyme is not commonly measured. It does have some value in nonhuman primates, but not in other species (Lohss, Federhen, and Kraft 1988).

3.4.1.10   Alpha-Glutathione S-Transferase (Alpha-GST)

This enzyme has been measured in a number of toxicology studies with hepatotoxins (Di Simplicio 1982; Beckett, Hunter, and Hayes 1986; Clarke et al. 1997; Kilty et al. 1998; van der Aar et al. 1998; Eaton and Bammier 1999; Coluccio et al. 2000; Giffen et al. 2002; Strelic et al. 2003; Awasthi 2006). However, it has yet to establish a place among the common enzyme measurements, possibly because of the short half-life (<90 minutes). Currently, alpha-GST may be measured by radioimmunoassay or enzyme immunoassays; given the complexity of the GST enzyme family, it may be more successful if new assays can be developed (see Chapter 2).

3.4.1.11   Cholinesterases and Paraoxanase

Neither of these enzymes (see Chapter 2) is widely used for the diagnosis of hepatotoxicity because, unlike the other enzyme measurements mentioned previously, their plasma levels decrease rather than increase. Also, the plasma enzyme activities are more variable than those of other enzymes. However, these enzymes are useful in assessing neurotoxicity (see Chapter 11).

3.4.2   Plasma Bilirubin and Bile Acids

Either plasma total bilirubin or plasma bile acids should be measured, but these are different measurements. Bile acids are more of a functional assay that is subject to more variation, particularly following food intake.

3.4.2.1   Bilirubin

Although it is possible to measure both total and conjugated (direct) bilirubin, measurement of total bilirubin is usually sufficient because plasma total bilirubin levels are lower in laboratory animals compared to humans. If plasma total bilirubin is markedly elevated, it imparts a visible yellow color to the plasma. Plasma total bilirubin values in rats and dogs are near the limit of detection by common colorimetric methods, which rely on diazotization reactions with bilirubin; concentrations in rats have been found to be less than 2 μmol/L by more sensitive methods (Rosenthal et al. 1981). Although subtracting the conjugated bilirubin value from the total provides a measure of unconjugated bilirubin, this is of limited use in species where the total bilirubin values may be low and close to the detection limit of the method.

When bilirubin production increases in hemolytic anemias, the unconjugated fraction of plasma bilirubin increases; the finding can be confirmed with evidence from the full blood count. Unconjugated plasma bilirubin may also increase as a consequence of impaired hepatic conjugation of bilirubin or uptake. When increases of plasma unconjugated bilirubin occur, the excess bilirubin will be bound to albumin and not be filtered through the renal glomeruli (i.e., bilirubinuria does not appear). In cholestasis, the conjugated bilirubin increases and raises the concentration of plasma conjugated bilirubin (which is water soluble and less firmly bound to albumin) so that, in severe cholestasis, the unconjugated bilirubin appears in the urine.

Hemolysis interferes with many of the common methods for determining bilirubin; this can be problematic when the hemolysis is due to a hemolytic anemia rather than to hemolysis caused by the sample collection procedure. Checking the hematological data and the quality of samples collected at the same time helps in identifying the cause of hemolysis. Blood samples must be protected from light because bilirubin level falls when exposed to light.

Plasma bilirubin may be increased due to drug-related inhibition of uridine diphosphate glucuronosyltransferase (Zucker et al. 2001) or inhibitors of hepatic bilirubin transporters. By contrast, plasma bilirubin concentration may fall following administration of some mixed-function oxidase inducers, which may enhance the metabolism and excretion of bilirubin.

3.4.2.2   Bile Acids

Plasma bile acids (total bile acids, TBAs) have been recommended as an alternative measurement to plasma bilirubin because TBAs can indicate biliary functionality in terms of the response to food intake. TBA values are dependent upon a number of factors, including stomach emptying; gall bladder contraction, where it exists; intestinal motility; intestinal absorption; hepatic uptake; and hepatic excretion. The enterohepatic circulation amplifies deficiencies in the hepatic transport system; this results in reduced secretion of bile acids into the bile. Studies with dogs have shown that timed postprandial measurements have greater diagnostic value than fasting or random samples (Center et al. 1991; Jensen and Poulsen 1992), but the collection of timed postprandial samples is more difficult.

In hamsters, beta-cyclodextrin (a vehicle sometimes used in oral toxicology studies) and cholestyramine have been reported to alter bile acid profiles in bile (Trautwein et al. 1999). Enzymatic methods measuring three alpha-hydroxy bile acids are available and used more frequently than the measurements of individual bile acids; although they are sometimes referred to as TBAs, these enzymatic methods do not include all bile acids (Mashige, Imai, and Osuga 1976; Gopinath et al. 1980; Woodman and Maile 1981; Hauge and Abdelkader 1984; Quereshi, Smith, and Murphy 1984; Center et al. 1985, 1991; Parraga and Kaneko 1985; Crampton and Walthen 1990; Jensen and Poulsen 1992; Azer et al. 1993; Hamdan and Stacey 1993;

Solter et al. 1994; Washizu et al. 1994; Azer, Klaessen, and Stacey 1997; Turgut et al. 1997; Neghab and Stacey 2005). Plasma bile acids have been measured individually using high-performance liquid chromatography or gas liquid chromatography electrospray tandem mass spectrometry (Lauff, Kasper, and Ambrose 1981; Rosenthal et al. 1981; Thompson et al. 1987; Wang and Stacey 1990; Gatti et al. 1997; Perwaiz et al. 2001).

There are species differences for the individual bile acids. Cholic acid is the major primary bile acid in most species. Muricholic acid is a major bile acid in the rat that increases rapidly during cholestasis (Hofmann 1988). More experimental work is needed to analyze the patterns of individual bile acids after various forms of chemically induced liver injury to see if these profiles can provide better diagnosis.

3.4.3   Urine Test Strips/Dipsticks for Bilirubin and Urobilinogen

Semiquantitative test strips for these two measurements are designed for use with human urine rather than that of laboratory animals and are of very limited value in toxicology studies. Elevation of urinary bilirubin in the urine is suggestive of hepatocellular dysfunction, but the test strips can react to give false positive results, particularly with rodent urine.

3.4.4   Lipids

The liver is a major site of cholesterol synthesis, so hepatic injury can cause abnormal accumulation of fat—mainly, triglycerides in the parenchymal cells. Initially, the fatty changes are found by the liposomes and then, at a later stage, the number of vacuoles containing fat increases in the hepatocytes (Lombardi 1966). These fatty changes may result from one of a number of mechanisms, including an imbalance between the body's fat requirements to supply energy and fat utilization; increased transport of fatty acids from adipose tissue to the liver; inhibition of PPAR receptors that, in turn, affect fatty acid beta-oxidation; or reduced transport of hepatic triglycerides (Reddy and Rao 2006). The accumulation of fat in the liver is generally associated with lower plasma triglyceride values. During cholestasis, cholesterol synthesis is increased, and this results in higher plasma concentrations of cholesterol and low density and very low density lipoproteins (LDL and VLDL).

3.4.4.1   Liver Fatty Acid Binding Proteins (L-FABP)

Hepatic fatty acid binding proteins have a molecular mass of about 15 kDa. These are involved in the transport of long chain fatty acids along a declining gradient from the portal to central zones (Bass et al. 1989; Glatz and van der Vusse 1996; also see Chapter 9).

3.4.5   Proteins

Many proteins are synthesized by the liver, and several measurements can be added to the basic measures of plasma total protein, albumin, and globulin. Reduced food intake due to hepato- or gastrointestinal toxicity will result in hypoproteinemia

(Hulsewe et al. 1997). Several of the plasma proteins that alter in hepatotoxicity include fibrinogen, haptoglobin, transferrin, ceruloplasmin, alpha$_2$-macroglobulin, coagulation cascade and complement proteins, secretory IgA, carbohydrate deficient transferrin (CDT), and protein F (see Chapter 8).

Following hepatocellular injury, protein synthesis may be reduced; however, this may not be evident immediately because the protein half-lives are relatively long compared to the half-lives of enzymes. The protein pattern seen following significant chronic hepatocellular damage is a hypoproteinemia with a reduction of albumin, accompanied by a relative increase of globulins. These two changes may counter-balance so that there is little or no change in the plasma total protein but a marked change in the ratio of albumin to globulin.

The injured liver may produce an acute-phase response due to stress or inflammation, with increased synthesis of the acute-phase proteins, which include C-reactive protein alpha$_2$-macroglobulin, a haptoglobin and fibrinogen. The changes caused by inflammation may stimulate the cytokines and the actions of the macrophages and Kupffer cells prior to hepatocellular injury or the injury may cause the release of interleukins (Sipe 1989; see Chapter 8). Changes of the acute-phase proteins are not always obvious from the total protein, albumin, and globulin concentrations, but several of the acute-phase response proteins can be measured in plasma samples from laboratory animals.

Hepatic injury can also alter the synthesis of the blood coagulation cascade and prolong prothrombin and activated partial thromboplastin times. These effects on vitamin K dependent coagulation factors II (prothrombin), VII, IX, and X and protein C, protein S, and protein Z tend to affect the prothombin time (PT) more frequently than the activated partial thromboplastin time (APTT): however in some cases of hepatotoxicity, the APTT changes may be more marked than those for PT (Pritchard et al. 1987).

Proteomic studies are adding to our knowledge of the changes to cellular proteins in hepatotoxicity, and this may lead to new protein measurements (Anderson et al. 1996; Amacher et al. 2005; Giometti et al. 2005). Although some protein measurements, such as haptoglobin, are useful in hepatotoxicity, they are not specific for the liver; even specific proteins such as protein F have not been widely measured (Foster, Goldin, and Oliviera 1989).

3.4.6 DYE EXCRETION (OR DYE BINDING) TESTS

A number of tests for liver functionality involve the administration of a dye or radiolabeled compound and measurements of these compounds at timed intervals after their administration. These compounds include bromsulfphthalein (BSP or sulfobromophthalein; Klaassen and Plaa 1967; Jablonski and Owen 1969; Cutler 1974; Meyer 1986; Fuiji 1997; Plaa and Charbonneau 2001), indocyanine green (ICG; Klaassen and Plaa 1969; Shibata and Odani 1991), lidocaine monoethylglycinexylide (MEGX; Kaneko et al. 2001), and galactose. These functional tests are rarely used in toxicology studies because they require additional procedures for administering these exogenous compounds and critical timings for sampling procedures; thus, the procedures are unsuitable when dealing with large numbers of animals. The compounds may be associated with irritability and tolerability and affect protein binding of the test compound, and they should not be used where there is cardiac or renal toxicity. These tests are seldom justified when hepatic injury is evident.

3.4.7 URINARY KETONES

Increased urinary excretion of ketones is an indication of perturbations of carbohydrate or impaired fatty acid oxidation. Acetoacetate and beta-hydroxybutyrate are the major compounds appearing in ketosis.

3.4.8 HEMATOLOGY

Examination of results from the full blood count may reveal evidence of hemolytic effects from the erythrocytic measurements and inflammatory effects from the leukocyte differential count. The possible effects on PT and APTT have been mentioned previously in Section 3.4.5.

3.4.9 OTHER SUPPLEMENTARY AND EMERGING TESTS

3.4.9.1 Taurine and Creatine

The amino acid taurine has been suggested as a marker of hepatotoxicity because it is involved in the conjugation of bile acids to bile acids, the conjugation of xenobiotics, and the detoxification of reactive metabolites. Taurine is a product of sulfur acid metabolism and may reflect protein synthesis. The measurement of urinary taurine in models of hepatotoxicity has been described (Sanins et al. 1990; Waterfield et al. 1993a, 1993b, 1993c; Timbrell, Seabra, and Waterfield 1995; Waterfield, Asker, and Timbrell 1996), but the measurement is reported to show diurnal variation, wide intra-animal variability, and less success at minor levels of hepatic injury (Maxuitenko, North, and Roebuck 1997).

Changes of both plasma and urine creatine have been reported in various models of hepatotoxicity and may be related to perturbations of cysteine and glutathione metabolism. However, the creatine changes also may be due to nutritional effects of hepatotoxins (Clayton et al. 2003, 2004). Neither taurine nor creatine measurements using high-performance liquid chromatography with fluorimetric or proton nuclear magnetic resonance (NMR) spectroscopy have been widely evaluated.

3.4.9.2 Tissue Glutathione

Glutathione can be measured by a variety of analytical techniques, including colorimetric assays, enzyme-linked immunoassays, high-performance liquid chromatography, and capillary electrophoresis. However, plasma glutathione constitutes less than 0.5% of the total blood concentration, with the greatest proportion present in erythrocytes. Buthionine sufoximine is a useful model compound for inducing glutathione depletion. The measurement should be considered if major alterations of glutathione occur with reduced red cell survival, and the measurement might help in mechanistic studies.

3.4.9.3   Tissue Microsomal P450 and Other Urinary Measures of Enzyme Induction

The methods for P450 measurements require the extraction of hepatic tissue at necropsy to obtain microsomal preparations for the measurement of some of the relevant cytochromes (Batt et al. 1992, 1994; Halpert et al. 1994; Ioannides 1996; Wang et al. 1999). The relationships of microsomal enzyme induction with liver pathology in dogs and rats have been described by Amacher and colleagues (1998, 2001).

Alternative measures for assessing enzyme induction include urinary 6-β-hydroxycortisol and urinary D-glucaric acid. The measurement of 6-β-hydroxycortisol is successful in nonhuman primates and dogs, but this measurement varies with species and is less suitable for rats and mice because the production of 6-β-hydroxycortisol is much lower in other species (Ohnaus and Park 1979; Totsuka et al. 1999; Galteau and Shamsa 2003). Although urinary D-glucaric acid has been used as a measure of enzyme induction, it has not been widely applied (Talafant, Hošková, and Pojerová 1976; Jung, Scholz, and Schreiber 1981; Apostoli et al. 2003).

3.4.9.4   Hepatic Fibrosis

Inflammatory processes in the liver increase production of cytokines, chemokines, and signaling molecules, which activate the stellate cells to produce a complex extracellular glycoprotein matrix (i.e., the development of fibrosis). The matrix formed includes collagen, elastin, fibronectin, and laminin. Several noninvasive tests can be used as nonspecific indicators of fibrosis, but these have not been widely applied in laboratory animals. These tests include the collagen markers type III procollagen, YKL-40, and hyaluronic acid; however, these tests have not been widely evaluated in laboratory animals (Cho and Lee 1998; Tran et al. 2000; Ding et al. 2001; Mardini and Record 2005).

3.4.9.5   Oxidative Stress

The effects of oxidative phosphorylation and redox potential are receiving increasing attention in metabolic disease and in assessing liver injury, particularly when there may be mitochondrial dysfunction (Pessayre et al. 1999; Otsyula et al. 2003; Berdanier 2005; Surh and Packer 2005). Among the emerging measurements are lipid peroxides, the aldehydes, malondialdehyde and 4-hydroxynonenal, and the isoprostanes. These additional measurements are of products resulting from oxidative stress because the direct measurements of the short-living active oxygen species are technically challenging. Other measurements include antioxidants (e.g., retinol, alpha-tocopherol, and ascorbate) and antioxidant enzymes (e.g., superoxide dismutase, catalase, and glutathione peroxidase). Nuclear magnetic resonance spectroscopy has been used to study hepatotoxic effects on fatty acid metabolism (Coen et al. 2003; Mortishire-Smith et al. 2004). The responses of neutrophils and macrophages may be monitored using plasma myeoperoxidase and elastase.

3.4.9.6   Ratio of Acetoacetate to 3-Hydroxybutyrate

The redox potential is a measure of oxidative phosphorylation maintained by the hepatic mitochondria. Changes of the redox potential are reflected by alterations to the ratio of acetoacetate to 3-hydroxybutyrate (also called the ketone body ratio). This ratio is dependent on mitochondrial 3-hydroxybutyrate dehydrogenase activity, which catalyzes the interconversion of acetoacetate and 3-hydroxybuyrate (Laun et al. 2001; Fukao, Lopaschuk, and Mitchell 2004; Hidaka 2004; Matsumoto et al. 2005). Major changes of hepatic energy production or demand are indicated by alterations to the ketone body ratio; these changes may be reflected by ketonuria.

3.5   SUMMARY

The detection of hepatotoxicity—particularly of idiosyncratic reactions—remains a major challenge. The core plasma assays form a cornerstone for detecting hepatotoxicity, although several of the assays are limited by their lack of organ and cellular specificity. Even tried and tested assays such as ALT may be elevated without good supporting histological evidence of cellular change. Some tests of liver function, such as dye binding tests, have been mentioned, but these are limited by the suitability of the procedures for many studies. The major areas of immune responses and mitochondrial dysfunction require the development of suitable assays that can be incorporated simply into toxicology studies.

REFERENCES

Batt, A. M., and L. Ferrari. 1995. Manifestations of chemically induced liver damage. *Clinical Chemistry* 41:1882–1887.

Beaune, P. H., and S. Lecoeur. 1997. Immunotoxicology of the liver: Adverse reactions to drugs. *Journal of Hepatology* 26 (Suppl 2): 37–42.

Berger, J., and D. E. Moller. 2002. The mechanisms of action of PPARs. *Annual Review of Medicine* 53:409–435.

Boelsterli, U. A. 1993. Specific targets of covalent drug–protein interactions and their toxicological significance in drug-induced liver injury. *Drug Metabolism Review* 25:395–451.

———. 2003. Disease-related determinants of susceptibility to drug-induced idiosyncratic hepatotoxicity. *Current Opinions in Drug Discovery and Development* 6:81–91.

Buratti, S., and J. E. Lavine. 2002. Drugs and the liver: Advances in metabolism, toxicity, and therapeutics. *Current Opinions in Pediatrics* 14:601–607.

Deleve, L. D. 1998. Glutathione defense in nonparenchymal cells. *Seminars in Liver Disease* 18:403–413.

Dobrinska, M. R. 1989. Enterohepatic circulation of drugs. *Journal of Clinical Pharmacology* 29:577–580.

Ferenci, P., G. Zollner, and M. Trauner. 2002. Hepatic transport systems. *Journal of Gastroenterology and Hepatology* 17 (Suppl): S106–S113.

Gibson, G. G., and B. G. Lake. 1993. *Peroxisomes: Biology and importance in toxicology and medicine.* London: Taylor & Francis.

Greaves, P. 2007. *Histopathology in preclinical toxicity studies: Interpretation and relevance in drug safety evaluation,* 3rd ed. Amsterdam: Elsevier Science.

Hardisty, J. F., and A. E. Brix. 2005. Comparative hepatic toxicity: Prechronic/chronic liver toxicity in rats. *Toxicology and Pathology* 33:35–40.

Iverson, S. L., and J. P. Uetrecht. 2001. Identification of a reactive metabolite of terbinafine: Insights into terbinafine-induced hepatotoxicity. *Chemical Research in Toxicology* 14:175–181.

Kaplowitz, N. 2002. Biochemical and cellular mechanisms of toxic liver injury. *Seminars in Liver Disease* 22:137–144.

Kaplowitz, N., and L. D. DeLeve. 2003. *Drug-induced liver disease.* New York: Marcel Decker Inc.

Klaassen, C. D., and A. M. Hood. 2001. Effects of microsomal enzyme inducers on thyroid follicular cell proliferation and thyroid hormone metabolism. *Toxicologic Pathology* 29:34–40.

Klaassen, C. D., and J. B. Watkins. 1984. Mechanisms of bile formation, hepatic uptake and biliary excretion. *Pharmacology Review* 36:1–67.

Kluwe, K. M. 1994. The relevance of hepatic peroxisome proliferation in rats to assessment of human carcinogenic risk for pharmaceuticals. *Regulatory Toxicology and Pharmacology* 20:170–186.

Kuipers, F., R. Havinga, H. Bosschieter, G. P. Toorop, F. R. Hindriks, and R. J. Vonk. 1985. Enterohepatic circulation in the rat. *Gastroenterology* 88:403–411.

Lee, W. M. 2003. Drug-induced hepatotoxicity. *New England Journal of Medicine* 349:474–485.

Luster, L. I., P. P. Simeonova, R. M. Gallucci, J. M. Matheson, and B. Yucesoy. 2000. Immunotoxicology: Role of inflammation in chemical-induced hepatotoxicity. *International Journal of Immunopharmacology* 22:1143–1147.

McGuire, E. J., J. A. Lucas, R. H. Gray, and F. A. Iglesia. 1991. Peroxisome induction potential and lipid-regulating activity in rats. *American Journal of Pathology* 139:217–229.

McKenzie, R. et al. 1995. Hepatic failure and lactic acidosis due to fialuridine (FIAU), an investigational nucleoside analogue for chronic hepatitis B. *New England Journal of Medicine* 333:1099–1105.

Moody, D. E., J. K. Reddy, B. G. Lake, J. A. Popp, and D. H. Reese. 1991. Peroxisome proliferation and nongenotoxic carcinogenesis: Commentary on a symposium. *Fundamental and Applied Toxicology* 16:233–248.

Parker, G. A., and C. A. Picut. 2005. Liver immunobiology. *Toxicologic Pathology* 33:52–62.

Plaa, G. L. 1991. Toxic responses of the liver. In *Casarett and Doull's toxicology: The basic science of poisons,* 4th ed., ed. M. O. Amdur, C. D. Klaassen, and J. Doull, pp. 334–353. New York: Pergamon Press.

Plaa, G. L., and M. Charbonneau. 2001. Detection and evaluation of chemically induced liver injury. In *Principles and methods of toxicology,* 4th ed., ed. A. W. Hayes, pp. 1145–1187. Philadelphia: Taylor & Francis.

Pohl, L. R., H. Satoh, D. D. Christ, and J. G. Kenna. 1988. The immunological and metabolic basis of drug hypersensitivities. *Annual Review of Pharmacology and Toxicology* 128:367–387.

Reichel, C., and T. Sauerbruch. 1995. Serum bile acids: Physiology and clinical relevance. *European Journal of Gastroenterology and Hepatology* 7:951–953.

Roberts, R. A., P. E. Ganey, C. Ju, L. M. Kamendulis, I. Rusyn, and J. E. Klaunig. 2007. Role of the Kupffer cells in mediating hepatotoxicity and carcinogenesis. *Toxicological Sciences* 96:2–15.

Sipe, J. D. 1989. The molecular biology of interleukin 1 and the acute phase response. *Advances in Internal Medicine* 34:1–20.

Spatzenegger, M., and W. Jaeger. 1995. Clinical importance of hepatic cytochrome P450 in drug metabolism. *Drug Metabolism Reviews* 27:397–417.

Stumvoll, M., and H. U. Haring. 2002. Glitazones: Clinical effects and molecular mechanisms. *Annals of Medicine* 34:217–224.

Uetrecht, J. P. 1999. New concepts in immunology relevant to idiosyncratic drug reactions: The "danger hypothesis" and innate immune system. *Chemical Research in Toxicology* 12:387–395.

Wang, R. S., T. Nakajima, and T. Honma. 1999. Different change patterns of the isozymes of cytochorm P450 and glutathione S-transferases in chemically induced liver damage in rats. *Industrial Health* 37:440–448.

Zimmerman, H. J. 1999. *Hepatotoxicity: The adverse effects of drugs and other chemicals on the liver,* 2nd ed. Chapters 4, 5, and 16. Philadelphia: Lippincott Williams and Wilkins.

Zucker, S. D., X. Qin, S. D. Rouster, F. Yu, R. M. Green, P. Kehavan, J. Feinberg, and K. E. Sherman. 2001. Mechanism of indinavir-induced hyperbilirubinemia. *Proceedings of the Society of National Academy of Sciences USA* 98:12671–12676.

Laboratory Tests

Amacher, D. E. 2002. A toxicologist's guide to biomarkers of hepatic response. *Human and Experimental Toxicology* 21:253–262.

Amacher, D. E., R. Adler, A. Herath, and R. R. Townsend. 2005. Use of proteomic methods to identify serum biomarkers associated with rat liver toxicity or hypertrophy. *Clinical Chemistry* 51:1796–1803.

Bondy, G. S., C. L. Armstrong, I. H. Curran, M. G. Barker, and R. Mehta. 2000. Retrospective evaluation of serum ornithine carbamyl transferase as an index of hepatotoxicity in toxicological studies with rats. *Toxicology Letters* 114:163–171.

Boone, L. et al. 2005. Selection and interpretation of clinical pathology indicators of hepatic injury in preclinical studies. *Veterinary Clinical Pathology* 34:182–188.

Carakostas, M. C., K. A. Gossett, G. E. Church, and B. L. Cleghorn.1986. Evaluating toxin-induced hepatic injury in rats by laboratory results and discriminant analysis. *Veterinary Pathology* 23:264–269.

Dufour, D. R., J. A. Lott, F. S. Nolte, D. R. Gretch, R. S. Koff, and L. B. Seeff. 2000. Diagnosis and monitoring of hepatic injury. II. Recommendations for use of laboratory tests in screening, diagnosis and monitoring. *Clinical Chemistry* 46:2050–2068.

FDA. 2000. *Nonclinical assessment of potential hepatotoxicity in man.* Rockville, MD: Center for Drug Evaluation and Research.

Fujii, T. 1997. Toxicological correlation between changes in blood biochemical parameters and liver histopathological findings. *Journal of Toxicological Science* 22:161–183.

Shah, R. R. 1999. Drug induced hepatotoxicity: Pharmacokinetic perspective and strategies for risk assessment. *Adverse Drug Reactions and Toxicological Reviews* 18:181–233.

Travlos, G. S., R. W. Morris, M. R. Elwell, A. Duke, S. Rosenblum, and M. B. Thompson. 1996. Frequency and relationships of clinical chemistry and liver and kidney histopathology findings in 13-week toxicity studies in rat. *Toxicology* 107:17–29.

Waring, J. F., R. A. Jolly, R. Ciurlionis, P. Lum, J. T. Praestgaard, D. C. Morfitt, B. Buratto, C. Roberts, E. Schadt, and R. G. Ulrich. 2001. Clustering of hepatotoxins based on mechanism of toxicity using gene expression profiles. *Toxicology and Applied Pharmacology* 175:28–42.

Weingand, K. et al. 1996. Harmonization of animal clinical pathology testing in toxicity and safety studies. The Joint Scientific Committee for International Harmonization of Clinical Pathology Testing. *Fundamental and Applied Toxicology* 29:198–201.

Zimmerman, H. J. 1999. *Hepatotoxicity: The adverse effects of drugs and other chemicals on the liver,* 2nd ed. Chapters 4, 5, and 16. Philadelphia: Lippincott Williams and Wilkins.

Enzymes

Abdelkader, S. V., and J. G. Hauge. 1986. Serum enzyme determination in the study of liver disease in dogs. *Acta Veterinaria Scandinavica* 27:58–70.

Amacher, D. E. 1998. Serum transaminase elevations as indicators of hepatic injury following the administration of drugs. *Regulatory Toxicology and Pharmacology* 27:119–130.

Awasthi, Y. C. 2006. *Toxicology of glutathione transferases.* Boca Raton, FL: CRC Press.

Balazs, T., T. M. Farber, and G. Feuer. 1978. Drug induced changes in serum alkaline phosphatase and alanine aminotransferase activities not related to hepatic injuries. *Archives of Toxicology* 1 (Suppl): 159–163.

Beckett, G. J., J. E. Hunter, and J. D. Hayes. 1986. Hepatic damage in the rat following administration of thyroxine or triodothyronine assessed by measurement of plasma glutathione S-transferase Ya Ya concentrations. *Clinica Chimica Acta* 161:69–70.

Bondy, G. S., C. L. Armstrong, I. H. Curran, M. G. Barker, and R. Mehta. 2000. Retrospective evaluation of serum ornithine carbamyl transferase as an index of hepatotoxicity in toxicological studies with rats. *Toxicology Letters* 114:163–171.

Boyd, J. W. 1962. The comparative activity of some enzymes in sheep cattle and rats—Normal serum and tissue levels and changes during experimental liver necrosis. *Research in Veterinary Science* 3:256–268.

Carakostas, M. C., K. A. Gossett, G. E. Church, and B. L. Cleghorn.1986. Evaluating toxin-induced hepatic injury in rats by laboratory results and discriminant analysis. *Veterinary Pathology* 23:264–269.

Clarke, H., D. A. Egan, M. Heffernan, S. Doyle, C. Byrne, C. Kilty, and M. P. Ryan. 1997. Alpha-glutathione s-transferase α-GST) release, an early indicator of carbon tetrachloride hepatotoxicity in the rat. *Human and Experimental Toxicology* 16:154–157.

Coluccio, D., R. Nicklaus, S. Schneider, M. Lewis, and L. Hall. 2000. Evaluation of the Biotrin® alpha-glutathione S-transferase (α-GST) enzyme immunoassay (EIA) in detecting liver changes compared to standard liver enzymes. *Clinical Chemistry* 46:A140.

Cornelius, C. E., G. M. Douglas, R. R. Gronwall, and R. A. Freedland. 1963. Comparative studies on plasma arginase and transaminases in hepatic necrosis. *Cornell Veterinarian* 53:181–191.

De Simplicio, P. 1982. Glutathione and glutathione S-transferases in rat liver and plasma after carbon tetrachloride and thioacetamide intoxication. *Pharmacological Research Communications* 14:909–920.

Dhami, M. S., R. Drangova., R. Farkas, T. Balazs, and G. Feuer. 1979. Decreased aminotransferase activity of serum and various tissues in the rat after cefazolin treatment. *Clinical Chemistry* 25:1263–1266.

Dooley, J. F., L. J. Turnquist, and L. Racich. 1979. Kinetic determination of serum sorbitol dehydrogenase activity with a centrifugal analyzer. *Clinical Chemistry* 25:2026–2029.

Eaton, D. L., and T. K. Bammier. 1999. Concise review of the glutathionine S-transferases and their significance in toxicology. *Toxicological Sciences* 49:156–164.

Evans, G. O. 1986: Further observations on plasma γ-glutamyltransferase activity after oral administration of α-napthylisothiocyanate. *Human Toxicology* 5:120–121.

Giffen, P. S., C. R. Pick, M. A. Price, A. Williams, and M. J. York. 2002. Alpha-glutathione S-transferase in the assessment of hepatotoxicity—Its diagnostic utility in comparison with other recognized markers in the Wistar Han rat. *Toxicological Pathology* 30:365–372.

Huseby, N. E., and V. Torstein. 1978. The activity of gamma glutamyl transferase after bile duct ligation in guinea pig. *Clinica Chimica Acta* 88:385–392.

Ikemoto, M., S. Tsunekawa, Y. Toda, and M. Totani. 2001. Liver-type arginase is a highly sensitive marker for hepatocellular damage in rats. *Clinical Chemistry* 47:946–948.

Keller, P. 1981. Enzyme activities in the dog: Tissue analyses, plasma values and intracellular distribution. *American Journal of Veterinary Research* 42:575–582.

Kilty, C., S. Doyle, B. Hassett, and F. Mannings. 1998. Glutathione S-transferases as biomarkers of organ damage: Applications of rodent and canine GST enzyme immunoassays. *Chemico-Biological Interactions* 111–112:123–135.

Kryszewski, A., J. B. Whitfield, D. W. Moss, and G. Neale. 1973. Enzyme changes in experimental biliary obstruction. *Gut* 14:419.

Leonard, T. B., D. A. Neptun, and J. A. Popp. 1984. Serum gamma glutamyl transferase as a specific indicator of bile duct lesions in the rat liver. *American Journal of Pathology* 116:262–269.

Lohss, E., C. Federhen, and W. Kraft. 1988. Die ornithin-carbamyl-transferase (OCT) 5′-Nucleotidase (5′-ND) und Leucinarylamidase (LAP) als diagnostika bei leberkrankheiten des hundes. *Journal of Veterinary Medicine A* 35:81–91.

Moss, D. W. 1982. Alkaline phosphatase isoenzymes. *Clinical Chemistry* 28:2007–2016.

Noonan, N. E., and D. J. Meyer. 1979. Use of plasma arginase and gamma-glutamyl transpeptidase as specific indicators of hepatocellular or hepatobiliary disease in the dog. *American Journal of Veterinary Research* 40:942–947.

O'Brien, P. J., M. R. Slaughter, S. R. Polley, and K. Kramer. 2002. Advantages of glutamate dehydrogenase as a blood marker of acute hepatic injury in rats. *Laboratory Animals* 36:313–321.

Rutgers, H. C., J. R. M. Batt, C. Vaillant, and J. E. Riley. 1995. Subcellular pathologic features of glucocorticoid-induced hepatopathy in dogs. *American Journal of Veterinary Research* 56:898–907.

Schlaeger, R., P. Haux, and R. Katterman. 1982. Studies on the mechanism of the increase in serum alkaline phosphatase activity in cholestasis. *Enzyme* 28:508–516.

Solter, P. F., W. F. Hoffmann, M. D. Chambers, D. J. Schaeffer, and M. S. Kuhlenschmidt. 1994. Hepatic total 3-alpha-hydroxy bile acid concentration and enzyme activity in prednisolone-treated dogs. *American Journal of Veterinary Research* 55:1086–1092.

Strelic, N. J., Z. S. Salcic, Z. M. Magic, M. B. Spasic, N. V. Trutic, and K. V. Krtolica. 2003. Aflatoxin B1-induced changes of glutathione–S-transferase activity in the plasma and liver of the rat. *Vojnosanitetski Pregled* 60:415–420.

Travlos, G. S., R. W. Morris, M. R. Elwell, A. Duke, S. Rosenblum, and M. B. Thompson. 1996. Frequency and relationships of clinical chemistry and liver and kidney histopathology findings in 13-week toxicity studies in rat. *Toxicology* 107:17–29.

van der Aar, E. M., K. T. Tan, J. N. M. Commandeur, and N. P. E. Vermeulen. 1998. Strategies to characterize the mechanism of action and active sites of glutathione S transferases: A review. *Drug Metabolism Reviews* 30:569–643.

Zimmerman, H. 1982. Chemical injury and its detection. In *Toxicology of the liver*, ed. G. Plaa and W. R. Hewitt. New York: Raven Press.

Bilirubin and Bile Acids

Azer, S. A., C. D. Klaassen, and N. H. Stacey. 1997. Biochemical assay of serum bile acids. *British Journal of Biomedical Science* 54:118–132.

Azer, S. A., M. Murray, G. C. Farrell, and N. H. Stacey.1993. Selectivity and sensitivity of changes in serum bile acids during induction of cirrhosis in rats. *Hepatotology* 18:1224–1231.

Center, S. A., B. H. Baldwin, H. N. Erb, and B. C. Tennant. 1985. Bile acid concentrations in the diagnosis of hepatobiliary disease in the dog. *Journal of the American Veterinary Medical Association* 187:935–940.

Center, S. A., T. ManWarren, M. R. Slater, and E. Wilentz. 1991. Evaluation of twelve-hour and two-hour postprandial serum bile acid concentrations for diagnosis of hepatobiliary disease in dogs. *Journal of the American Veterinary Medical Association* 199:145–154.

Crampton, D. J., and L. K. Walthen. 1990. HPLC assay for quantifying serum bile acids in several species. *Clinical Chemistry* 36:2142–2143.

Gatti, R., A. Roda, C. Cerre, D. Bonazzi, and D. Cavrini. 1997. HPLC-fluorescence determination of individual free and conjugated bile acids in human serum. *Biomedical Chromatography* 11:11–15.

Gopinath, C., D. E. Prentice, A. E. Street, and D. Crook. 1980. Serum bile acid concentration in some experimental liver lesions of rat. *Toxicology* 15:113–127.

Hamdan, H., and N. H. Stacey. 1993. Mechanism of trichloroethylene-induced elevation of serum bile acids. 1. Correlation of trichloroethylene concentrations to bile acids in rat serum. *Toxicology and Applied Pharmacology* 121:291–295.

Hauge, J. G., and S. V. Abdelkader. 1984. Serum bile acids as an indicator of liver disease in dogs. *Acta Veterinaria Scandinavica* 25:495–503.

Hofmann, A. F 1988. Bile acids. In *The liver: Biology and pathobiology,* ed. I. M. Arias, W. B. Jakoby, M. Popper, D. Schachter, and D. A. Shafritz, pp. 553–572. New York: Raven Press.

Jensen, A. L., and J. S. Poulsen. 1992. Evaluation of diagnostic tests using relative operating characteristic (ROC) curves and the differential positive rate. An example using total serum bile acid concentration and alanine aminotransferase activity in the diagnosis of canine hepatobiliary disease. *Zentralblatt für Veterinarmedizin. Reihe A* 39:656–668.

Klaassen, C. D., and J. B. Watkins. 1984. Mechanisms of bile formation, hepatic uptake and biliary excretion. *Pharmacology Review* 36:1–67.

Lauff, J. J., H. E. Kasper, and R. T. Ambrose. 1981. Separation of bilirubin species in serum and bile by high-performance liquid chromatography. *Journal of Chromatography* 226:629–639.

Mashige, F., K. Imai, and T. Osuga. 1976. A simple and sensitive assay of total serum bile acids. *Clinica et Chimica Acta* 70:79–86.

Neghab, M., and N. H. Stacey. 2005. Serum bile acids as a sensitive biological marker for evaluating hepatic effects of organic solvents. *Biomarkers* 5:81–108.

Parraga, M. E., and J. J. Kaneko. 1985. Total serum bile acids and the bile acid profile as tests of liver function. *Veterinary Research Communications* 9:9–88.

Perwaiz, S., B. Tuchweber, D. Mignault, T. Gilat, and I. M. Yousef. 2001. Determination of bile acids in biological fluids by liquid chromatography–electrospray tandem mass spectrometry. *Journal of Lipid Research* 42:114–119.

Quereshi, M. Y., S. M. Smith, and G. M. Murphy. 1984. Colorimetric enzymatic measurement of serum total 3α-hydroxy bile acid concentrations without extraction. *Journal of Clinical Pathology* 37:317–320.

Reichel, C., and T. Sauerbruch. 1995. Serum bile acids: Physiology and clinical relevance. *European Journal of Gastroenterology and Hepatology* 7:951–953.

Rosenthal, S. M., N. Blankaert, P. M. Kabra, and M. M. Thaler. 1981. Liquid chromatographic determination of bilirubin and its conjugates in rat serum and human amniotic fluid. *Clinical Chemistry* 27:1704–1707.

Solter, P. F., W. F. Hoffmann, M. D. Chambers, D. J. Schaeffer, and M. S. Kuhlenschmidt. 1994. Hepatic total 3-alpha-hydroxy bile acid concentration and enzyme activity in prednisolone-treated dogs. *American Journal of Veterinary Research* 55:1086–1092.

Thompson, M. B., P. C. Blair, R. W. Morris, D. A. Neptun, D. F. Deyo, and J. A. Popp. 1987. Validation and application of a liquid-chromatographic/enzymatic assay for individual bile acids in the serum of rats. *Clinical Chemistry* 33:1856–1862.

Trautwein, E. A., K. Forgbert, D. Rieckhoff, and H. F. Erbersdobler. 1999. Impact of beta-cyclodextrin and resistant starch on bile acid metabolism and fecal steroid excretion in regard to their hypolipidemic action in hamsters. *Biochimica et Biophysica Acta* 1437:1–12.

Turgut, K., C. Demir, M. Ok, and K. Çiftçi. 1997. Pre- and postprandial total serum bile acid concentration following acute liver damage in dogs. *Journal of Veterinary Medicine A* 44:25–29.

Wang, G., and N. H. Stacey. 1990. Elevation of individual bile acids on exposure to trichlorethylene or α-napthylisothiocyanate. *Toxicology and Applied Pharmacology* 105:209–215.

Washizu, T., T. Ishida, M. Wshizu, and J. J. Kaneko. 1994. Changes in bile acid composition of serum and gallbladder bile in bile duct ligated dogs. *Journal of Veterinary Medical Science* 56:299–303.
Woodman, D. D., and P. Maile. 1981. Bile acid assay as an index of cholestasis. *Clinical Chemistry* 27:846–848.
Zucker, S. D., X. Qin, S. D. Rouster, F. Yu, R. M. Green, P. Kehavan, J. Feinberg, and K. E. Sherman. 2001. Mechanism of indinavir-induced hyperbilirubinemia. *Proceedings of the Society of National Academy of Science USA* 98:12671–12676.

Lipids

Bass, N. M., M. E. Barker, J. A. Manning, A. L. Jones, and R. K. Ockner. 1989. Acinar hetero-geneity of fatty acid-binding protein in the livers of male, female and clofibrate treated rats. *Hepatology* 9:12–21.
Glatz, J. F., and van der Vusse, G. J. 1996. Cellular fatty acid binding proteins: Their function and physiological significance. *Progress in Lipid Research* 3:243–282.
Lombardi, B. 1966. Considerations on the pathogenesis of fatty liver. *Laboratory Investigation* 15:1–20.
Reddy, J. K., and M. S. Rao. 2006. Lipid metabolism and liver inflammation. II. Fatty liver disease and fatty acid oxidation. *American Journal of Physiology. Gastrointestinal and Liver Physiology* 290:G852–858.

Proteins

Amacher, D. E., R. Adler, A. Herath, and R. R. Townsend. 2005. Use of proteomic methods to identify serum biomarkers associated with rat liver toxicity or hypertrophy. *Clinical Chemistry* 51:1796–1803.
Anderson, N. L. J. Taylor, J-P. Hofmann, R. Esquer-Blasco, S. Swift, and N. G. Anderson. 1996. Simultaneous measurement of hundreds of liver proteins: Application in assess-ment of liver function. *Toxicologic Pathology* 24:72–76.
Foster, G. R., R. D. Goldin, and D. B. Oliviera. 1989. Serum F protein: A new sensitive and specific marker for hepatocellular damage. *Clinica Chimica Acta* 184:85–92.
Giometti, C. S., S. L. Tollaksen, X. Liang, and M. L. Cunningham. 2005. Proteomics and two-dimensional electrophoresis. A comparison of liver protein changes in mice and hamsters treated with peroxisome proliferator Wy-14, 643. *Electrophoresis* 19:2498–2505.
Hulsewe, K. W., N. E. Deutz, I. De Blaauw, R. R. van der Hulst, M. M. von Meyenfeldt, and P. B. Soeters. 1997. Liver protein and glutamine metabolism during cachexia. *Proceedings of the Nutrition Society* 56:801–806.
Pritchard, D. H., M. G. Wright, S. Sulsh, and W. H. Butler. 1987. The assessment of chemi-cally induced liver injury in rats. *Journal of Applied Toxicology* 7:229–236.
Sipe, J. D. 1989. The molecular biology of interleukin 1 and the acute phase response. *Advances in Internal Medicine* 34:1–20.

Dye Excretion or Binding Tests

Cutler, M. G. 1974. The sensitivity of function tests in detecting liver damage in the rat. *Toxicology and Applied Pharmacology* 28:349–357.
Fujii, T. 1997. Toxicological correlation between changes in blood biochemical parameters and liver histopathological findings. *Journal of Toxicological Science* 22:161–183.
Jablonski, P., and J. A. Owen. 1969. The clinical chemistry of bromosulfophthalein and other cholephilic dyes. *Advances in Clinical Chemistry* 12:309–386.

Kaneko, H., Y. Otsuka, M. Katagiri, T. Maeda, M. Tsuchiya, A. Tamura, T. Ishii, S. Takagi, and
T. Shiba. 2001. Reassessment of monoethylglycinexylidide as preoperative liver function test in a rat model of liver cirrhosis and man. *Clinical and Experimental Medicine*
1:19–26.

Klaassen, C. D., and G. L. Plaa. 1967. Species variation in metabolism, storage and excretion
of sulfobromophthalein. *American Journal of Physiology* 213:1322–1326.

———. 1969. Plasma clearance and biliary excretion of indocyanine green in rats, rabbits and
dogs. *Toxicology and Applied Pharmacology* 15:374–384.

Meyer, D. J. 1986. Liver function tests in dogs with portosystemic shunts: Measurement of
serum bile acid concentraton. *Journal of the American Veterinary Medical Association*
188:168–169.

Plaa, G. L., and M. Charbonneau. 2001. Detection and evaluation of chemically induced liver
injury. In *Principles and methods of toxicology,* 4th ed., ed. A. W. Hayes, pp. 1145–1187.
Philadelphia: Taylor & Francis.

Shibata, H., and N. Odani. 1991. Blood clearances of 99mTc-phytate and indocyanine green in
carbon tetrachloride treated dogs. *Journal of Toxicological Science* 16:145–154.

Taurine and Creatine

Clayton, T. A., J. C. Lindon, J. R. Everett, C. Charuel, G. Hanton, J-L. Le Net, J-P. Provost, and
J. K. Nicholson. 2003. An hypothesis for a mechanism underlying hepatotoxin-induced
hypercreatinuria. *Archives of Toxicology* 77:208–217.

———. 2004. Hepatotoxin-induced hypercreatinemia and hypercreatinuria: Their relationship to one another, to liver damage and to weakened nutritional status. *Archives of
Toxicology* 78:86–96.

Maxuitenko, Y. Y., W. G. North, and R. D. Roebuck. 1997. Urine taurine as a noninvasive marker
of aflatoxin B1-induced hepatotoxicity: Success and failure. *Toxicology* 118:159–169.

Sanins, S. M., J. K. Nicholson, C. Elcombe, and J. A. Timbrell. 1990. Hepatotoxin-induced
hypertaurinuria: A proton NMR study. *Archives of Toxicology* 64:407–411.

Timbrell, J. A., V. Seabra, and C. J. Waterfield. 1995. The in vivo and in vitro protective properties of taurine. *General Pharmacology* 26:453–462.

Waterfield, C. J., D. S. Asker, and J. A. Timbrell. 1996. Does urinary taurine reflect changes in
protein metabolism? A study with cycloheximide in rats. *Biomarkers* 1:107–114.

Waterfield, C. J., J. A. Turton, M. D. Scales, and J. A. Timbrell. 1993a. Effects of various nonhepatic
compounds on urinary and liver taurine levels in rats. *Archives of Toxicology* 67:538–546.

———. 1993b. Reduction of liver taurine in rats by β-alanine treatment increases carbon tetrachloride toxicity. *Toxicology* 77:7–20.

———. 1993c. The correlation between urinary and liver taurine levels and between predose
taurine and liver damage. *Toxicology* 77:1–5.

Enzyme Induction

Amacher, D. A., S. J. Schomaker, and J. E. Burkhardt. 1998. The relationship among
microsomal enzyme induction, liver weight and histological change in rat toxicology
studies. *Food and Chemical Toxicology* 36:831–839.

———. 2001.The relationship among microsomal enzyme induction, liver weight and histological change in beagle dog toxicology studies. *Food and Chemical Toxicology*
39:817–825.

Apostoli, P., A. Mangili, S. Carasi, and M. Manno. 2003. Relationships between PCBs in
blood and D-glucaric acid in urine. *Toxicology Letters* 144:17–26.

Batt, A. M., J. Magdalou, M. Vincent-Viry, M. Ouzzine, S. Fournel-Gigleux, M. M. Galteau, and
G. Siest. 1994. Drug metabolizing enzymes related to laboratory medicine: Cytochromes
P-450 and UDP-glucuronsyltransferases. *Clinica Chimica Acta* 226:171–190.

Batt, A. M., G. Siest, J. Magdalou, and M. M. Galteau. 1992. Enzyme induction by drugs and toxins. *Clinica Chimica Acta* 209:109–121.

Galteau, M. M., and F. Shamsa. 2003. Urinary 6-β-hydroxycortisol: A validated test for evaluating drug induction or drug inhibition mediated through CYP3A in humans and animals. *European Journal of Clinical Pharmacology* 59:713–733.

Halpert, J. R., F. P. Guengerich, J. R. Bend, and M. A. Correia. 1994. Selective inhibitors of cytochromes P450. *Toxicology and Applied Pharmacology* 125:163–175.

Ioannides, C. 1996. *Cytochromes P450: Metabolic and toxicological aspects.* Boca Raton FL: CRC Press.

Jung, K., D. Scholz, and G. Schreiber. 1981. Improved determination of D-glucaric acid in urine. *Clinical Chemistry* 27:422–426.

Ohnaus, E. E., and B. K. Park. 1979. Measurement of urinary 6-β-hydroxy cortisol excretion as an in vivo parameter in the clinical assessment of the microsomal enzyme-inducing capacity of antipyrine, phenobarbitone and rifampicin. *European Journal of Clinical Pharmacology* 15:139–145.

Talafant, E., A. Hošková, and A. Pojerová. 1976. Serum glutamyl transpeptidase activity and urinary D-glucaric acid excretion in newborns in the first week of life; effects of phenobarbital and nicethamide combination. *Acta Paediatrica* 65:85–88.

Totsuka, S., T. Wanatabe, F. Koyanagi, K. Tanaka, M. Yasuda, and S. Manabe. 1999. Increase in urinary excretion of 6-β-hydroxycortisol in common marmosets as a marker of hepatic CYP3A induction. *Archives of Toxicology* 73:203–207.

Wang, R. S., T. Nakajima, and T. Honma. 1999. Different change patterns of the isozymes of cytochrome P450 and glutathione S-transferases in chemically induced liver damage in rats. *Industrial Health* 37:440–448.

Fibrosis

Cho, J-J., and Y-S. Lee. 1998. Enzyme linked immunosorbent assay for serum procollagen type III peptide in rats with hepatic fibrosis. *Journal of Veterinary Medical Science* 60:1213–1220.

Ding, H., Y. Chen, X. Feng, D. Liu, A. Wu, and L. Zhang. 2001. Correlation between liver fibrosis stage and serum liver fibrosis markers in patients with chronic hepatitis B. *Chung Hua Kan Tsang Ping Tsa Chih* 9:78–80.

Mardini, H., and C. Record. 2005. Detection, assessment and monitoring of hepatic fibrosis: Biochemistry or biopsy? *Annals of Clinical Biochemistry* 42:441–447.

Tran, A. et al. 2000. Chondrex (YKL-40), a potential new serum fibrosis marker in patients with alcoholic disease. *European Journal of Gastroenterology and Hepatology* 12:989–993.

Oxidative Stress

Berdanier, C. D. 2005. *Mitochondria in health and disease.* Boca Raton, FL: CRC Press.

Coen, M., E. M. Lenz, J. K. Nicholson, I. D. Wilson, F. Pognan, and J. C. Lindon. 2003. An integrated metabonomic investigation of acetaminophen toxicity in the mouse using NMR spectroscopy. *Chemical Research in Toxicology* 16:295–303.

Mortishire-Smith, R. J., G. L. Skiles, J. W. Lawrence, S. Spence, A. W. Nicholls, B. A. Johnson, and J. K. Nicholson. 2004. Use of metabonomics to identify impaired fatty acid metabolism as the mechanism of drug induced-toxicity. *Chemical Research in Toxicology* 17:165–173.

Otsyula, M., M. S. King, T. G. Ketcham, R. A. Sanders, and J. B. Watkins. 2003. Oxidative stress in rats after 60 days of hypergalactosemia or hyperglycemia. *International Journal of Toxicology* 22:423–427.

Pessayre, D., A. Mansouri, D. Haouzi, and B. Fromenty. 1999. Hepatotoxicity due to mitochondrial dysfunction. *Cell Biology and Toxicology* 15:367–373.

Surh, Y-J., and L. Packer. 2005. *Oxidative stress, inflammation and health,* vol. 18. Boca Raton, FL: CRC Press.

Ketones

Fukao, T., G. D. Lopaschuk, and G. A. Mitchell. 2004. Pathways and control of ketone body metabolism: On the fringes of lipid metabolism. *Prostaglandins Leukotrienes and Essential Fatty Acids* 70:243–251.

Hidaka, H. 2004. Ketone bodies: Measurement and its clinical significance. *Nippon Rinsho* 62 (Suppl. 11): 676–678.

Laun, R. A., B. Rapsch, W. Abel, O. Schroder, H. D. Roher, A. Ekkernkamp, and K. M. Schulte. 2001. The determination of ketone bodies: Preanalytical, analytical and physiological considerations. *Clinical and Experimental Medicine* 1:201–209.

Matsumoto, K., A. Takuwa, A. Terashi, I. Ui, A. Okajo, and K. Endo. 2005. Correlation between ketone body level in selenium-deficient rats and oxidative damages. *Biological and Pharmaceutical Bulletin* 28:1142–1147.

4 Assessment of Nephrotoxicity

4.1 STRUCTURE, PHYSIOLOGY, AND BIOCHEMISTRY

The kidneys are complex multifunctional organs that have major roles in the regulation of whole-body homeostasis and excretion of the waste metabolic products. Each kidney is formed from many basic functional units called nephrons (approximately 35,000 nephrons per kidney in adult rats); each nephron has a single glomerulus where ultrafiltration of blood occurs. The remainder of the nephron is formed by several continuing tubular structures formed by the proximal convoluted tubule, the loop of Henlé, the distal tubule, and the collecting ducts; thus, along the nephron, there are at least 10 different types with structural and functional differences (Berndt 1976).

The kidney can be divided into two main anatomic areas: the major outer part—the cortex and the inner medulla, with the glomeruli, proximal convoluted tubules, and distal convoluted tubules located within the cortex—and the remaining parts of the nephrons lying within the medulla. The collecting ducts extend through the medulla to the renal papillae, which drain via the renal pelvises into the ureters and thence to the bladder, where fluid is stored prior to urination. There are some differences between species, and not all are related to body size and its proportionality (Davies and Morris 1993) (Table 4.1).

The proximal tubules are divided into the convoluted section: the pars convoluta and the straight portion of the tubule descending into the medulla, the pars recta. The pars recta is sometimes referred to as the S3 segment of the proximal tubules; the other two segments, S1 and S2, form the convoluted part of the tubule.

From the kidney surface (cortex) to its inner portion (medulla), there exists an osmolarity gradient associated with higher concentrations of many solutes. As a broad rule across species, urine concentrating ability declines with increasing body mass, and the relative thickness of the medulla relative to the kidney declines with body size, although larger mammals have longer nephrons compared to smaller animals (Schmidt-Nielsen and O'Dell 1961; Corman, Pratz, and Poujeol 1985; Beuchat 1990a, 1990b; Knepper, Chou, and Layton 1993). The urine composition is affected by other organs (and toxic effects on these organs); these effects include alterations of hepatic function (e.g., protein, carbohydrate, and fatty acid metabolism) and renal blood flow.

Within the proximal tubules, the tubules are lined with epithelial cells that have microvillous brush borders that provide the absorptive surfaces of these tubules. The longer loops of Henlé extend into the medulla, and the relative lengths of these loops vary between species, with longer loops found in animals that normally inhabit dry

TABLE 4.1

Some Renal Parameters in Mouse, Rat, Dog, and Man

Parameter	Mouse	Rat	Dog	Man
Body mass (kg)	0.02	0.25	10	70
Kidney mass (g)	0.32	2.0	50	310
Total body water (mL)	14.5	167	6,036	42,000
Plasma volume (mL)	1.0	7.5	515	3,000
Renal blood flow (mL/min)	1.3	9.2	216	1,240
Urine flow rate (mL/24h)	1.0	50	300	1,400
GFR (mL/min)	0.3	1.3	61	125
Maximum urine osmolality (mosmol/kg body water)	>2,500	>2,500	>2,500	1,400

areas, which helps normal fluid conservation processes. The epithelial cells of the distal tubules do not have a brush border, but there are intercalated cells that can excrete acids.

The kidney receives about 20–25% of the cardiac blood output at rest via the renal arteries, which deliver blood to the afferent arterioles of the glomeruli. Following filtration, blood is returned via the efferent arterioles; both of these arterioles form the vascular element of the glomeruli. The renal artery also supplies blood to the adrenal glands.

Blood is returned to the heart via series of veins connecting to the renal vein and then to vena cava. Renal perfusion with nutrients and oxygen is essentially for normal renal functions and this is dependent on adequate renal blood flow. This balance is controlled by several factors, including systemic blood pressure, glomerular capillary hydrostatic pressure, afferent/efferent arteriolar vasoconstriction, edema, plasma total protein and albumin concentration, glomerular ultrafiltration rates, and permeability—all of which also will affect the glomerular filtration rate.

The glomerular filtrate is formed by the passage of fluid though fenestrations in the endothelial lining cells and then through the basement membrane. The sizes of the endothelial fenestrations do not normally allow a significant passage of the blood erythrocytes, leukocytes, and platelets. Many of the plasma proteins do not pass into the glomerular filtrate because of their size and anionic charge, and these largely mechanical controls involve the basement membrane and podocytes (Lund et al. 2003). The concept that all of the plasma proteins are sieved into the glomerular filtrate on the basis of size does not explain the passage of some proteins but not others of a similar molecular size; however, most filtered proteins are generally less than 68 kDa. For example, albumin has a molecular mass of about 68 kDa (Russo, Bakris, and Comper 2002). Xenobiotics strongly bound to molecules with a mass > 70 kDa will normally not cross this glomerular barrier.

Within the proximal tubules, the bulk of filtered solutes (e.g., glucose, amino acids, bicarbonate, potassium) and a large proportion of filtered sodium are reabsorbed with water. The luminal portion of the tubular cells is equipped with numerous transport systems and the absorption of solutes requires these active mechanisms, including ion channels, cotransporters, and ion pumps. On the basolateral side of these cells, there are transport systems for weak organic acids and bases, and some filtered proteins are taken into the tubular cells by endocytosis (Marshansky et al. 1997). Separate renal secretory mechanisms exist for both anionic and organic cationic compounds (Inui, Masuda, and Saito 2000; Masereeuw and Russel 2001), and there are also nucleoside and P-glycoprotein transporters. Some transport mechanisms have a limited capacity and may not be able to deal with very high concentrations of a solute (e.g., glucose); generalized dysfunction of proximal tubules will result in the appearance in the urine of many natural metabolites normally reabsorbed in the proximal tubule.

Within the descending and ascending parts of the loop of Henlé, there is active transport of primarily sodium and chloride, and the fluid passing from the loop of Henlé becomes more hypertonic as it passes through the medulla as water is conserved by the body (Schmidt-Nielsen and O'Dell 1961; Beuchat 1990a, 1990b; Knepper et al. 1993). Tubular glomerular feedback mechanisms govern the fluid flow through glomeruli and tubules. In the distal convoluted tubules, sodium reabsorption and secretion of potassium and hydrogen ions occur largely under the influence of aldosterone. Reabsorption of water through the collecting dusts occurs through the action of vasopressin; very small amounts of sodium are reabsorbed in exchange for hydrogen and potassium.

The kidneys play important roles in regulating acid–base balance, water and electrolyte balance, blood volume, and blood pressure by interacting with blood hormones. For example, any major change of plasma osmolality is detected by the hypothalamus, which relays messages to the posterior pituitary gland, which then alters the secretion of antidiuretic hormones. Some metabolites (e.g., amino acids and glucose, which are filtered by the glomeruli) are reabsorbed by the tubules and conserved for recirculation.

The metabolic processes within the cortex and medulla differ. Within the cortex, the major processes include gluconeogenesis, fatty acid utilization, prostaglandin catabolism, cytochrome P450 metabolism, and vitamin D metabolism; within the medulla, the metabolic processes include glycolysis, lipogenesis, prostaglandin synthesis, oxidation of xenobiotics, and synthesis of glycosaminoglycans. The proportions of individual P450 cytochromes present in cortical microsomes differ from those found in the liver, and the bioactivations of xenobiotics are generally lower than similar reactions in the liver. Adequate supplies of glutathione are essential for normal renal function (Lash 2005).

In addition, the kidneys have direct endocrine functions. Because they are a major site of synthesis of several hormones, including erythropoietin and 1,25-dihydroxy-cholecalciferol, the kidneys indirectly influence the regulation of blood pressure and vasopressor activity via the renin–angiotensin, prostaglandins, and kallekrein–kinin systems, which exert a regulatory effect on water and electrolyte homeostasis (Harris 1992; Parekh et al. 1993; Gonzalez et al. 1998; Câmpean et al. 2003; see also Chapters 6 and 10).

4.2 RENAL TOXICITY

Nephrotoxic effects can range from mild to severe cell necrosis, and changes in functionality can also range from minor alterations of tubular function (e.g., glucosuria) to severe renal failure with reduced urine output (decreased—oliguria or absent—anuria) and electrolyte imbalance. Renal tubular damage can lead to the loss of cells of the nephron into the tubule (e.g., tubular epithelial cells that subsequently appear in the urine); the loss of renal function can have an impact on major organs such as the heart and liver.

Renal tissue metabolism and transport mechanisms play important roles in the excretion and detoxification of xenobiotics (and/or their metabolites). Although the kidneys play an important part in the detoxification of xenobiotics, renal tissue may produce or increase the amounts of toxic metabolites received via the renal blood supply by metabolism (e.g., mixed-function oxidase reactions or concentrating effects within the nephron) (Piperno 1981; Commandeur and Vermeulen 1990; Goldstein 1994; Diamond and Zalups 1998; Endou 1998; Tarloff and Lash 2004).

Given the relatively high blood volume supplied to the kidneys and the ability of the kidneys to concentrate solutes, renal exposure to xenobiotics is relatively high compared to other body tissues; it commences at the glomerulii and then within the renal cortex before reaching the medulla. Although pharmacologically mild and reversible changes can be used to advantage in therapeutics (e.g., diuretics and renin–angiotensin inhibitors), adverse irreversible nephrotoxic effects have serious consequences, even given the large functional reserve capacity of the kidneys. Vasoconstriction induced by xenobiotics may lead to changes of glomerular function and permeability or effects on tubular reabsorption or excretion. In addition to the acute renal failure caused by nephrotoxins, other factors can contribute to producing acute renal failure; these factors include decreased cardiac output, hypovolemia associated with hemorrhage or gastrointestinal fluid loss, diuresis, and some alteration of autoregulation of renal blood flow (e.g., the action of angiotensin converting enzyme inhibitors).

The elimination of xenobiotics and/or their metabolites involves the unidirectional glomerular filtration and the opposing mechanisms of tubular reabsorption and tubular secretion (Bendayan 1996; Dantzler and Wright 1997; Pritchard and Miller 1997; Russel, Masereeuw, and Van Aubel 2002). Glomerular injury can impair the retention of proteins of high molecular weight, such as albumin; damaged or dead renal cells can release enzymes and other proteins into the urine. Some nephrotoxicants alter the glomerular anionic filtration characteristics and produce morphological changes (e.g., of the podocytes), which lead to increased proteinuria, such as doxorubicin and puromycin.

Proximal tubular injury due to nephrotoxicants occurs more frequently than other nephrotoxic effects, and this probably reflects a combination of the proportion of the total renal blood supply received by the renal cortex and the number of xenobiotics reabsorbed and excreted within the proximal tubule. Xenobiotics can alter or inhibit the transport processes of passive diffusion and/or carrier transporters for both anionic/base and cationic molecules.

Aminoglycosides exemplify compounds that enter the proximal tubular cells by endocytosis and then are stored in secondary lysosomes, which have a lamellate appearance with aminoglycosides. Low molecular weight proteins can also enter the same tubular cells by endocytosis and accumulate in lysosomes. A number of compounds cause a male rat-specific nephrotoxicity that results from the accumulation of the male rat major urine protein (MUP)—alpha$_{2u}$-globulin—in secondary lysosomes of the renal tubules and with the development of hyaline droplet formation. This accumulation of alpha$_{2u}$-globulin can give angular appearances to the secondary lysosomes (Alden 1986; Lock et al. 1987; Borghoff, Short, and Swenberg 1990; Lehman-McKeeman and Caudill 1992). Some compounds (e.g., cisplatin) inhibit protein endocytosis (Takano et al. 2002).

The phase I reactions of the cytochrome P450 cytochrome mono-oxygenase hydroxylate lipophilic compounds, increasing their polarity solubility and then facilitating their excretion; phase II conjugation reactions increase the excretion of some compounds. In addition, renal metabolism may produce toxic metabolites, such as free radicals or electrophilic compounds, which then bind to other large molecules that may be eliminated more slowly or retained in the tissues. Thus, there may be an opposing effect to renal detoxifying actions.

Some nephrotoxicants generate reactive oxygen species (ROS) and these ROS can oxidize sulfhydryl or amino groups of cellular enzymes, cause DNA damage, and induce lipid peroxidation (Bach et al. 1991; Ichikawa, Kiyama, and Yoshioka 1994; Theilemann, Rodrigo, and Videla 1999; Bach and Thanh 1998). The peroxidation of membrane lipids and decomposition of lipid hydroperoxides cause alterations to cellular membranes and organelle and cellular dysfunction. Changes of intracellular calcium may be associated with changes of plasma membrane phospholipids via calcium-dependent phospholipases, or altered intracellular calcium homeostasis may change cellular integrity.

The renal concentrating mechanisms can increase by the concentration of a nephrotoxicant in the glomerular filtrate and/or lead to an accumulation of a compound within the proximal tubular cells, which can be several fold times the levels found in the plasma; thus both or either of these factors can lead to cellular toxicity. These compounds, which are concentrated as they move down the nephron, can cause injury to the renal medulla and papilla (e.g., phenacetin). Some compounds may alter renal function by relatively simple processes, such as tubular obstruction by crystal formation (e.g., some antiviral compounds) (Izzedine, Launay-Vacher, and Deray 2005) or altering the renal ability to acidify urine (e.g., amphotericin).

If the test chemical or its metabolites are present in the urine at high concentrations, it or they may precipitate from solution and form solid aggregates visible on examination. This may result in irritation or mechanical abrasion, or cause inflammation of the kidney, ureters, or bladder, with findings of erythrocytes, leukocytes, and/or hemoglobin in the urine.

4.3   LABORATORY INVESTIGATIONS

Although some plasma measurements are very important tests of glomerular function (e.g., creatinine), most laboratories will include some urinalysis in study designs. Urinalysis is essential for the detection of tubular injury, and several plasma and urinary tests have been proposed for detecting nephrotoxicity in preclinical studies (Kluwe 1981; Price 1982, 2002; Bovee 1986; Fent, Mayer, and Zbinden 1988; Lauwerys and Bernard 1989; Stonard 1990, 1996; Price et al. 1996, 1999; Zalups and Lash 1996; Bernard et al. 1997; Mueller, Lash et al. 1997; Mueller, Price, and Porter 1997; Loeb 1998; Raab 1998; Price 2000). Although some tools for investigating nephrotoxicity are available, the exact localization and quantification of renal injury remain as a challenge. Much of the effort in developing markers for nephrotoxicity has focused on proteins, enzymes, and some markers of general metabolism (e.g., glucose, amino acids, and electrolytes).

A tiered approach is useful for the detection of nephrotoxicity. In addition to plasma creatinine and urea in the core plasma measurements (see Chapter 1; IHCPT 1996), the measurements of plasma electrolytes and proteins may be indicative of renal dysfunction. For urinalysis, many laboratories use urinary test strips (dipsticks) as a screening method, with measures of urine volume and concentration and possible inclusion of microscopy of the urinary sediment. As a minimum, the first tier of testing should include the following tests:

plasma creatinine and urea (blood urea nitrogen) and, for urinalysis:
    abnormal color and appearance (clarity/turbidity);
    volume;
    relative concentration/density, either as osmolality or specific gravity;
    protein;
    glucose;
    blood;
    pH (or hydrogen ion concentration); and
    microscopy of urine sediment.

Additional tests can be included when there is a suspicion or evidence that the xenobiotic and/or metabolite causes nephrotoxicity. Many of the additional tests used to detect nephrotoxicity are aimed at measures of tubular dysfunction rather than glomerular function and either supplement or replace some of the qualitative test strips. These additional tests may be divided into:

second tier:
    quantitative urinary glucose;
    urinary proteins;
    urinary enzymes; and
    urinary electrolytes
third tier:
    concentration and dilution tests;
    renal blood or plasma flow;
    glomerular filtration rate determinations (other than by plasma creatinine);
    tubular transport measurements;
    proteomics;
    metabonomics; and
    acid/base measurements.

Some of these additional tests may be included as part of separate safety pharmacology studies of renal function that generally include urine measurements of protein, creatinine, electrolytes, volume, relative concentration/density, and pH over timed collection periods. When further investigations of nephrotoxicity are required, urine should be collected more frequently than in the regulatory study designs discussed in Chapter 1. Some correction of urinary excretions for urine concentration should be considered either for the collection period or for random samples. Current renal tests are generally directed at detecting changes of glomerular filtration and tubular injury.

4.3.1 Plasma Creatinine, Urea (Blood Urea Nitrogen), and Cystatin C

These plasma tests are used as indirect measurements of the glomerular filtration rate (GFR); to some extent, these endogenous tests supplement each other despite having different limitations. Plasma creatinine, urea, and cystatin C are normally filtered from the plasma, and they are reabsorbed or secreted by the proximal tubules to a minor extent, which differs between species. Tubular secretion leads to overestimation of GFR and it is higher in laboratory animals than in man. These secretions/reabsorption mechanisms may change as a consequence of major tubular injury. In addition to renal injury, the GFR may be altered by changes of renal hemodynamics or extracellular dehydration.

4.3.1.1 Plasma Creatinine

Creatinine is a product of the degradation of creatine and creatine phosphate, which are present mainly in muscle and in food. Plasma creatinine is dependent on muscle mass and can be lowered in severe myopathy. Although plasma levels are less affected by diet compared to urea, malnutrition may lower plasma creatinine (Evans 1987; Braun, Lefebvre, and Watson 2003). Plasma creatinine is normally filtered from the plasma, and it is reabsorbed and secreted by the proximal tubules to a minor extent, although secretion is higher in rodents compared to humans. Elevated plasma creatinine is a reliable indicator of impaired glomerular filtration or alterations in renal blood flow, but severe tubular dysfunction can also increase plasma creatinine.

Plasma creatinine is a better marker of glomerular function than urea, and these two measurements are not always simultaneously increased or normal (Prause and Grauer 1998; Medaille et al. 2004). For measurements of plasma creatinine and urea to change, there has to be significant loss of renal function (i.e., a 50% loss of GFR capacity leads to a doubling of these plasma values), and these relationships are not linear. To a lesser extent, both plasma creatinine and urea show variation with age (Gray 1977; Corman et al. 1985; Goldstein 1990).

Plasma and urinary creatinine are commonly measured by the colorimetric alkaline picrate method of Jaffé or by alternative enzymatic methods. Enzymatic methods use creatinine amidohydrolase or creatinine iminohydrolase and are more specific for creatinine. The measurement of plasma creatinine may be affected by endogenous noncreatinine chromogens (e.g., bilirubin and ketones); this can overestimate plasma creatinine in dogs by up to 45% and to an even greater extent in rats and mice (Evans 1986; Jung et al. 1987; Palm and Lundblad 2005). Some xenobiotics (e.g., cephalosporins) may interfere with assay (Grotsch and Hajdu 1987).

4.3.1.2   Plasma Urea (BUN: Blood Urea Nitrogen)

Urea is produced by protein catabolism and is primarily hepatic in origin (see Chapter 3), although generalized tissue catabolism also leads to increased plasma urea. Plasma urea levels are altered by food intake and the food protein content. Urea is partially reabsorbed by the renal tract. In addition to glomerular changes, plasma urea may be increased by toxic effects on the renal tubules, renal parenchyma, cardiac injury, and blockage of the urinary outflow tract by crystalluria, calculi, or other obstructions. Heavy blood loss from the upper gastrointestinal tract produces nitrogenous breakdown products, which are reabsorbed; these can produce increases of plasma urea (Prause and Grauer 1998).

4.3.1.3   Plasma Cystatin C

This protein is one of the latest small molecular weight proteins to be considered and used as a measure of GFR. Cystatin C a member of the cystine protease inhibitor superfamily found in a wide variety of tissues with a molecular mass of 13.5 kDa (Schaeffer et al. 1994; Laterza, Price, and Scott 2002; Curhan 2005). Although the cystatin C is freely filtered through the glomerulus, some evidence now suggests that the protein is not secreted but, rather, is partially reabsorbed in the proximal tubules. Plasma cystatin C levels may be reduced in malnutrition; the level of plasma cystatin also seems to be subject to the tubular mechanisms for handling low molecular mass proteins, the rate of hepatic protein synthesis, and thyroid dysfunction. The protein can be measured using antibodies to human cystatin because the protein shows approximately 70% homology with other species of laboratory animals (Bøkenkamp, Ciarimboli, and Dieterich 2001; Almy et al. 2002; Braun et al. 2002). Some studies of this assay suggest that the imprecision of the assay is greater than for creatinine.

4.3.1.4   Glomerular Filtration Rate (GFR)

In addition to using plasma creatinine (or cystatin C) as an indicator of GFR, several other methods for estimating GFR can be expressed as

$$\text{GFR ml/min} = \frac{\text{Urine analyte concentration}}{\text{Plasma analyte concentration}} \times \text{Urine flow rate ml/min}$$

where both plasma and urine concentrations are expressed in the same unitage (e.g., micromoles per liter or millimoles per liter for creatinine). The methods to determine GFR using endogenous or exogenous compounds include (DiMeola et al. 1974; Cronin et al. 1980; Finco, Coulter, and Barsanti 1981; Kampa et al. 2003):

    endogenous creatinine
    exogenous compounds: inulin
        radiolabeled inulin
        radiolabeled ^{125}I iothalamate

radiolabeled ^{51}Cr ethylenediamine tetraacetic acid
radiolabeled ^{99m}Tc diethylenetriamine-pentaacetic acid
iohexol.

All endogenous and exogenous methods of determining GFR require careful timing and sample collection. The requirements for additional procedures, blood sampling, use of radioisotopes, and, in some cases, anesthesia make most of these tests unsuitable for inclusion in general screening for nephrotoxicity in rodents. The simplest and commonest endogenous method is to use plasma and urine creatinine concentrations to determine the creatinine clearance, which then may be adjusted for body mass. Although methods using inulin to determine GFR are generally regarded as the reference method, this method is not ideal because it requires continuous infusion of inulin for accurate determinations. Older analytical methods for inulin required a heating hydrolysis step and were not simple to automate; however, these measurements have been improved by the use of inulase (Delanghe et al. 1991).

4.3.2 URINE

4.3.2.1 Urine Sample Collection
The methods used for urine collection should be designed to avoid fecal and other contamination (Figure 4.1). For smaller laboratory animals, well-designed metabolic cages (bowls) with fecal separators can be used to house the animals

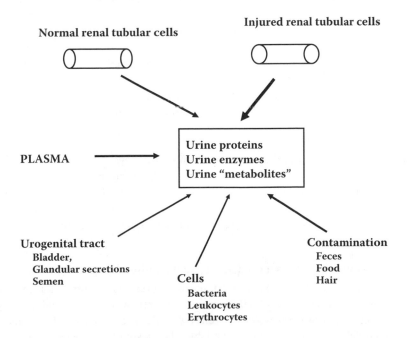

FIGURE 4.1 Sources of contaminants of urine.

during collection. In some laboratories, urethral catheterization is used to collect random samples from larger animals such as dogs; here, the collection procedure should be designed and performed so as not to cause injury to the renal tract. Timed collection periods give more meaningful results than random collections, where there is more variability. It is preferable to acclimatize animals to the metabolism cages prior to the collection period; when more detailed studies are required, predosing urine samples should be taken on several occasions to provide some indication of intra- and interanimal variability. The use of liquid preservatives such as toluene and mineral oil is not recommended for the majority of urine collections; sodium azide may be used to inhibit bacterial growth in longer-term urine collections. The collection vessel may be chilled with ice for some urine collections, particularly enzymes. When metabolic cages are used, diet food should be removed to reduce sample contamination; additionally, water intake may be restricted. Water loading by gavage is not recommended for general studies. When food and/or water is restricted, the procedures should be designed so as not to cause significant body weight loss, and the procedures should meet the local requirements for animal care. All urine samples should be thoroughly mixed following collection.

4.3.2.2   Urine Color and Appearance

Although it is valuable to record abnormal colors and appearance, recording the varying yellow shades of urine due to urochromes adds little value. The majority (>95%) of urine will appear as shades of yellow in color; some appearing brownish if contaminated with feces. Urine of watery appearance may be due to contamination from water bottle spillage. Abnormal urine colors may be due to the xenobiotics (e.g., orange with rifamicin) or administered dyes (e.g., methylene blue). Red colors may be due to hematuria or porphyria, and urine may appear brown when methemoglobin is present. Some compounds impart fluorescence to the urine. Urine turbidity is generally associated with phosphates and urates, and if the urine is turbid and brownish in appearance, it often reflects fecal contamination. Crystalluria due to xenobiotics or metabolites is sometimes found on visual inspection.

4.3.2.3   Urine Volume

Urine volume on timed period collections should always be recorded, and water intake data or clinical observations of increased drinking must always be considered when interpreting changes of urine volumes. Excessive fluid loss by vomitus or diarrhea also will affect urine output. Some laboratories use additional water loads to achieve urine collection, but enforced diuresis can alter the excretion of urinary enzymes and metabolites.

4.3.2.4   Osmolality or Specific Gravity Determined by Refractometry

Osmolality is dependent on the number of particles present in solution; it is measured by freezing point depression or vapor pressure and results are expressed as milliosmoles per kilogram of body water (Sweeney and Beauchat 1993). When urine and plasma osmolality measurements are available, the plasma-to-urine ratio can be used as a broad indication of the glomerular filtrate to urine ratio. Handheld refractometers are used to measure the urinary refractive index, which is then converted to specific gravity (SG) using calibrated scales (George 2001). The SG values for most laboratory animal urine lie in the range of 1.015–1.050. SG measurements using test strips are unsuitable for laboratory animals (Allchin and Evans 1986; Allchin et al. 1987).

4.3.2.5 Urine Test Strips

Several of these screening tests are performed using test strips (dipsticks) designed for use with human urine, and it should not be assumed that these tests perform in exactly the same way with urine collected from laboratory animals. The presence of oxidizing or reducing agents may affect the glucose and blood test strips using a peroxidase-based method, and several xenobiotics can give false positive or negative reactions with other areas of the test strips. Oxidizing or reducing agents can interfere with the diazotization reaction used for urobilinogen, bilirubin, and leukocytes by producing a color different from the expected positive reaction results.

Some test strips detect the presence of leukocytes indicated by positive nitrite reactions. The reading times of the test strips are critical, and observer error is reduced by using automated test strip readers. This enforces the timing required to read results after dipping the strips into urine. Significant delays in reading test strips after dipping them into urine can lead to false positive results for protein, blood, glucose, and pH. Most manufacturers of test strips give some information on the limitations of these measurements.

4.3.2.5.1 Protein

The urinary protein composition varies between species. Albumin is the major urinary protein in dogs and nonhuman primates, but in male rats the major urinary protein is alpha$_{2u}$-globulin. Mice have differing protein patterns (Finlayson and Baumann 1958; Roy and Neuhaus 1967; Groen and Lagerwerf 1979; Adams and Sawyer 1990; Cavaggioni and Mucignat-Caretta 2000). After puberty, male rats excrete more proteins than females, and the amount of protein increases with age (Neuhaus and Flory 1978; Alt et al. 1980). Most test strips have a lower limit of detection of approximately 300 mg/L protein and are designed to detect albumin, so these test strips are insensitive to the major urinary proteins (MUPs) in rodents and are unable to detect minor glomerular or tubular proteinuria (Evans and Parsons 1986). Urine samples with high concentrations of ammonia or high bacterial content can cause high alkalinity, leading to false positive results for protein.

4.3.2.5.2 Glucose

Glucosuria may be detected using test strips using glucose oxidase methods, although these may be affected by several interferents, including endogenous ascorbate (Taylor and Neal 1982). Quantitative methods can be used to confirm the presence and degree of glycosuria. The glucose filtered through the glomeruli is normally reabsorbed in the renal proximal tubules, and urinary glucose is present in trace amounts. When there is profound hyperglycemia, urinary glucose will increase as the active transport reabsorption mechanisms are overloaded, or urinary glucose may be increased due to impaired reabsorption by the proximal tubules.

4.3.2.5.3   Blood

A positive test strip result for the presence of blood that is not accompanied by the intact red blood cells (detected by microscopy) suggests the presence of free hemoglobin or myoglobin. This can be supported by the hematologic findings and the presence of free hemoglobin in plasma, or when free hemoglobin is absent, myoglobinuria may be present. Delays in analyzing urine may lead to the lysis of intact red blood cells, particularly in alkaline urine. Blood contamination of urine samples from intravenous lines, bites, and superficial injuries on paws, etc. should always be considered as a possible explanation for blood in urine. Hematuria associated with proteinuria suggests a glomerular change, although these findings can occur when there is severe proximal tubular injury.

4.3.2.5.4   Hydrogen Ion Concentration, pH

Despite the introduction of SI unitage (Appendix B), many investigators prefer to use pH values for urine. Bacterial growth may increase urinary pH if analyses are delayed. For critical decisions concerning pH, measurements should be made using a pH meter in preference to a reagent strip or dipstick (Heuter, Buffington, and Chew 1998). Urinary pH values for rodents tend to be on the alkaline side of pH 7, whereas canine urine tends to be below a pH of 7.

The pH of urine is dependent on the cationic and anionic composition, with the cationic products of normal metabolism buffered by the renal handling of bicarbonate and dietary protein content affecting urinary pH. In catabolic states associated with severe toxicity, the urinary pH may be lowered. Thus, changes of pH may reflect major metabolic perturbations, changes in tubular function, or the presence of xenobiotics and/or their metabolites in urine.

4.3.2.6   Urinary Sediment and Celluria

Crystals may be detected microscopically in urine sediments and their presence is largely pH dependent (e.g., phosphates or urates); the degree of crystalluria often increases on storage at lower temperatures. Crystalluria may be due to high concentrations of a xenobiotic or metabolite, where their solubility in urine has been exceeded (Izzedine et al. 2005). With some xenobiotic-induced crystalluria, the crystals are not observed in renal sections because of their solubilization during tissue processing, although there may be evidence of histological injury.

Microscopic examination of urine sediment may reveal the presence of erythrocytes, leucocytes, renal epithelial cells, bladder cells, spermatozoa, etc. The sediment may be examined unstained or stained to help distinguish renal epithelial cells and leucocytes (Prescott and Brodie 1964; Hardy 1970; Gheilli et al. 1998). The methodologies used for the collection, centrifugation, and preparation of urine deposits for semiquantitative analyses are not standardized, often relying on a final semiquantitative resuspension of sediment prior to subjective microscopic examination. The background findings of celluria differ from one species to another, and these findings are also dependent on the collection procedures; celluria is increased by some invasive collection techniques. Bacteria, occasional parasites, and evidence of feces, hair, and food may also be found in the urine sediment. Occasionally, fat droplets may be observed, and it should be established that these droplets are not due to a lubricating agent used for catheterization.

Celluria can indicate proximal tubular injury (Davies and Kennedy 1967; Prescott and Ansari 1969), but it does not occur in every case. Celluria may occur after an initial delay following dosing peak and then be absent even during continued treatment or rechallenge. Cellular examinations do not appear to be useful when investigating chronic tubular injury and acute distal tubular damage except to confirm hematuria.

4.3.3 Urinary Enzymes and Proteins

The second tier of tests is often implemented when there is suspicion or evidence of a nephrotoxic effect gained either from the initial urinalysis or histopathology. The focus is mainly on characterizing and identifying the affected regions of the using proteins, enzymes, electrolytes, or metabolites. A combination of protein, enzyme, and metabolite measurements can help to localize the site of renal injury.

4.3.3.1 Stability

Urine pH, temperature, and the presence of inhibitors can have adverse effects on urinary enzymes and proteins, and contradictory evidence has been published concerning cold storage effects on proteins including albumin and low molecular weight proteins (e.g., beta$_2$-microglobulin) (Schultz et al. 2000). Levels of several enzymes (e.g., urine GGT) fall rapidly when frozen (Stokke 1974) and urine GST enzymes require the addition of stabilizers to retain their activities (Matteucci et al. 1991; Matteucci and Giampietro 1994; Berg et al. 1998). Ideally, urine samples should not be frozen and should be analyzed promptly to avoid any protein degradation. Again, it is essential to minimize contamination of urine samples for these additional measurements of enzymes, proteins, and electrolytes; fecal contamination of urine can cause increases of enzyme (see Figure 4.1; Plummer and Wright 1970), protein, and electrolyte values.

4.3.3.2 Proteins

Various proteins occur normally in urine, but the term *proteinuria* is used generally to indicate increased urine protein content. Proteinuria is a consequence of the glomerular filtration of plasma proteins, reabsorption of the filtered proteins in the renal tubules, and protein secretion in the tubular and distal urinary tract.

The urine proteins may be divided into low molecular weight (LMW) and high molecular weight (HMW) proteins, although there is no strict definition for this classification. Many of the LMW proteins have a molecular mass of less than 50 kDa and include beta$_2$-microglobulin, alpha$_1$-microglobulin, retinol binding protein, and cystatin C. Some of the proteins of interest are listed in Table 4.2.

The glomerular filtration barrier generally restricts the filtration of protein molecules that are larger than albumin (68 kDa), but it allows the LMW proteins to be filtered. In the proximal renal tubule, filtered proteins are reabsorbed by endocytosis and the megalin/cubulin transport systems. Although albumin is primarily filtered by the glomeruli and excreted unchanged, endocytosis and the lysosomal production of albumin fragments also occur. Uromodulin (also known

TABLE 4.2
Some Proteins and Their Approximate Molecular Masses

Protein	Molecular Mass, kDa	Protein	Molecular Mass, kDa
Beta-2-microglobulin	11.8	Transferrin	66
Cystatin	13	Albumin	68
Myoglobin	14	Uromodulin (Tamm–Horsfall glycoprotein)	85
Lysozyme (muramidase)	14.5	Immunoglobulin G	150
Alpha-$_{2u}$-globulin	18	Alpha-2-macroglobulin	720
Retinol binding protein	21 .5	Immunoglobulin M	900
Alpha-1-microglobuln	31		
Alpha-2-microglobulin	30		

as Tamm–Horsfall mucoprotein) is a specific renal protein with a molecular monomeric mass of 85 kDa that is localized on the membrane of the thick part of the loop of Henlé. This protein forms large aggregates in the urine (Gokhale, Glenton, and Khan 1997; Raila, Forterre, and Schweigert 2005; Devuyst, Dahan, and Pirson 2005).

Albumin is the major urinary protein in many species; however, rodents have other MUPs that exhibit polymorphism. These proteins are synthesized by the liver and filtered into the urine of adult male mice and rats; adult female rats excrete much smaller amounts of these proteins. Alpha$_{2u}$-globulin found in male rat urine with a molecular mass of approximately 18 kDa is freely filtered at the glomerulus and can be reabsorbed in the proximal tubule. This protein is also found in female rat urine, but at much lower concentrations. Proteinuria is common among aging rats as a result of progressive nephropathy, and this may complicate interpretation of results during the second year of a chronic study.

Although test strips offer a simple method of assessing albuminuria, they do not detect changes of LMW urine proteins. A quantitative method for total urinary proteins and some assessment of the relative proportion and size of the urine proteins should be made.

4.3.3.2.1 Quantitative Measurement of Total Urinary Protein
Of a number of quantitative methods for estimating total urinary protein (Pesce 1974; McElderry, Tarbit, and Cassells-Smith 1982; Dilena, Penberthy, and Fraser 1983), several are subject to interference from xenobiotics. No single method is ideal because all suffer from a lack of sensitivity to increased low molecular weight proteins. However, methods using pyrogallol red appear to be robust, although they are affected by the inclusion of sodium dodecyl sulfate as a solubilizer (Le Bricon 2001).

Several of the individual urinary proteins (e.g., albumin, immunoglobulins) can be measured by quantitative immunochemical methods when suitable antisera and calibration proteins are available (Woo et al. 1978; Bernard, Vyskocil, and Lauwerys

1981; Viau et al. 1986; Pressler et al. 2002). By measuring several specific proteins of different molecular sizes, the proteinuria can, to some extent, be characterized as glomerular or tubular in origin (Maachi et al. 2004).

4.3.3.2.2 Electrophoretic Separation of Proteins

A variety of methods is available using different electrophoretic support media and buffers (Boesken et al. 1973; Allchin and Evans 1986; Kshirsagar and Wiggins 1986; Stonard et al. 1987; Bianchi-Bosisio et al. 1991; Hofmann et al. 1992; Kolaja et al. 1992), which can be used to identify the relative proportions of high and low molecular mass proteins. Some investigators express the proportions of LMW and HMW proteins as a ratio to help in characterizing the proteinuric pattern. This further testing can be performed by several available separation techniques: methods using unidirectional agarose electrophoresis or sodium dodecyl sulfate/polyacrylamide gel electrophoresis (SDS-PAGE) are convenient techniques.

Thus, proteinuria may be due to an alteration in the structural integrity of the glomerular filtration barrier, injury to the tubular cells, saturation of the reabsorptive mechanisms of the tubular cells, injury to other parts of the renal tract, protein overload from the plasma (e.g., myoglobinuria in acute renal failure following rhabdomyolysis), or renal hemodynamic effects at the glomeruli (Bernard and Lauwerys 1991; Schurek 1994). The broad patterns of proteinuria may be summarized as

glomerular proteinuria, with increased albumin reflecting the changes of glomerular filtration;

tubular proteinuria, with increased excretion of LMW proteins reflecting changes in the tubular reabsorption and secretion of LMW proteins, which may be adaptive responses or indicative of tubular injury;

mixed proteinuria, reflecting both glomerular and tubular changes;

selective glomerular proteinuria;

selective LMW proteinuria (e.g., myoglobinuria); and

other proteinurias, with proteins derived from within the nephron, sometimes associated with increased cellular or cell fragment proteins, hematuria, or uromodulin.

High levels of protein in the urine may also be associated with the presence of casts; hyaline casts contain protein alone, and cellular casts consist of aggregated erythrocytes, leukocytes, or epithelial cells. The formation of some casts is associated with uromodulin.

All of the information obtained on the amounts and patterns of urinary proteins should be interpreted, together with plasma measurements—particularly for evidence of glomerular filtration changes—and altered hepatic protein synthesis. For example, loss of large amounts of urinary albumin may result in hypoalbuminemia, or the hypoalbumineamia may reflect reduced hepatic synthesis with no evidence of marked changes of renal clearance of albumin.

4.3.3.2.3   Other Techniques for Evaluation of Urinary Proteins:
Proteomics and Renal Cell Antigens

Proteomic studies extend the characterization of the pattern of urinary excretion by measuring the relative abundance of many additional proteins not separated by simpler electrophoretic techniques and identifying more of these proteins by mass and immunochemistry (Hampel et al. 2001; Nedlekov and Nelson 2001; Bandara et al. 2003; Idborg-Björkman et al. 2003; Thongboonkerd and Klein 2003; Forterre, Raila, and Schweigert 2004; Hewitt, Dear, and Star 2004; Witzmann and Li 2004). Although considerable investment and effort have been made in proteomics, very few additional markers of renal toxicity that can be measured by less expensive technologies have been developed.

In addition to the specific protein measurements, studies using monoclonal antibodies to antigenic structures in rat proximal and distal tubules, papillary and cortical collecting ducts, and the loop of Henlé have been evaluated (Bomhard, Falkenberg, and Loof 1994; Hildebrand et al. 1999). The excretion of some of these antigens can be performed by enzyme-linked immunoassays, but these assays have not been widely evaluated.

Some proteins identified more recently that have yet to be evaluated widely as potential markers include renal papillary antigen 1 (RPA-1), Kim-1 (Han et al. 2002; Ichimura et al. 2004), and apolipoprotein-J (Clusterin), a sulfated glycoprotein (Aulitzky et al. 1992; Eti et al. 1993) generally distributed in the nephron, and neutrophil gelatinase associated lipocalin (NGal: an alpha-2-microglobulin of approximately 22–25 kDa).

4.3.3.3   Enzymes

A few urinary enzymes have been found to be useful as potential markers of kidney dysfunction, although more than 40 enzymes have been evaluated (Raab 1972) and plasma enzyme measurements have little value in detecting nephrotoxicity. The choice of urine enzyme measurements should be based on the location of the enzyme along the nephron and the intracellular location of the enzyme (e.g., lysosomal, mitochondrial, cytoplasm, or the cellular brush border). The distribution of enzymes is associated with differing cell types, but there is considerable overlap in their regional distribution (Amador et al. 1963; Heinle, Wendel, and Schmidt 1977; Lehir, Dubach, and Guder 1980; Guder and Ross 1984; Bomhard et al. 1990). Many of the enzymes studied for the detection of nephrotoxicity show higher concentrations in the proximal tubules and cortex than in the renal papilla and cortex; with lower levels in the medulla, this has limited the use of many enzymes in identifying these specific regions. The enzymes may be partially divided into those associated with lysosomes, cytoplasm, microsomes, and the cellular brush border. Most urinary enzymes with a molecular mass greater than albumin have a renal tubular origin, although many of these enzymes are found in plasma but not used to monitor glomerular injury (Lovett et al. 1982). When only urinary enzymes of cytoplasmic origin are increased and there is no evidence of lysosomal or brush border enzymes increasing, this may be due to an adaptive response rather than a response to injury.

Several reviews of urinary enzymes and their use in assessing nephrotoxicity have been published (Raab 1972, 1980; Mattenheimer 1977; Stroo and Hook 1977; Price 1982; Hofmeister, Bhargava, and Gunzel 1986; Jung, Mattenheimer, and Burchardt 1992; Clemo 1998; Turecky and Uhlikova 2003), as well as many studies (Plaa and Larson 1965; Prescott and Ansari 1969; Wright, Leathwood, and Plummer 1972; Ellis, Price, and Topham 1973; Wright and Plummer 1974; Ellis and Price 1975; Plummer, Leathwood, and Blake 1975; Cottrell et al. 1976; Bhargava, Khater, and Gunzel 1978; Whiting and Brown 1996; Marchewka and Dugosz 1998; Bomhard, Maruhn, and Rinke 1999).

The flow rate can affect the measurement of urine enzymes, proteins, and metabolites. Diuresis increases enzymuria, which may reflect incomplete reabsorption of these enzymes (Jung, Schultz, and Reinholdt 1986). Water loading (i.e., additional water given by gavage) can increase urine flow, but it can also introduce effects due to diuresis and is an additional experimental procedure. Several enzymes show diurnal and temporal variations (Pariat et al. 1990) and this, together with differing temporal responses to dosing reference, makes the timings for urine collection periods important. Urine collection at several time points after dosing provides valuable information of the site of injury and mechanisms of toxic injury, together with information on glomerular function and urine protein excretion patterns.

Some urinary enzymes are inhibited by endogenous molecules in the urine, and these inhibitors require removal by gel filtration, dialysis, or ultrafiltration prior to analysis (Werner, Maruhn, and Atoba 1969; Werner and Gabrielson 1977). In some instances, the effects of inhibitors are reduced by the use of smaller sample volumes in proportion to the reagent volume, compared to the methods used in older studies. The distribution of enzymes may vary between the cellular sediment and supernatant, and here the cellular enzymes may be released by sonication.

Urine enzyme values may be expressed per liter or per collection period or be adjusted by using urine creatinine. The calculation based on creatinine makes broad assumptions that creatinine accurately reflects urine concentration and is relatively constant. The second assumption is incorrect because tubular secretion of creatinine may change and result in an overestimation of enzyme values where urine creatinine is reduced (Jung 1991).

Interferences with the enzyme measurements due to xenobiotics can be a potential problem when the compound is present in high concentrations in the urine sample. To eliminate this as a potential effect, urine from animals not receiving the test compound can be spiked with the compound and the mixture examined for potential effects.

In most studies, a combination of more than two or three enzymes has provided better information than the measurement of a single enzyme, with measurements based on regional and cellular location. Urinary enzymes have been particularly useful in detection of acute renal damage and, specifically, proximal tubular damage; however, they are correspondingly less valuable in providing information about chronic injury.

Although increased excretion of some enzymes appears to be a measure of nephrotoxicity, there is no current agreement on which enzymes should be measured in animal studies. In published studies, the enzymes that have been measured more frequently include:

cytosolic
lactate dehydrogenase (LDH) (an enzyme that has a widespread renal
   distribution)
proximal tubular brush border enzymes
   alanine aminopeptidase (AAP)
   leucine arylamidase
   gamma glutamyl transferase (GGT: also microsomal)
   alpha-glutathione S-transferase (YaYc GST)
distal tubular enzyme
   rat tau-glutathione S-transferase (Yb1, GST)
lysosomal enzyme
   N-acetyl-beta-glucosaminidase (NAG)

Although the aminotransferases AST and ALT are present in urine, they have not proved to be useful in monitoring nephrotoxic effects. The measurement of lysozyme (muramidase), which could be useful in monitoring lysosomal protein turnover, is limited by changes during urinary tract and other infections because this enzyme is secreted from phagocytic cells, macrophages, and monocytes. Therefore, it is an equivocal marker.

The glutathione S-transferases have been reported to increase in a number of acute studies, but the enzymes have short half-lives and are unstable, requiring stabilizers to be added prior to analysis (Bomhard et al. 1990; Saduka, Shimuzi, and Takino 1994; Sundberg et al. 1994; Moser et al. 1995; Kharash et al. 1998; Kilty et al. 1998; Usuda et al. 1999; Dote et al. 2000). Some markers may be specific for smaller segments of nephron. Intestinal alkaline phosphatase (IALP) shows specificity for the S3 segment of proximal tubules (Wright et al. 1972; Nuyts, Verpooten, and de Broe 1992), but this test has not been widely applied in animals, and in renal tissue other alkaline phosphatases are widely distributed. In rats with mercury nephropathy at low dosages, the S3 segment was affected and IALP increased, but at higher dosages the tubular injury spread to the preceding two segments and IALP was not useful as a segmental marker (Diamond and Zalups 1998).

Among the various published observations for enzyme measurements, evidence has been provided for several enzymes; however, none of these suggestions have been widely applied. These observations include the differing distributions of LDH and NAG isoenzymes along the nephron; these have also been suggested as regional markers of nephron toxicity used to differentiate between proximal and distal tubular injury (Bomhard et al. 1990; Morita et al. 1998).

There are marked sex differences for urinary N-acetyl-beta-glucosaminidase (NAG), with higher values in male mice and dogs (Funakawa et al. 1984; Grotsch et al. 1985; Clemo 1998). NAG is found in the proximal tubules, papilla, glomerulus, and plasma, but it remains a useful enzyme for detecting nephrotoxicity (Price 1982). Renal papillary toxicity is often accompanied by large volumes of dilute urine and increased N-acetyl-beta-glucosaminidase excretion prior to any subsequent effects on renal tubules (Ellis and Price 1975; Bach and Hardy 1985; Stonard et al. 1987).

4.3.4   WATER DEPRIVATION AND CONCENTRATION TESTS

When the body is deprived of water for a period exceeding several hours, the urinary osmolality and SG normally increase as the body tries to conserve fluid; however, these indices do not increase to the same extent when there is tubular dysfunction, Conversely, when the body accumulates water or the animal is given a water load, the osmolality and SG normally decrease along with an increase in urine flow.

In severe tubular disease, the urine tends to remain at a uniform solute concentration, irrespective of whether the urine is formed under conditions of water deficit or excess. Using plasma and urine osmolality measurements, a concentration or dilution test can measure the capacity of the distal tubules, the loop of Henlé, and the action of antidiuretic hormones to respond to water loading or deprivation by the ability or inability of an animal to concentrate urine (Sharratt and Fraser 1963; Diezi and Biollaz 1979; Kluwe 1981). The procedures should be designed so that the dehydration period does not cause severe changes of body weight and meets local regulations for animal welfare (Kulick et al. 2005). When animals are given a water load, osmolality and SG normally decrease along with an increase in urine volume. When there is tubular dysfunction, there is little or minor change of these measurements, but the water loading test is less useful than the water deprivation test. General observations in the animal house on water intake and urination patterns sometimes can indicate renal tubular changes.

4.3.5   OTHER TESTS OF TUBULAR DYSFUNCTION

Quantitative measurements of osmolality and electrolytes provide a useful second tier of tests for distal proximal tubular injury because tubular dysfunction may be associated with changes in the excretion of glucose, sodium, potassium, calcium, phosphate, amino acids, and organic acids. The latter two have received particular attention through nuclear magnetic resonance (NMR) spectroscopy technology. Quantitative glucose measurements can confirm test strip findings of glucosuria.

4.3.6   RENAL PLASMA FLOW

Several techniques using injected substances such as radiolabeled ortho-iodohippurate, p-aminohippurate, or tetraethylammonium bromide are available to determine renal plasma flow (Tune, Burg, and Patlak 1969; Mann and Kinter 1993). However, they are not suitable for inclusion in general toxicity studies. These compounds, filtered by the glomeruli and secreted by the renal proximal tubules, provide an estimate of total renal plasma flow. Because some of the blood passing through the kidneys flows through other tissues such as the medulla and capsular regions, the measurements are, in effect, of plasma flow to the cortex and are therefore termed the effective renal plasma flow (ERPF).

4.3.7 OTHER TUBULAR FUNCTION TESTS

The administration of tetraethylammonium (TEA) and the organic anionic phenol-sufonphthalein (PSP) can be used as indices of cationic tubular transport systems (Klaassen and Plaa 1966). However, these tests are not included in general toxicity studies. Again, these tests require administration of the compound and carefully timed sample collections (Poutsiaka et al. 1962).

4.3.8 METABONOMICS

These studies use proton NMR spectroscopy to measure amino acids and other metabolites. The changes of the individual components of the NMR profile can yield information on the regional effects in the kidney (Holmes, Bonner, and Nicholson 1997; Holmes et al. 1998; Lindon, Holmes, and Nicholson 2004; Robertson et al. 2005). Several investigators have applied principal component analysis to improve the identification of affected regions of the nephron. As for other renal tests, the timing and collection procedures are critical to the application; in addition, several of the measured metabolites are affected by other organ toxicities, particularly hepatotoxicity.

REFERENCES

Structure, Physiology, and Biochemistry

Berndt, W. O. 1976. Renal function tests: What do they mean? A review of renal anatomy, biochemistry and physiology. *Environmental Health Perspectives* 15:55–71.

Beuchat, C. A. 1990a. Metabolism and the scaling of urine concentrating ability in mammals: Resolution of a paradox? *Journal of Theoretical Biology* 143:113–122.

———.1990b. Body size, medullary thickness and urine concentrating ability in mammals. *American Journal of Physiology* 258:R298–308.

Câmpean, V., F. Theilig, A. Paliege, M. Breyer, and S. Bachmann. 2003. Key enzymes for renal prostaglandin synthesis: Site-specific expression in rodent kidney (rat, mouse). *American Journal of Physiology* 285:F19–32.

Corman, B., J. Pratz, and P. Poujeol. 1985. Changes in the anatomy, glomerular filtration rate and solute excretion in aging rat kidney. *American Journal of Physiology* 248:282–287.

Davies, B., and T. Morris. 1993. Physiological parameters in laboratory animals and humans. *Pharmaceutical Research* 10:1093–1095.

Gonzalez, J. D., M. T. Llinas, E. Nava, L. Ghiadoni, and F. J. Salazar. 1998. Role of nitric oxide and prostaglandins in the long-term control of renal function. *Hypertension* 32:33–38.

Harris, K. 1992. The role of prostaglandins in the control of renal function. *British Journal of Anesthesiology* 69:233–235.

Inui, K. I., S. Masuda, and H. Saito. 2000. Cellular and molecular aspects of drug transport in the kidney. *Kidney International* 58:944–958.

Knepper, M. A., C-L. Chou, and H. E. Layton. 1993. How urine is concentrated by the renal inner medulla. In *Moving points in nephrology. Contributions in nephrology,* vol. 102, pp.144–160. Basel, Switzerland: Karger.

Lash, L. H. 2005. Role of glutathione transport processes in kidney function. *Toxicology and Applied Pharmacology* 204:392–342.

Lund, U., A. Rippe, D. Venturoli, O. Tenstad, A. Grubb, and B. Rippe. 2003. Glomerular filtration rate dependence of sieving of albumin and some neutral proteins in rat kidneys. *American Journal of Physiology* 284:F1226–1234.

Marshansky, V., S. Bourgoin, I. Londono, M. Bendayan, B. Maranda, and P. Vinay. 1997. Receptor-mediated endocytosis in kidney proximal tubules: Recent advances and hypothesis. *Electrophoresis* 18:2661–2676.

Masereeuw, R., and F. G. Russel. 2001. Mechanisms and clinical implications of renal drug excretion. *Drug Metabolism Reviews* 33:299–351.

Parekh, N., A. P. Zou, I. Jungling, K. Endlich, J. Sadowksi, and M. Steinhausen. 1993. Sex differences in control of renal outer medullary circulation in rats: Role of prostaglandins. *American Journal of Physiology* 264:F629–636.

Russo, L. M., G. L. Bakris, and W. D. Comper. 2002. Renal handling of albumin: A critical review of basic concepts and perspective. *American Journal of Kidney Disease* 39:899–919.

Schmidt-Nielsen, B., and R. O'Dell. 1961. Structure and concentrating mechanism in the mammalian kidney. *American Journal of Physiology* 200:1119–1124.

Renal Toxicity

Alden, C. L. 1986. A review of unique male rat hydrocarbon nephropathy. *Toxicologic Pathology* 14:109–111.

Bach, P. H., D. J. Scholey, L. Delacruz, M. Moret, and S. Nichol. 1991. Renal and urinary lipid changes associated with an acutely induced renal papillary necrosis in rats. *Food and Chemcal Toxicology* 29:211–219.

Bach, P. H., and T. K. Thanh. 1998. Renal papillary necrosis—40 years on. *Toxicologic Pathology* 26:73–91.

Bendayan, R. 1996. Renal drug transport. *Pharmacotherapy* 1996:971–985.

Borghoff, S. J., B. G. Short, and J. A. Swenberg. 1990. Biochemical mechanisms and pathobiology of alpha-2u-globulin nephropathy. *Annual Review of Pharmacology and Toxicology* 30:349–367.

Commandeur, J. N., and N. P. Vermeulen. 1990. Molecular and biochemical mechanisms of chemically induced nephrotoxicity: A review. *Chemical Research in Toxicology* 3:171–194.

Dantzler, W. H., and S. H. Wright. 1997. Renal tubular secretion of organic anions. *Advanced Drug Delivery Reviews* 25:217–230.

Diamond, G. L., and R. K. Zalups. 1998. Understanding renal toxicity of heavy metals. *Toxicologic Pathology* 26:92–103.

Endou, H. 1998. Recent advances in molecular mechanisms of nephrotoxicity. *Toxicology Letters* 102–103:29–33.

Goldstein, R. 1994. *Mechanisms of injury in renal disease and toxicity.* Boca Raton, FL: CRC Press.

Ichikawa, I., S. Kiyama, and T. Yoshioka. 1994. Renal antioxidant enzymes: Their regulation and function. *Kidney International* 45:1–9.

Izzedine, H., V. Launay-Vacher, and G. Deray. 2005. Antiviral drug-induced nephrotoxicity. *American Journal of Kidney Disease* 45:804–817.

Lehman-McKeeman, L. D., and D. Caudill. 1992. Biochemical basis for mouse resistance to hyaline droplet nephropathy: Lack of relevance of the α_{2u}-globulin protein superfamily in this male rat specific syndrome. *Toxicology and Applied Pharmacology* 112:214–221.

Lock, E. A., M. Charbonneau, J. Strasser, J. A. Swenberg, and J. S. Bus. 1987. 2,2,4-Trimethylpentane-induced nephropathy. II. The reversible binding of a TMP metabolite to a renal protein fraction containing alpha-2u globulin. *Toxicology and Applied Pharmacology* 91:182–192.

Piperno, E., 1981. Detection of drugs induced nephrotoxicity with urinalysis and enzymuria assessment. In *Toxicology of the kidney,* ed. J. B. Hook, pp. 31–55. New York: Raven Press.

Pritchard, J. B., and D. S. Miller. 1997. Renal secretion of organic cations: A multistep process. *Advanced Drug Delivery Reviews* 25:231–242.

Russel, F. G., R. Masereeuw, and R. A. Van Aubel. 2002. Molecular aspects of renal anionic drug transport. *Annual Review of Physiology* 64:563–594.

Takano, M., N. Nakanishi, Y. Kitahara, Y.Sasaki, T. Murakami, and J. Nagai. 2002. Cisplatin-induced inhibition of receptor-mediated endocytosis of protein in the kidney. *Kidney International* 62:1707–1717.

Tarloff, J. B., and L. H. Lash. 2004. *Toxicology of the kidney. Target organ toxicology series,* 3rd ed. Boca Raton, FL: CRC Press.

Theilemann, L. E., R. A. Rodrigo, and L. A. Videla. 1999. Changes in antioxidant enzyme activities and lipid peroxidation related to bromoethylamine-induced renal toxicity. *Archives of Medical Research* 30:14–18.

Laboratory Assessment

Bernard, A., H. Stolte, M. E. de Broe, P. W. Mueller, H. Mason, L. H. Lash, and B. A. Fowler. 1997. Urinary biomarkers to detect significant effects of environmental and occupational exposure to nephrotoxins. IV. Current information on interpreting the health implications of tests. *Renal Failure* 19:553–556.

Bovee, K. C. 1986. Renal function and laboratory evaluation. *Toxicologic Pathology* 14: 26–26.

Fent, K., E. Mayer, and G. Zbinden. 1988. Nephrotoxicity screening in rats: A validation study. *Archives of Toxicology* 61:349–358.

Kluwe, W. M. 1981. Renal function tests as indicators of kidney injury in subacute toxicity studies. *Toxicology and Applied Pharmacology* 57:414–424.

Lauwerys, R., and A. Bernard. 1989. Preclinical detection of nephrotoxicity: Description of the test and appraisal of their health significance. *Toxicology Letters* 46:13–29.

Loeb, W. F. 1998. The measurement of renal injury. *Toxicologic Pathology* 26:26–28.

Mueller, P. W., L. Lash, R. G. Price, H. Stolte, E. Geipi, J. Maack, and W. O. Berndt. 1997. Urinary biomarkers to detect significant effects of environmental and occupational exposure to nephrotoxins. 1. Categories of tests for detecting effects of nephrotoxins. *Renal Failure* 19:505–521.

Mueller, P. W., R. G. Price, and G. A. Porter. 1997. Proceedings of the Joint US/EU workshop: Urinary biomarkers to detect significant effects of environmental and occupational exposure to nephrotoxins. *Renal Failure* 19:501–504.

Price, R. G. 1982. Urinary enzymes, nephrotoxicity and renal disease. *Toxicology* 23:99–134.

———. 2002. Early markers of nephrotoxicity. *Comparative Clinical Pathology* 11:2–7.

Price, R. G. et al. 1996. Development and validation of new screening tests for nephrotoxic effects. *Human and Experimental Toxicology* 15 (Suppl. 1): S10–19.

Price, R. G. et al. 1999. Urinary biomarkers: Roles in risk assessment to environmental and occupational nephrotoxins: Monitoring of effects and evaluation of mechanisms of toxicity. *Renal Failure* 21:3–4; xiii–xviii.

Price, R. G. 2000. Urinalysis to exclude and monitor nephrotoxicity. *Clinica Chimica Acta* 297:173–182.

Raab, H. 1998. Evaluation of urinary markers in acute renal failure. *Current Opinion in Nephrology and Hypertension* 7:681–685.

Stonard, M. D. 1990. Assessment of renal function and damage in animal species. *Journal of Applied Toxicology* 10:267–274.

———. 1996. Assessment of nephrotoxicity. In *Animal clinical chemistry. A primer for toxicologists,* ed. G. O. Evans, pp. 87–98. London: Taylor & Francis Ltd.

Zalups, R. K., and L. H. Lash. 1996. *Methods in renal toxicology.* Boca Raton, FL: CRC Press.

Plasma Creatinine, Urea, Cystatin C, and GFR

Almy, F. S., M. M. Christopher, D. P. King, and S. A. Brown. 2002. Evaluation of cystatin C as an endogenous marker of glomerular filtration rate in dog. *Journal of Veterinary Internal Medicine* 16:45–51.

Bøkenkamp, A., G. Ciarimboli, and C. Dieterich. 2001. Cystatin C in a rat model of end-stage renal failure. *Renal Failure* 23:431–438.

Braun, J-P., H. P. Lefebvre, and A. D. J. Watson. 2003. Creatinine in the dog: A review. *Veterinary Clinical Pathology* 32:162–176.

Braun, J-P., A. Perxachs, D. Péchereau, and F. de La Farge. 2002. Plasma cystatin C in the dog: Reference values and variations with renal failure. *Comparative Clinical Pathology* 11:44–49.

Corman, B., J. Pratz, and P. Poujeol. 1985. Changes in the anatomy, glomerular filtration rate and solute excretion in aging rat kidney. *American Journal of Physiology* 248:282–287.

Cronin, R. E., R. E. Bulger, P. Southern, and W. L. Henrich. 1980. Natural history of amonoglycoside nehrotoxicity in the dog. *Journal of Laboratory and Medical Medicine* 95:463–474.

Curhan, G. 2005. Cystatin C: A marker of renal function or something more? *Clinical Chemistry* 51:293–294.

Delanghe, J., J. Bellon, M. De Buyzere, G. Van Daele, and G. Leorux-Roels.1991. Elimination of glucose interference in enzymatic determination of inulin. *Clinical Chemistry* 37:2017–2018.

DiMeola, H. J., N. J. Siegel, J. M. Kaufman, and J. P. Hayslett. 1974. Evaluation of the constant-infusion technique to determine inulin clearance in the rat. *Journal of Applied Physiology* 36:261.

Evans, G. O. 1986. The use of an enzymatic kit to measure plasma creatinine in the mouse and three other species. *Comparative Biochemistry and Physiology* 85B:193–195.

———. 1987. Postprandial changes in canine plasma creatinine. *Journal of Small Animal Practice* 28:311–315.

Finco, D. R., D. B. Coulter, and J. A. Barsanti. 1981. Simple, accurate method for clinical estimation of glomerular filtration rate in the dog. *American Journal of Veterinary Research* 42:1874–1877.

Goldstein, R. S. 1990. Drug-induced nephrotoxicity in middle-aged and senescent rats. In *Basic science in toxicology,* ed. G. N. Volans, J. Sims, F. M. Sullivan, and P. Turner, pp. 412–421. London: Taylor & Francis.

Gray, J. E. 1977. Chronic nephrosis in the albino rat. *CRC Critical Reviews in Toxicology* 5:115–144.

Grotsch, H., and P. Hajdu. 1987. Interference by the new antibiotic cefipirome and other cephalosporins in clinical laboratory tests, with specific regard to the Jaffe reaction. *Journal of Clinical Chemistry and Clinical Biochemistry* 25:49–52.

Jung, K., C. Wesslau, F. Priem, G. Schreiber, and A. Zubek. 1987. Specific creatinine determination in laboratory animals using the enzymatic test kit "Creatinine–PAP." *Journal of Clinical Chemistry and Clinical Biochemistry* 25:357–361.

Kampa, N., I. Boström, P. Lord, U. Wennstrom, P. Öhagen, and E. Maripuu. 2003. Day-to-day variability in glomerular filtration rate in normal dogs by scintographic technique. *Journal of Veterinary Medicine A* 50:37–41.

Laterza, O. F., C. P. Price, and M. G. Scott. 2002. Cystatin C: An improved estimator of glomerular filtration rate? *Clinical Chemistry* 48:699–707.

Medaille, C., C. Trumel, D. Concordet, F. Vergez, and J. P. Braun. 2004. Comparison of plasma/serum urea and creatinine concentrations in the dog: A 5-year retrospective study in a commercial veterinary clinical pathology laboratory. *Journal of Veterinary Medicine A* 51:119–123.

Palm, M., and A. Lundblad. 2005. Creatinine concentration in plasma from dog, rat and mouse: A comparison of three different methods. *Veterinary Clinical Pathology* 34:232–236.

Prause, L. C., and G. F. Grauer. 1998. Association of gastrointestinal hemorrhage with increased blood urea nitrogen and BUN/creatinine ratio in dogs: A literature review and a retrospective study. *Veterinary Clinical Pathology* 27:107–111

Schaeffer, L., U. Gilge, A. Heidland, and R. M. Schaeffer. 1994. Urinary excretion of cathepsin B and cystatins as parameters of tubular damage. *Kidney International* 46 (Suppl. 47): S64–67.

Osmolality or Specific Gravity Determined by Refractometry

Allchin, J. P., and G. O. Evans. 1986. A comparison of three methods for determining the concentration of rat urine. *Comparative Biochemistry and Physiology* 85A:771–773.

Allchin, J. P., G. O. Evans, and C. E. Parsons. 1987. Pitfalls in the measurement of canine urine concentration. *Veterinary Record* 120:256–257.

George, J. W. 2001. The usefulness and limitations of handheld refractometers in veterinary laboratory medicine: An historical and technical review. *Veterinary Clinical Pathology* 30:201–210.

Sweeney, T. E., and C. A. Beauchat. 1993. Limitations of method of osmometry: Measuring the osmolality of biological fluids. *American Journal of Physiology* 264:R469–480.

Test Strips

Adams, P., and L. Sawyer. 1990. Structure of rodent urinary proteins. *Biochemical Society Transactions* 18:936–937.

Alt, J. M., H. Hackbarth, F. Deerberg, and H. Stolte. 1980. Proteinuria in rats in relationship to age-dependent renal changes. *Laboratory Animals* 14:95–101.

Cavaggioni, A., and C. Mucignat-Caretta. 2000. Major urinary proteins alpha (2U) globulins and aphrodism. *Biochimica et Biophysica Acta* 1482:218–228.

Evans, G. O., and C. E. Parsons. 1986. Potential errors in the measurement of total protein male rat urine using test strips. *Laboratory Animals* 20:27–31.

Finlayson, J. S., and C. A. Baumann. 1958. Mouse proteinuria. *American Journal of Physiology* 192:69–72.

Groen, A., and A. J. Lagerwerf. 1979. Genetically determined electrophoretic variants of the major urinary protein (Mup) complex in mouse urine. *Animal Blood Groups and Biochemical Genetics* 10:107–114.

Heuter, K. J., T. Buffington, and D. J. Chew. 1998. Agreement between two methods for measuring urine pH in cats and dogs. *Journal of American Veterinary Medical Association* 213:996–998.

Neuhaus, O. W., and W. Flory. 1978. Age-dependent changes in the excretion of urinary proteins by the rat. *Nephron* 22:570–576.

Roy, A. K., and O. W. Neuhaus. 1967. Androgenic control of a sex-dependent protein in the rat. *Nature* 214:618–620.

Taylor, D. M., and D. L. Neal. 1982. False negative hyperglucosuria test-strip reactions in laboratory mice. *Laboratory Animals* 16:192–197.

Urinary Sediment and Celluria

Davies, D. J., and A. Kennedy. 1967. The excretion of renal cells following necrosis of the proximal convoluted tubule. *British Journal of Experimental Pathology* 48:45–50.

Gheilli, M., W. Verstrepen, K. de Greef, S. Vercauteren, D. Ysebaert, E. Nouwen, and M. de Broe. 1998. Inflammatory cells in renal pathology. *Néphrologie* 19:59–67.

Hardy, T. L. 1970. Identification of cells exfoliated from the rat kidney by experimental nephrotoxicity. *Annals of the Rheumatic Diseases* 29:64–66.

Izzedine, H., V. Launay-Vacher, and G. Deray. 2005. Antiviral drug-induced nephrotoxicity. *American Journal of Kidney Disease* 45:804–817.

Prescott, L. F., and S. Ansari. 1969. The effects of repeated administration of HgCI on exfoliation of renal tubular cells and urinary glutamic-oxaloacetic transaminase activity in the rat. *Toxicology and Applied Pharmacology* 14:97–107.

Prescott, L. F., and D. E. Brodie. 1964. A simple differential stain for urinary sediment. *Lancet* 288:940.

Stability

Berg, K. J. et al. 1998. Reference ranges of some enzymes and proteins in untimed overnight urine and their stability after freezing. *Clinica Chimica Acta* 272:225–230.

Matteucci E., G. Gregori, L. Pellegrini, R. Navalesi, and O. Giampietro. 1991. How can storage time and temperature affect enzymic activities in urine? *Enzyme* 45:116–120, p. 79.

Matteucci, E., and O. Giampietro. 1994. To store urinary enzymes: How and for how long? *Kidney International* (Suppl. 47): S58–59.

Plummer, D. T., and P. J. Wright. 1970. The collection of rat urine free of fecal contamination. *Journal of Physiology* 209 (Suppl.): 16.

Schultz, C. J., R. N. Dalton, C. Turner, H. A. W. Neil, and D. B. Dunger. 2000. Freezing method affects the concentration and variability or urine proteins and the interpretation of data on microalbuminuria. *Diabetic Medicine* 17:7–14.

Stokke, O. 1974. Preservation of gamma glutamyl transpeptidase in human urine. *Clinica Chimica Acta* 57:143–148.

Quantitative Protein Measurements

Bernard, A. M., A. Vyskocil, and R. Lauwerys. 1981. Determination of beta 2-microglobulin in human urine and in serum by latex immunoassay. *Clinical Chemistry* 27:832–837.

Devuyst, O., K. Dahan, and Y. Pirson. 2005. Tamm–Horsfall protein or uromodulin: New ideas about an old molecule. *Nephrology, Dialysis, Transplantation* 20:1290–1294.

Dilena, B. A., L. A. Penberthy, and C. G. Fraser. 1983. Six methods for determining urinary protein compared. *Clinical Chemistry* 29:553–557.

Gokhale, J. A., P. A. Glenton, and S. R. Khan. 1997. Biochemical and quantitative analysis of Tamm–Horsfall protein in rats. *Urology Research* 25:347–354.

Le Bricon, T. 2001. Exporation biologique de la protéinurie au laboratoire d'analyses: Aspects quantitatifs. *Annales de Biologie Clinique* 59:710–715.

Maachi, M., S. Fellahi, A. Regeniter, M-E Diop, J. Capeau, J. Rossert, J-P. Bastard. 2004. Patterns of proteinuria: Urinary sodium dodecyl sulfate electrophoreses versus immunonephelometric protein marker measurement following interpretation of knowledge base system MDI-Lablink. *Clinical Chemistry* 50:1834–1837.

McElderry, L. A., I. F. Tarbit, and A. J. Cassells-Smith. 1982. Six methods of urinary protein compared. *Clinical Chemistry* 28:356–360.

Pesce, A. J. 1974. Methods used for the analysis of proteins in the urine. *Nephron* 13:93–104.

Pressler, B. M., S. L. Vaden, W. A. Jensen, and D. Simpson. 2002. Detection of canine microalbuminuria using semiquantitative test strips designed for use with human urine. *Veterinary Clinical Pathology* 31:56–60.

Raila, J., S. Forterre, and F. J. Schweigert. 2005. Physiologische und pathophysiologische grundlagen der proteinurie. *Berliner und Munchener Tierarztliche Wochenschrift* 118:229–239.

Viau, C., A. Bernard., A. A. Ouled, and R. Lauwerys. 1986. Determination of rat beta-2-microglobulin in urine and in serum. II. Application of its urinary determination to selected nephrotoxicity models. *Journal of Applied Toxicology* 6:191–195.

Woo, J., M. Floyd, D. C. Cannon, and B. Kahan. 1978. Radioimmunassay for urinary albumin. *Clinical Chemistry* 24:1464–1467.

Separations of Proteins

Allchin, J. P., and G. O. Evans. 1986. A comparison of three methods for determining the concentration of rat urine. *Comparative Biochemistry and Physiology* 85A:771–773.

Bernard, A., and R. R. Lauwerys. 1991. Proteinuria: Changes and mechanisms in toxic nephropathies. *Critical Reviews in Toxicology* 21:373–405.

Bianchi-Bosisio, A., F. D'Agrosa, F. Gaboardi, E. Gianazza, and P. G. Righetti. 1991. Sodium dodecyl sulphate electrophoresis of urinary proteins. *Journal of Chromatography* 569:243–260.

Boesken, W. H., K. Kopf, and P. Schollmeyer. 1973. Differentiation of proteinuric diseases by disc electrophoretic molecular weight analytes of urinary proteins. *Clinical Nephrology* 1:311–318.

Hofmann, W., B. Rossmuller, W. G. Guder, and H. H. Edel. 1992. A new strategy for characterizing proteinuria and hematuria from a single pattern of defined proteins in urine. *European Journal of Clinical Chemistry and Clinical Biochemistry* 30:707–712.

Kolaja, G. J., D. A. Vandermeer, W. H. Packwood, and P. S. Satoh. 1992. The use of sodium dodecyl sulfate-polyacrylamide gel electrophoresis to detect renal damage in Sprague–Dawley rats treated with gentamicin sulfate. *Toxicologic Pathology* 20:603–607.

Kshirsagar, B., and R. C. Wiggins. 1986. A map of urine proteins based on one-dimensional SDS-polyacrylamide gel electrophoresis and Western blotting using one microliter of unconcentrated urine. *Clinica Chimica Acta* 158:13–22.

Schurek, H-J. 1994. Mechanisms of glomerular proteinuria and hematuria. *Kidney International* 46 (Suppl. 47): S12–16.

Stonard, M. D., C. W. Gore, G. J. A. Oliver, and I. K. Smith. 1987. Urinary enzymes and protein patterns as indicators of injury to different regions of the kidney. *Fundamental and Applied Toxicology* 9:339–351.

Proteomics

Bandara, L. R., M. D. Kelly, E. A. Lock, and S. Kennedy. 2003. A correlation between a proteomic evaluation and conventional measurements in the assessment of renal proximal tubular toxicity. *Toxicological Sciences* 73:195–206.

Forterre, S., J. Raila, and F. J. Schweigert. 2004. Protein profiling of urine from dogs with renal disease using ProteinChip analysis. *Journal of Veterinary Diagnostic Investigation* 16:271–277.

Hampel, D. J., C. Sansome, M. Sha, S. Brodsky, W. E. Lawson, and M. S. Goligorsky. 2001. Towards proteomics in uroscopy: Urinary protein profiles after radio contrast medium administration. *Journal of American Society of Nephrology* 12:1026–1035.

Hewitt, S. M., J. Dear, and R. A. Star. 2004. Discovery of protein biomarkers of renal diseases. *Journal of the American Society of Nephrology* 15:1677–1689.

Idborg-Björkman, H., P-O. Edlund, O. M. Kvalein, I. Schuppe-Koistinen, and S. P. Jacobsen. 2003. Screening of biomarkers in rat urine using LC/mass electrospray ionization-MS and two-way data analysis. *Analytical Chemistry* 75:4784–4792.

Nedlekov, D., and R. W. Nelson. 2001. Analysis of human urine protein biomarkers via bimolecular interaction analysis mass spectrometry. *American Journal of Kidney Disease* 38:481–487.

Thongboonkerd, V., and J. B. Klein, eds. 2003. *Proteomics in nephrology. Contributions to nephrology.* Basel, Switzerland: S. Karger AG.

Witzmann, F. A., and J. Li. 2004. Proteomics and nephrotoxicity. *Contributions to Nephrology* 141:104–123.

Other Renal Antigens

Aulitzky, W. K., P. N. Schlegel, D. F. Wu, C. Y. Cheng, C. L. Chen, P. S. Li, M. Goldstein, M. Reidenberg, and C. W. Bardin. 1992. Measurement of urinary clusterin as an index of nephrotoxicity. *Proceedings of the Society for Experimental Biology and Medicine* 199:93–96.

Bomhard, E. M., F. W. Falkenberg, and I. Loof. 1994. Changes in urinary enzymes and kidney-derived antigens after acute renal papillary necrosis in rats. *Kidney International* 47 (Suppl.): 60–63.

Eti, S., C. Y. Cheng, A. Marshall, and M. M. Reidenberg. 1993. Urinary clusterin in chronic nephrotoxicity of the rat. *Proceedings of the Society for Experimental Biology and Medicine* 202:487–490.

Han, W. K., V. Bailly, R. Abichandani, R. Thadhani, J. V. Bonventre, et al. 2002. Kidney injury molecule-1 (KIM-1). *Kidney International* 62:237–244.

Hildebrand, H., M. Rinke, G. Schlüter, E. Bomhard, and F. W. Falkenberg. 1999. Urinary antigens as markers of papillary toxicity. II. Application of monoclonal antibodies for the determination of papillary antigens in rat urine. *Archives of Toxicology* 73:233–245.

Ichimura, T., C. C. Hung, S. A. Yang, J. L. Stevens, and J. V. Bonventre. 2004. Kidney injury molecule-1, a tissue and urinary biomarker for nephrotoxicant-induced renal injury. *American Journal of Renal Physiology* 286:F552–563.

Enzymes

Amador, E., T. S. Zimmerman, and W. E. C. Wacker. 1963. Urinary alkaline phosphatase activity. II. An analytical validation of the assay method. *Journal of the American Medical Association* 185:953–957.

Bach, P. H., and T. L. Hardy. 1985. Relevance of animal models to analgesic-associated papillary necrosis in humans. *Kidney International* 28:605–613.

Bhargava, A. S., A. R. Khater, and P. Gunzel. 1978. The correlation between lactate dehydrogenase activity in urine and serum and experimental renal damage in the rat. *Toxicology Letters* 1:319–323.

Bomhard, E., D. Maruhn, and M. Rinke. 1999. Time course of chronic oral cadmium nephrotoxicity in Wistar rats: Excretion of urinary enzymes. *Drug and Chemical Toxicology* 22:679–703.

Bomhard, E., D. Maruhn, O. Vogel, and H. Magel. 1990. Determination of urinary glutathione S-transferase and lactate dehydrogenase for differentiation between proximal and distal nephron damage. *Archives of Toxicology* 64:269–278.

Clemo, F. A. 1998. Urinary enzyme evaluation of nephrotoxicity in the dog. *Toxicologic Pathology* 26:29–32.

Cottrell, R. C., C. E. Agrelo, S. D. Gangolli, and P. Grasso. 1976. Histochemical and biochemical studies of chemically induced acute kidney damage in the rat. *Food Cosmetics Toxicology* 14:593–598.

Diamond, G. L., and R. K. Zalups. 1998. Understanding renal toxicity of heavy metals. *Toxicological Pathology* 26:92–103.

Dote, T., K. Kono, K. Usuda, H. Nishiura, and T. Tagawa. 2000. Acute renal damage dose response in rats to intravenous infusion of sodium fluoride. *Fluoride Quarterly Report* 33:210–217.

Ellis, B. G., and R. G. Price. 1975. Urinary enzyme excretion during renal papillary necrosis induced in rats with ethyleneimine. *Chemico-Biological Interactions* 11:473–482.

Ellis, B. G., R. G. Price, and J. C. Topham. 1973. The effect of tubular damage by mercuric chloride on kidney function and some urinary enzymes in the dog. *Chemico-Biological Interactions* 7:101–113.

Funakawa, S., T. Itoh, K. Miyata, Y. Tochino, and M. Nakamura. 1984. Sex difference of N-acetyl-beta-glucosaminidase activity in the kidney, urine and plasma of mice. *Renal Physiology* 7:124–128.

Grotsch, H., M. Hropot, E. Klaus, V. Malerczyk, and H. Mattenheimer. 1985. Enzymuria of the rat: Biorhythms and sex differences. *Journal of Clinical Chemistry and Clinical Biochemistry* 23:343–347.

Guder, W. G., and B. D. Ross. 1984. Enzyme distribution along the nephron. *Kidney International* 26:101–111.

Heinle, H., A. Wendel, and U. Schmidt. 1977. The activities of the key enzymes of the gamma-glutamyl cycle in microdissected segments of the rat nephron. *FEBS Letters* 73:220–224.

Hofmeister, R., A. S. Bhargava, and P. Gunzel. 1986. Value of enzyme determinations in urine for the diagnosis of nephrotoxicity in rats. *Clinica Chimica Acta* 160:163–167.

Jung, K. 1991. Enzyme activities in urine: How should we express their excretion? A critical literature review. *European Journal of Clinical Chemistry and Clinical Biochemistry* 29:725–729.

Jung, K., H. Mattenheimer, and U. Burchardt, eds. 1992. *Urinary enzymes in clinical and experimental medicine.* Berlin: Springer–Verlag.

Jung, K., G. Schultz, and C. Reinholdt. 1986. Diuresis dependent excretion of urinary enzymes: N-acetyl-beta-D-glucosaminidase, alanine aminopeptidase, alkaline phosphatase and gamma-glutamyltransferase. *Clinical Chemistry* 32:529–532.

Kharash, E. D., G. M. Hoffman, D. Thorning, D. C. Hankins, and C. G. Kilty. 1998. Role of renal cysteine conjugate β-lyase pathway in inhaled compound A nephrotoxicity in rats. *Anesthesiology* 88:1624–1633.

Kilty, C., S. Doyle, B. Hassett, and F. Manning. 1998. Glutathione S-transferases as biomarkers of organ damage: Applications of rodent and canine GST immunoassays. *Chemico-Biological Interactactions* 111–112:123–135.

Lehir, M., U. C. Dubach, and W. G. Guder. 1980. Distribution of acid hydrolases in the nephron of normal and diabetic rats. *International Journal of Biochemistry* 12:41–45.

Lovett, D. H., J. L. Ryan, M. Kashgarian, and R. B. Sterzel. 1982. Lysosomal enzymes in glomerular cells of the rat. *American Journal of Pathology* 107:161–166.

Marchewka, Z., and A. Dugosz. 1998. Enzymes in urine as markers of nephrotoxicity of cytostatic agents and aminoglycoside antibiotics. *International Urology and Nephrology* 30:339–348.

Mattenheimer, H. 1977. Enzymes in renal diseases. *Annals of Clinical and Laboratory Science* 7:422–432.

Morita, A., Y. Numata, Y. Kosigi, A. Noto, N. Takeuchi, and K. Uchida. 1998. Stabilities of N-acetyl-β-D-glucoaminidase isoenzymes: Advantage of NAG isoenzyme B measurement in clinical applications. *Clinica Chimica Acta* 278:35–43.

Moser, R., T. D. Oberley, D. A. Daggett, A. L. Friedman, J. A. Johnson, and F. L. Siegel. 1995. Effects of lead administration on developing rat kidney. 1. Glutathione S-transferase isoenzymes. *Toxicology and Applied Pharmacology* 131:85–93.

Nuyts, G. D., G. F. Verpooten, and M. E. de Broe. 1992. Intestinal alkaline phosphatase as an indicator of effects on the S3-segment of the human proximal tubule. *European Journal of Clinical Chemistry and Clinical Biochemistry* 30:713–715.

Pariat, C. L., P. Ingrand, J. Cambar, E. de Lemos, A. Piriou, and P. T. Courtois. 1990. Seasonal effects on the daily variations of gentamicin-induced nephrotoxicity. *Archives of Toxicology* 64:205–209.

Plaa, G. L., and R. E. Larson. 1965. Relative nephrotoxic properties of chlorinated methane, ethane and ethylene derivatives in mice. *Toxicology and Applied Pharmacology* 7:37–44.

Plummer, D. T., P. D. Leathwood, and M. E. Blake. 1975. Urinary enzymes and kidney damage by aspirin and phenacetin. *Chemico-Biological Interactions* 10: 277–284.

Prescott, L. F., and S. Ansari. 1969. The effects of repeated administration of HgCI on exfoliation of renal tubular cells and urinary glutamic-oxaloacetic transaminase activity in the rat. *Toxicology and Applied Pharmacology* 14:97–107.

Price, R. G. 1982. Urinary enzymes, nephrotoxicity and renal disease. *Toxicology* 23:99–134.

Raab, W. P. 1972. Diagnostic value of urinary enzyme determinations. *Clinical Chemistry* 18:5–25.

————. 1980. Nephrotoxicity of drugs, evaluated by renal enzyme excretion studies. *Archives of Toxicology* 4 (Suppl): 194–200.

Saduka, Y., Y. Shimuzi, and Y. Takino. 1994. Role of glutathione S-transferase isoenzymes in cisplatin-induced nephrotoxicity in the rat. *Toxicology Letters* 70:211–222.

Stonard, M. D. 1990. Assessment of renal function and damage in animal species. *Journal of Applied Toxicology* 10:267–274.

Stonard, M. D., C. W. Gore, G. J. A. Oliver, and I. K. Smith. 1987. Urinary enzymes and protein patterns as indicators of injury to different regions of the kidney. *Fundamental and Applied Toxicology* 9:339–351.

Stroo, W. E., and J. B. Hook. 1977. Enzymes of renal origin in urine as indicators of nephrotoxicity. *Toxicology and Applied Pharmacology* 39:423–434.

Sundberg, A. G. M., E-L. Appelkvist, L. Backman, and G. Dallner. 1994. Urinary π-class glutathione transferase as an indicator of tubular damage in the human kidney. *Nephron* 67:308–316.

Turecky, L., and E. Uhlikova. 2003. Diagnostic significance of urinary enzymes in nephrology. *Bratislavske Lekarske Listy* 104:27–31.

Usuda, K., K. Kono, T. Dote, H. Nisbiura, and T. Tagawa. 1999. Usefulness of the assessment of urinary enzyme leakage in monitoring acute fluoride nephrotoxicity. *Archives of Toxicology* 73:346–351.

Werner, M., and D. Gabrielson. 1977. Ultrafiltration for improved assay of urinary enzymes. *Clinical Chemistry* 23:700–704.

Werner, M., D. Maruhn, and Atoba M. 1969. Use of gel filtration in the assay of urinary enzymes. *Journal of Chromatography* 40:254–263.

Whiting, P. H., and P. A. Brown. 1996. The relationship between enzymuria and kidney enzyme activities in experimental gentamicin nephrotoxicity. *Renal Failure* 18:899–909.

Wright, P. J., P. D. Leathwood, and D. T. Plummer. 1972. Enzymes in rat urine: Alkaline phosphatase. *Enzymologia* 42:317–327.

Wright, P. J., and D. T. Plummer. 1974. The use of urinary enzyme measurements to detect renal damage caused by nephrotoxic compounds. *Biochemical Pharmacology* 23:65–73.

Functional Tests

Diezi, J., and J. Biollaz. 1979. Renal function tests in experimental toxicity studies. *Pharmacology and Therapeutics* 5:135–145.

Klaassen, C. D., and G. L. Plaa. 1966. Relative effects of various chlorinated hydrocarbons on liver and kidney function in mice. *Toxicology and Applied Pharmacology* 9:139–151.

Kluwe, W. M. 1981. Renal function tests as indicators of kidney injury in subacute toxicity studies. *Toxicology and Applied Pharmacology* 57:414–424.

Kulick, L. J., D. J. Clemmons, R. L. Hall, and M. A. Koch. 2005. Refinement of the urine concentration test in rats. *Contemporary Topics in Laboratory Animal Science* 44:46–49.

Mann, W. A., and L. B. Kinter. 1993. Characterization of the renal l handling of p-aminohippurate (PAH) in the beagle dog (*Canis familiaris*). *General Pharmacology* 24:367–372.

Poutsiaka, J. W., C. H. Keysser, B. G. Thomas, and C. R. Linegar. 1962. Simultaneous deter-
    mination in dogs of liver and kidney functions with bromosulfalein and phenolsulfo-
    nephthalein. *Toxicology and Applied Pharmacology* 4:55–59.
Sharatt, M., and A. C. Frazer. 1963. The sensitivity of function tests in detecting renal damage
    in the rat. *Toxicology and Applied Pharmacology* 5:36–48.
Tune, B. M., M. B. Burg, and C. S. Patlak. 1969. Characteristics of PAH transport in proximal
    renal tubules. *American Journal of Physiology* 217:1057–1063.

Metabonomics

Holmes, E., F. W. Bonner, and J. K. Nicholson. 1997. ^{1}H NMR spectroscopic and histo-
    pathological studies on propylene-induced renal papillary necrosis in the rat and the
    multimammate desert mouse (*Mastomys natalensis*). *Comparative Biochemistry and
    Physiology* 116C:125–134.
Holmes, E., J. K. Nicholson, A. W. Nicholls, J. C. Lindon, S. C. Connor, S. Polley, and J.
    Connelly. 1998. The identification of novel biomarkers of renal toxicity using automatic
    data reduction techniques and PCA of proton NMR spectra of urine. *Chemometrics and
    Intelligent Laboratory Systems* 44:245–255
Lindon, J. C., E. Holmes, and J. K. Nicholson. 2004. Metabonomics: System biology in phar-
    maceutical research. *Current Opinion in Molecular Therapeutics* 6:265–272.
Robertson, D. G., J. Lindon, J. K. Nicholson, and E. Holmes. 2005. *Metabonomics in toxicity
    assessment.* Boca Raton, FL: CRC Press.

5 Assessment of Gastrointestinal and Pancreatic Toxicities

5.1 STRUCTURE, PHYSIOLOGY, AND BIOCHEMISTRY

The disposition of xenobiotics can be considered to occur in four interrelated phases (i.e., absorption, distribution, metabolism, and excretion, collectively abbreviated as ADME). The major routes for the absorption of xenobiotics include skin, lungs (or gills), and the parenteral routes—intravenous (i.v.), intraperitoneal (i.p.), subcutaneous (s.c.), and intramuscular (i.m.). The commonest route for administration in toxicology studies is per oral (p.o.) administration, with absorption of the test compound via the gastrointestinal (GI) tract; the per-oral route is also the commonest route for exposure to a wide variety of environmental xenobiotics by fluid or food intake.

In the upper part of the GI tract, the structure of the keratinized epithelium of the mouth and esophagus in rodents differs from the nonkeratinized epithelium found in nonhuman primates (NHPs) and humans. Rodents have two distinct parts of the stomach—a nonglandular stomach and a glandular stomach; these differ from NHPs and humans, where there is one stomach. Within the glandular stomach lining are three types of secreting cells: the parietal cells secreting hydrochloric acid, the chief cells secreting digestive proenzymes (e.g., pepsinogen), and mucous secreting cells. A glycoprotein (the intrinsic factor), which is essential for vitamin B_{12} absorption, is produced by the parietal cells of the stomach. The acidic pH of the stomach contents favors the cleavage of pepsinogen to pepsin. The hormone gastrin is secreted by the G-cells of the stomach and it is released in response to vagal stimulation. Some of the hormones associated with the gastrointestinal tract and pancreas are shown in Table 5.1 (see also Woodman 1997).

Gastric contents flow through to the duodenum via the pyloric sphincter, which is controlled by the action of several hormones and the nervous system in response to the volume, localized irritation, and chemical contents of the duodenum. The ducts of the liver (bile duct), pancreas, and exocrine glands empty into the upper part of the duodenum, which then leads to the small intestine, where many compounds can be absorbed. In the following larger intestine, the main function is the absorption of water.

Serving the GI tract is an important blood circulatory system, and a main feature is the flow from veins (serving the regions from the esophagus to near the end of the rectum) into the portal vein, which delivers blood to the hepatic sinusoids before blood flows into the general circulation. This is portal venous blood flow and is

TABLE 5.1

Hormones of the Gastrointestinal Tract and Pancreas

Hormone and Location	Function
Gastric Antrum and Duodenum	
Gastrin	Stimulates H+ secretion and trophic effect on gastrointestinal tract in some species
Gastric releasing peptide	Stimulates gastrin release
Ghrelin	Increases food appetite
Duodenum and Jejunum	
Cholecystokinin (CCK)	Stimulates secretion of pancreatic enzymes and gall bladder contraction where present, inhibits gastric emptying
Gastric inhibitory peptide (GIP) (or glucose dependent insulinotrophic peptide)	Stimulates postprandial release of insulin, inhibits gastric motility
Secretin	Stimulates pancreatic secretion of bicarbonate and water
Motilin	Stimulates intestinal motor activity and gastric smooth muscle
Pancreas	
Insulin	Stimulates glycogen synthesis and glucose uptake and inhibits lipolysis
Glucagon	Opposes actions to insulin
Pancreatic polypeptide	Inhibits release of pancreatic enzymes and counteracts actions of CCK
Ileum and Colon	
Glucagon-like peptide (enteroglucagon)	Increases small intestinal mucosal growth and retards intestinal transit rate
All Regions of GI Tract	
Vasoactive intestinal polypeptide (VIP)	Affects secretomotor actions, vasodilation, relaxation of intestinal smooth muscle
Somatostatin	Inhibits the actions of gastrin, motilin, secretin, CCK, GIP enteroglucagon, pancreatic polypeptide, and insulin

described as the "first pass," where xenobiotics are delivered to the liver and may be subjected to metabolic modifications that either detoxify or activate the xenobiotic prior to general circulation. Some circulating xenobiotics absorbed into the systemic circulation may be excreted by biliary excretion, and species differ, with the rat and dog showing greater ability to use this excretory pathway compared to rabbits, guinea pigs, and NHPs.

The pancreas gland has an exocrine function secreting the pancreatic juice, which contains digestive enzymes, and is an endocrine organ producing a number of hormones, including insulin and glucagons. The functioning of the exocrine pancreas is influenced by the hormones gastrin and secretin secreted by the cells of the stomach and duodenum. In the pancreatic juice, there are more than 20 different enzymes, including serine protease precursors—trypsinogen, chymotrypsinogen, proelastase, and kallikinogens (prekallikreins)—and exopeptidases—prophospholipase A2 and procarboxypeptidase. To prevent protease action on the pancreas (i.e., autodegradation, which might cause pancreatitis), several of the enzymes are produced as the precursors; intestinal enterokinase cleaves trypsinogen to the active trypsin, and trypsin then acts to convert chymotrypsinogen to chymotrypsin. Trypsin and chymotrypsin act as peptidases and elastases. Amylase, lipase, cholesterol ester hydrolase, colipase, bicarbonate, and chloride are also found in the pancreatic juice; amylase degrades glycogen, cellulose, and other carbohydrates. Lipase (triacylglycerol lipase) hydrolyzes triglycerides into fatty acids and glycerol. These digestive enzymes are produced by the acinar cells of the exocrine pancreas and mixed with a salt- and bicarbonate-rich fluid from the ductal cells, which is secreted into the lumen of the acini and then into the intralobular ducts, pancreatic duct, and, finally, the duodenum. The pancreatic juice neutralizes the acidic chyme from the stomach fluid, and pancreatic enzymes aid food digestion.

The pancreatic endocrine functions are associated with the cell clusters known as the islets of Langerhans, and the cells can be classified by their hormonal secretions: the alpha-cells secrete glucagons, the beta-cells secrete insulin and amylin, the δ-cells (also called the delta or D cells) secrete somatostatin, the PP cells (also called F cells) secrete pancreatic polypeptide, and the ε (epsilon)-cells secrete ghrelin (Woodman 1997). There are a number of autocrine and paracrine feedback mechanisms between these four cells types, with insulin activating beta-cells but inhibiting alpha-cells, and glucagon activating alpha-cells, which in turn activate beta- and delta-cells; somatostatin inhibits both alpha- and beta-cells (Motta et al. 1997). In most species, insulin is associated with a single-copy gene, but the rat has two non-allelic genes, so there are two proinsulins. These are cleaved to form type I and II insulins. Insulins have two polypeptide chains connected by disulphide bridges and approximate molecular mass of 6 kDa. Within the Golgi apparatus of the cells, the proinsulins are cleaved to release the insulin and a peptide (C-peptide) that connects the two polypeptide chains of the proinsulin. The key target tissues for insulin are liver, muscle, and adipose tissue through insulin receptors, ensuring that glucose is stored as glycogen in the liver and muscle while increasing the synthesis of fatty acids and their esterification and reducing gluconeogenesis. Glucagon is a linear peptide that has opposing effects to those of insulin because it stimulates hepatic glycogen catabolism and gluconeogenesis.

Body glucose is mainly confined to the extracellular fluid; glucose enters the body pool by nutrition or by hepatic glycogenolysis with small, freely exchangeable amounts in the liver and erythrocytes. Although this glucose pool is generally constant in laboratory animals, its levels vary more than in humans. The liver plays a key role in maintaining glucose homeostasis, removing approximately 70% of the glucose load via the portal circulation and storing this as glycogen. In addition, the precursors—lactate, glycerol, pyruvate, and alanine—resulting from tissue metabolism are converted into glucose by hepatic gluconeogenesis.

Absorption of many nutrients and xenobiotics occurs primarily in the small intestine, with some exceptions such as iron in the duodenum and bile salts in the ileum. A number of intestinal disaccharidases hydrolyze disaccharides into monosaccharides; these enzymes include lactase, maltase, sucrase, and trehalase. Thus, the absorption of both nutrients and xenobiotics depends on the differing pH ranges of the GI contents, the rate of movement of the contents through the GI tract, and the concentration and physicochemical properties of the xenobiotics (and/or metabolites), with molecular structure and mass, ionic charge, and hydrophobic properties (or lipid solubility) influencing absorption (Timbrell 2001). The mechanisms for absorption include active energy transport systems, which allow simple diffusion through lipid membranes, absorption though the lymphatics, and pinocytosis of macromolecules. The simple diffusion processes permit the absorption of non-ionic hydrophilic compounds with small molecular mass. Lipophilic compounds such as barbiturates, food additives, and some industrial chemicals are absorbed by passive diffusion; absorption mechanisms involving carrier proteins and cell transporters also enable the absorption of xenobiotics.

Other factors that affect absorption from the GI tract include its microflora and food content. The microflora of the GI tract, particularly in the large intestine, can play important roles in the activation of chemicals to toxic, mutagenic, or carcinogenic metabolites and in detoxifying mechanisms. The GI tract microflora differ between species and the flora can be affected following the administration of oral antibiotics or poorly soluble compounds. The presence of food in the GI tract may cause the absorption of compound to be reduced, delayed, or increased, or it can have no effect.

5.2   TOXIC EFFECTS

Adverse gastrointestinal events are not uncommon in early clinical trials because one objective of these studies is to assess tolerability; however, these effects are not always related to the pharmacology of the compound. Of the top 100 most frequently prescribed medications, 44 have been implicated in episodes of acute pancreatitis (Trivedi and Pitchumoni 2005). There is an objective to improve assessment of gastrointestinal toxicities by biochemical analyses in addition to enhancing safety pharmacology studies. Many of the mechanisms that cause gastrointestinal and pancreatic toxicity are poorly understood.

Given the diverse tissues of the GI tract and the differences both in anatomy and drug metabolism, it is not surprising to see different toxicological effects between species (Mallory and Kern 1980; Banerjee, Patel, and Grainger 1989; Biour, Daoud, and Salem 2005; Pour 2005; Badalov et al. 2007; Gad 2007). Some compounds are irritants to parts of the GI tract and the injury can be simply demonstrated by histopathology; when the inflammation is severe, this may cause blood and protein loss from the inflammatory site. Severely irritant xenobiotics, which produce toxic effects by direct action on the walls of the GI tract, often produce these effects in several species, but the observations of severe effects in rodents may stop administration of the test compound to another species.

Test formulations and the vehicle are usually manufactured so as not to cause severe injury due to the pH of the administered formulation. Although aqueous vehicles such as water or saline may be preferred, some less soluble materials may be administered with other vehicles such as oils or organic solvents, which may exert separate effects (e.g., ingestion of significant quantities of corn oil can increase the flow of lymph and affect uptake of lipophilic compounds). Supposedly inert suspension materials may cause minor changes to biochemical measurements when tested alone. It is important to delineate the effects due to a vehicle from those of the test compound, particularly when the vehicle is novel or used infrequently. The vomiting reflex varies between species; although it is stimulated by the nervous system in dogs and nonhuman primates, it is almost absent from rats and rabbits. In animals that can exhibit this reflex, it is sometimes difficult to ensure that correct doses of test compound are administered and retained, and frequent emesis can affect biochemical measurements.

In animal toxicological studies, there is an opportunity to obtain data on food and fluid intake during the treatment period and then to use these data (for the different treatment groups and controls) as indicators of gastrointestinal function and relate them to the clinical chemistry findings. When the gavage tube is correctly sited in the stomach of the animal, this generally avoids exposure and injury to the esophagus, particularly in rodents where regurgitation into the esophagus does not occur. It is also well recognized that dosing by inhalation may occasionally result in secondary exposure via the gastrointestinal tract.

5.3 LABORATORY INVESTIGATIONS

In general toxicology studies and for detecting gastrointestinal toxicity, the common clinical chemistry tests are generally focused on fluid and electrolyte balance supported by some measures of carbohydrate, lipid, and protein metabolism. However, few of the common tests recommended for regulatory studies are specific for gastrointestinal toxicity. When gastrointestinal toxic effects are prolonged, marked reductions in the intake of essential nutrients such as vitamins (e.g., folate), iron, and amino acids may occur and this may lead to other measurements. In addition to the investigations discussed in later paragraphs, drug-induced pancreatitis may be accompanied by gross plasma lipid changes and hypocalcemia due to excessive loss of pancreatic secretion with increases of acute phase proteins indicative of inflammation.

5.3.1 ENZYMES

Although several enzyme measurements are available for assessing gastrointestinal function, these assays are not frequently used; amylase and/or lipase are perhaps measured more often than other enzymes in order to evaluate pancreatic toxicity. Some enzyme measurements require the invasive collection of gastric, pancreatic, and intestinal fluids, or tissues and therefore are not suitable for many toxicological studies.

Enzyme changes occur in several gastrointestinal conditions, such as intestinal infarction or obstruction, parasitic infections, obstruction of the biliary system, and contraction of the sphincter of Oddi by drugs such as morphine, withdrawal of food, and age-related changes.

5.3.1.1 Amylase

This enzyme with a molecular mass of approximately 45 kDA is found in greatest abundance in the pancreas, but amylase is also found in other tissues, including the liver, salivary glands, and intestine. There are wide differences in the tissue distribution and plasma levels of amylase between species (Rajasingham, Bell, and Baron 1971; MacKenzie and Messer 1976; Jacobs, Hall, and Rogers 1982; McGeachin and Akin 1982; Murtaugh and Jacobs 1985). The reported number of isoenzymes in different species varies and appears to be partly dependent on the separation method. There are four plasma amylase isoenzymes in the rat, where the isoenzymes 1 and 2 are found in pancreatic tissue, and four isoenzymes are found in salivary glands and the liver. Amylase is present in much higher concentration in the salivary glands of rats and mice than in many other species, and increased plasma salivary amylase may be caused by sialoadenosis in the rat with increases of two of the isoenzymes (Robinovitch and Sreebny 1972; Arglebe, Bremer, and Chilla 1978). The pancreatic amylase is denoted P and the salivary amylase S to indicate their different tissue origins. The half-life of amylase is short, varying from less than 2 h in the mouse to 5 h in the dog. Urinary amylase is generally increased when plasma amylase is increased (Mályusz et al. 1990), but it offers no major diagnostic advantage over plasma measurements because it is also affected by renal injury and diuresis.

Total plasma amylase can be measured using chromogenic methods with one of several nitrophenyl-linked synthetic substrates, although not all substrates are suitable for use with samples from laboratory animals (Braun et al. 1990; Medaille and Breind-Marchal 2004), and the methods used for human samples may need to be adjusted by reducing the reaction sample volumes because the levels of plasma amylase are much higher in laboratory animals. Assays using monoclonal antibodies are now available to measure pancreatic (P) lipase, and these are suitable for use with some laboratory animals.

5.3.1.2 Lipase

This enzyme (triacylglycerol acyl-hydrolase) has a molecular mass of approximately 42 kDa (Hide, Chan, and Li 1992) and a short half-life of about 1–3 h in dogs. Pancreatic lipase is secreted in its active form, and this activity is enhanced by colipase and bile salts; the enzyme hydrolyzes triglycerides to monoglycerides. Other lipases—phospholipase a, phospholipase b, and cholesterol ester hydrolase—are also secreted by the pancreas.

Methods using oil suspension emulsions (Cherry–Crandall method) are largely obsolete and have been replaced by more convenient methods using chromogenic or immunological methods, thus leading to the increasing application of measuring both lipase and amylase (Walter, McGraw, and Tvedten 1992; Graca et al. 2005; Steiner, Rutz, and Williams 2006). There is some debate about whether one or another of these enzymes is more suitable for detecting pancreatitis, and published literature may have been biased by the limitations of lipase assays. Some drugs, such as dexamethasone in dogs, have been reported to alter serum lipase more than serum amylase (Parent 1982). If possible, both amylase and lipase should be measured when pancreatic toxicity is being investigated.

Example compounds causing increased plasma amylase and lipase associated with pancreatitis include tributylin (Sparmann et al. 1997; Merkord et al. 2001), cholecystokinin (Seo et al. 2005), cerulein (Abe et al. 1995; Mazzon et al. 2006), 3-aminobenzamide (Mazzan et al. 2006), dimethoate (Kamath, Joshi, and Rajini 2008), l-arginine (Ramos et al. 2005), cyanohydroxybutene (Wallig et al. 1992), and surgically induced ischemia (Sokolowski, Spormann, and Letko 1987).

Example compounds reported to inhibit amylase include extract of white kidney beans (Tormo et al. 2004), tetracyclin, enalapril, and captopril in vitro (Hamdan, Afifi, and Taho 2004).

5.3.1.3 Trypsin and Trypsinogen

Trypsin circulates in plasma bound to α-1-antitrypsin and α-2-macroglobulin and as trypsinogen; this provides some control and protection from the circulating protease action of trypsin. Both trypsin and trypsinogen have short half-lives of about 0.5 h. Trypsinogen has two major isoenzymes: trypsinogens-1 and -2. Trypsin activation peptide (TAP) is a pentapeptide released when active pancreatic trypsin is produced from trypsinogen. The number of methods described for measuring trypsin continues to increase and indicates some of the complexities of assaying this enzyme. Plasma trypsin may be altered due to lung injury.

A variety of methods has been described for measuring trypsin trypsinogen-like immunoreactivity (TLI) and that measure both trypsin and trypsinogen, trypsinogen-2, and trypsinogen activated peptide using colorimetric methods with benzoyl arginine-p-nitroanilide or other benzoyl napthylamide substrates, enzyme immunoassay, immunofluorescence, and radioimmunoassay. Older methods employ a preincubation step with enterokinase to release trypsin from the trypsinogen. Enzyme immunoassays specific for mouse and rat trypsin and trypsinogen are available (Geokas et al. 1981; Reddy et al. 1985; Fletcher, Tsukamoto, and Largman 1986; Williams and Batt 1988; Hedstrom et al. 1996; Archer, Kerr, and Houston 1997; Schmidt et al. 1999; Wilberg, Nurmi, and Westermarck 1999; Waritani et al. 2002; John-Baptiste et al. 2004).

5.3.1.4 Other Enzymes

Alkaline phosphatase. The effects of food intake on plasma alkaline phosphatase in the rat have been mentioned in Chapter 2. For this species with a much larger proportion of intestinal isoenzyme in plasma, changes of plasma alkaline phosphatase can indicate gastrointestinal toxicities.

Pepsinogen. This precursor of the proteolytic enzyme pepsin is secreted by gastric parietal cells; pepsinogen activities may be increased following peptic ulceration and by parasitic infections. The enzyme may be measured in plasma or gastric fluid using colorimetric, fluorimetric, or radioimmunometric methods and ELISA methods (Will et al. 1984; Ford et al. 1985; Tani et al. 1987; Lynch et al. 2004).

5.3.2   TESTS FOR CARBOHYDRATE METABOLISM

5.3.2.1   Plasma, Serum or Blood Glucose, and Urinary Glucose

The measurements of plasma and urinary glucose act as broad indicators of the severity of any disturbance to carbohydrate metabolism. Glucose measurements are of particular pharmacological interest when testing xenobiotics designed as hypo- or hyperglycemic agents. The homeostatic mechanisms for maintaining blood glucose are influenced by intestinal absorption and both hepatic and tissue metabolism. The balance is influenced by several hormones in addition to insulin and glucagon, and these other hormones include corticosteroids, growth hormones, adrenocorticotrophic hormone, and biogenic amines. Hypoglycemia may be due to malnourishment, malabsorption, hepatotoxicity, or mild to moderate toxicity associated with loss of body weight; increased plasma glucose levels may be more commonly caused by excitement, stress, blood collection procedures, or recent food intake rather than toxic effects on the pancreas. Plasma glucose levels below 1.7 mmol/L would give rise to clinical signs of hypoglycemia in humans, but these levels do not appear to produce similar adverse effects in some other nonhuman primates. Some nonhuman primates store food in their buccal pouches, which often prevents the true measurement of their "fasting" plasma glucose. With rodents, animals have to be fasted for much longer periods (>24–48 h) to deplete hepatic glycogen stores, which then results in significant changes of plasma glucose.

Glucose measurements are commonly made using glucose oxidase/peroxidase-linked chromogenic methods or hexokinase methods. Plasma or serum should be rapidly separated after collection to avoid the effects of erythrocytic glycolysis; if delays between sample collection and separation are anticipated, sodium fluoride should be used as an anticoagulant to inhibit glycolysis. Blood glucose values measured with dry film/test strip systems may be erroneous when the hematocrit values are outside the ranges specified by the supplier. It is rarely necessary to use glucose tolerance tests as part of toxicological studies.

5.3.2.2   Urinary Glucose

Test strips (or dipsticks) commonly used for measuring urinary glucose are based on glucose oxidase/chromogenic systems where color blocks indicate the relative concentrations for urinary glucose. Semiquantitative methods using a tablet form of alkaline copper sulfate reagent can also be used, and these tests will detect reducing substances other than glucose. Automated quantitative methods for urinary glucose similar to those used for plasma glucose are a suitable confirmation of test strip results. The presence of glucosuria in the absence of hyperglycemia may indicate renal tubular injury rather than effects on the pancreas.

5.3.2.3   Glycated (or Glycosylated) Hemoglobin

The additional measurement of glycated hemoglobin can be useful when monitoring the effects of proposed hypoglycemic agents or in longer-term studies where effects on the pancreas or carbohydrate metabolism are indicated. Hemoglobins combine via amino groups with glucose and other sugars to form glycated hemoglobins, including

HbA1a, HbA1b, and HbA1c; glycation is now preferred as a descriptive term, replacing glycosylation or glucosylation. Erythrocytes are permeable to glucose and a fraction of hemoglobin is glycated during the life span of erythrocytes. Glycated hemoglobin values alter if the erythrocyte life span shortens or when significant blood loss occurs. Glycated hemoglobin measurements are being used increasingly to monitor long-term glucose homeostasis, particularly in the evaluation of antidiabetic agents.

There are now more than 30 different methodologies for measuring human glycated hemoglobins, and a vigorous debate about international standardization and reporting unitage in human medicine continues. Existing analytical methods include ion exchange chromatography, electrophoresis, affinity chromatography immunoassay, high-performance liquid chromatography, and enzymatic techniques; not all methods are suitable for laboratory animals due to heterogeneity of the glycated hemoglobins in different species. Some ion exchange chromatography and immunochemical methods do not appear to give satisfactory results with animal samples, but affinity boronate chromatography appears to be suitable for rats (Nagisa et al. 2003; Evans, unpublished data, 2004). Glycated hemoglobins have been measured in mice, rats, dogs, and monkeys (Higgins, Garlick, and Bunn 1982; Rendell et al. 1985; Srinivas et al. 1986; Kondo et al. 1989; Hasegawa et al. 1991; Yue et al. 1992; Cefalu, Wagner, and Bell-Farrow 1993; Hooghuis, Rodriguez, and Castano 1994; Dan et al. 1997; Ukarapol et al. 2002).

5.3.2.4 Fructosamine (Glycated Plasma Protein or Glycated Plasma Albumin)

Fructosamine is a ketamine product of protein glycation that offers a simpler alternative methodology to glycated hemoglobin because it can be measured by most automated bioanalyzers (Rendell et al. 1985; Johnson et al. 1991; Cefalu et al. 1993; Levi and Werman 1998; Loste and Marca 2001; Çakatay and Kayali 2006). However, it reflects glucose homeostasis over a shorter time than glycated hemoglobin. Conversion factors between glycated hemoglobin and fructosamine used for human samples should not be applied to animal samples because the degree of glycation differs.

5.3.2.5 Ketones

In severe disturbances of carbohydrate metabolism, test strip results for urine ketones can show varying degrees of positive results. Because the test strips are designed for testing human urine, the tester should be aware of some species differences (e.g., it is not uncommon to see slight ketonuria as detected by the test strips in rodent urine from control animals). The main constituents of the ketone bodies are 3-β-hydroxybutyrate, acetone, and acetoacetate, and test strip results may be confirmed if necessary by measuring 3-β-hydroxybutyrate (Laffel 1999).

5.3.3 FLUID AND ELECTROLYTE BALANCE

Disturbances of gastrointestinal function are often accompanied by electrolyte imbalance due to fluid losses by emesis (vomiting), volvulus (dilation), diarrhea, or other perturbations of many varied mechanisms for electrolyte and fluid homeostasis (see

Chapter 6). Prolonged or excessive losses of fluid via the GI tract will affect packed cell volume (hematocrit), plasma total protein, albumin, electrolytes, acid–base balance, and osmolality values as the circulating blood volume adjusts to the fluid loss. Excessive and prolonged salivation may also cause electrolyte perturbations, but to a much smaller extent. Hypo- or hypernatremia may occur depending on the proportional losses of electrolyte to water; these electrolyte changes are also reflected by plasma osmolality. There may be significant differences between the measured and calculated plasma osmolality in the presence of hyperlipidemia and hyperproteinemia.

The pancreatic secretion of chloride varies inversely to the bicarbonate concentration, which in turn varies directly with the flow rate; the sum of these two anions tends to remain constant under physiological conditions, with the electrolyte concentrations of the pancreatic secretions tending to parallel blood pH and electrolytes. Excessive losses of pancreatic fluid can be monitored by plasma chloride measurements. Hypocalcemia may also accompany severe pancreatic toxicity, probably due to the formation of insoluble salts with fatty acids.

5.3.4 Lipids

Xenobiotic-induced pancreatitis may be accompanied by gross plasma lipid changes that may result from marked changes of carbohydrate metabolism (see Chapter 9). The observation of the presence of gross macroscopic fecal fat content (steatorrhea) can indicate effects on pancreatic function, biliary dysfunction, or intestinal malabsorption. In longer-term studies, malabsorption of fat-soluble vitamins may be reflected by the clinical condition of vitamin-deficient animals.

5.3.5 Fecal (Occult) Blood Tests

This test can be useful when gastrointestinal bleeding is suspected but blood cannot be seen macroscopically in the feces (e.g., with some nonsteroidal anti-inflammatory compounds). The sampling procedures and their timing are important, particularly when the bleeding may be intermittent.

A number of procedures for the detection of occult blood are available, and the majority of colorimetric qualitative tests are based on the pseudoperoxidase activity of hemoglobin. These tests can be performed using guaiac/peroxide detection systems or some tests using immunochemical detection methods. Although antihuman hemoglobin antibodies react with canine hemoglobin, immunochemical assays should be checked to establish suitable cross-reactivities with laboratory animal blood (Jinbo et al. 1998). Methods using the detection of peroxidase activity are subject to interference from the presence of other peroxidases in the diet and degradation of hemoglobin in the intestine, yielding false positive results (Johnson 1989; Cook et al. 1992; Rice and Ihle 1994). Some compounds (or metabolites) may impart a red color to feces, and it is important to exclude xenobiotic-induced porphyria as a possible cause of red coloration. Small amounts of blood may be naturally lost in the feces, so it may be necessary to adjust the sensitivity of the tests for each species by altering the proportions of the reagents (Dent 1973). Techniques using radio-labeled isotopes for the measurement of blood loss from the gastrointestinal tract are rarely used in toxicology studies.

5.3.6 HORMONES

The availability of hormone assays for laboratory animals has improved over the last decade, and this has been accompanied by a shift from radio-immunometric to nonisotopic assays using enzyme-linked immunosorbance, immunofluorescence, or chemiluminescence. Although these developments are welcome—particularly in the continuing search for therapies for diabetes, gastrointestinal hormones are not commonly measured in toxicology studies because these hormones have relatively short half-lives and their measurement requires carefully designed investigational studies (Woodman 1997).

Plasma gastrins have varied molecular structure across the species and have relatively short half-lives of less than 1 h. Measurement is mainly of use as an efficacy biomarker in compounds that have potential anti-ulcer properties (e.g., histamine receptor antagonists and proton pump inhibitors) (Larsson et al. 1986; Ishikawa et al. 1999; Morita et al. 2001; Jainu, Srinvasulu, and Devi 2005; Khayyal et al. 2006; Mao et al. 2008). Plasma cholecystokinin (CCK) is a hormone that has been given attention in pancreatic toxicities and as a biomarker for appetite suppressants (Axelson et al. 1996; Obourn, Frame, Bell, et al. 1997; Obourn, Frame, Chiu, et al. 1997; Rehfeld 1998a, 1998b; Wang et al. 1998). The molecular structures of the pancreatic hormones insulin (Stockham, Nachreiner, and Krehbiel 1983; Cartañá and Arola 1992; Chevenne, Trivin, and Porquet 1999; Hagar and Fahmy 2002; O'Hagan and Menzel 2003) and glucagon vary with animal species (Fletcher et al. 1988; Janssen et al. 2000). This prevents the universal application of immunoassays across different species; these hormone measurements are used primarily in animal models of diabetes.

5.3.7 OTHER TESTS OF GASTROINTESTINAL AND PANCREATIC FUNCTION

Three emerging fecal tests are for elastase, calprotectin, and adipsin, but these have yet to be tested widely in toxicology studies. The fecal elastase test has been developed as a noninvasive measurement of exocrine insufficiency, and fecal elastase does not appear to be increased in dogs with intestinal inflammation (Domínguez-Muñoz et al. 1995; Stein et al. 1996; Goldberg 2000; Battersby et al. 2005; Schneider et al. 2005). Adipsin is serine protease and has been shown to be increased in gastrointestinal toxicity associated with some gamma secretase inhibitors (Searfoss et al. 2003). Calprotectin is a calcium-binding protein (granulocyte marker protein) of approximately 37 kDa found mainly in neutrophils, and fecal calprotectin could be a surrogate marker for the migration of neutrophils through inflamed intestinal mucosae (Roseth et al. 1992; Kristensson et al. 1999).

Pancreatic function tests include the use of synthetic peptide N-benzoyl-1-tyrosyi-4-aminobenzoic acid (BT-PABA) tests, fluoroscein dilaurate, disaccharide tolerance, fat absorption, and stimulation of pancreatic enzyme secretion by cholecystokinin-pancreozymin (CCK-PZ) or the Lundh test meal. Because the exocrine pancreas is a target for toxicity from oxygen free radicals, other measurements for oxidative injury to assess the effect of these free radicals may be used in mechanistic studies (Braganza and Foster 1999).

Intestinal permeability may be measured following the administration of polyethylene glycol polymers (Walsh 2001), by the urinary excretion of orally administered sucrose as a marker of gastroduodenal damage and 51Cr-EDTA as markers of gastroduodenal and intestinal permeability (Yanez et al. 2003), or by other markers (Bjarnason, MacPherson, and Hollander 1995; Ford, Martin, and Houston 1995).

The use of these functional and other tests is rare in toxicological studies, although these tests are used in veterinary medicine. The tests often require additional invasive procedures and the administration of test substances, so they should be considered only for additional investigational studies.

REFERENCES

General

Badalov, N., R. Baradarian, K. Iswara, J. Li, W. Steinberg, and S. Tenner. 2007. Drug-induced acute pancreatitis: An evidence based review. *Clinical Gastroenterology and Hepatology* 5:648–661.

Banerjee, A. K., K. J. Patel, and S. L. Grainger. 1989. Drug induced pancreatitis. *Medical Toxicology and Adverse Drug Experiments* 4:186–189.

Biour, M., H. Daoud, and C. B. Salem. 2005. Pancreatotoxicite des medicaments. Seconde mise a jour du fichier bilographique des atteintes pancreatiques et des medicaments responsables. *Gastroenterology and Clinical Biology* 29:353–359.

Braganza, J. M., and J. R. Foster. 1999. Toxicology of the pancreas. In *General toxicology,* 2nd ed., ed. B. Ballantyne, T. Marrs, and T. Syversen, pp. 663–715. Basingstoke, England: Macmillan Reference Ltd.

Gad, S. C. 2007. *Toxicology of the gastrointestinal tract. Target organ toxicology series,* vol. 24. Boca Raton, FL: CRC Press.

Mallory, A., and J. Kern. 1980. Drug induced pancreatitis: A critical review. *Gastroenterology* 78:813–820.

Motta, P. M., G. Macchiarelli, S. A. Nottola, and S. Correr. 1997. Histology of the exocrine pancreas. Review. *Microscopy Research Techniques* 37:384–398.

Pour, P. M. 2005. *Toxicology of the pancreas. Target organ toxicology series,* vol. 21. Boca Raton, FL: CRC Press.

Rattner, D. W. 1999. Experimental models of acute pancreatitis and their relevance to human disease. *Scandinavian Journal of Gastroenterology* 31:6–9.

Timbrell, J. 2001. *Introduction to toxicology,* 3rd ed. London: Taylor & Francis.

Trivedi, C. D., and C. S. Pitchumoni. 2005. Drug-induced pancreatitis: An update. *Journal of Clinical Gastroenterology* 39:709–716.

Woodman, D. D. 1997. *Laboratory animal endocrinology,* pp. 310–447. Chichester, England: John Wiley & Sons.

Amylase and Lipase

Abe, T., T. Shimosegawa, A. Satoh, R. Abe, Y. Kikuchi, M. Koizumi, and T. Toyota. 1995. Nitric oxide modulates pancreatic edema formation in rat caerulein-induced pancreatitis. *Journal of Gastroenterology* 30:636–642.

Arglebe, C., K. Bremer, and R. Chilla. 1978. Hyperamylasemia in isoprenaline-induced experimental sialoadenosis in the rat. *Archives of Oral Biology* 23:997–999.

Braun, J. P., G. Ouedraogo, B. Thorel, C. Medaille, and A. G. Rico. 1990. Determination of plasma alpha-amylase in the dog: A test of the specificity of the new methods. *Journal of Clinical Chemistry and Clinical Biochemistry* 28:493–495.

Graca, R., J. Messick, S. McCullough, A. Barger, and W. Hoffmann. 2005. Validation and diagnostic efficacy of a lipase assay using the substrate 1,2-dilauryl-rac-glyceroglutaric acid (6′-methyl resorufin)-ester for the diagnosis of acute pancreatitis in dogs. *Veterinary Clinical Pathology* 34:39–43.

Hamdan, I. I., F. Afifi, and M. O. Taho. 2004. In vitro alpha amylase inhibitory effect of some clinically used drugs. *Pharmazie* 59:799–801.

Hide, W. A., L. Chan, and W. H. Li. 1992. Structure and evolution of the lipase superfamily. *Journal of Lipid Research* 33:167–178.

Jacobs, R. M., R. L. Hall, and W. A. Rogers. 1982. Isoamylases in clinically normal and diseased dogs. *Veterinary Clinical Pathology* 11:26–32.

Kamath, V., A. K. Joshi, and P. S. Rajini. 2008. Dimethoate induced biochemical perturbations in rat pancreas and its attenuation by cashew nut skin extract. *Pesticide Biochemistry and Physiology* 90:58–65.

MacKenzie, P. I., and M. Messer. 1976. Studies on the origin and excretion of serum α-amylase in the mouse. *Comparative Biochemistry and Physiology* 54B:103–106.

Mályusz, M., P. Wrigge, D. Caliebe, and J. Das. 1990. Differences in the renal handling of pancreatic and salivary amylase in the rat. *Enzyme* 43:129–136.

Mazzon, E. et al. 2006. Effects of 3-aminobenzamide, an inhibitor of poly (ADP-ribose) polymerase in a mouse model of acute pancreatitis induced by cerulein. *European Journal of Pharmacology* 549:149–156.

McGeachin, R. L., and J. R. Akin. 1982. Amylase levels in the tissues and body fluids of several primate species. *Comparative Biochemistry and Physiology* 72A:267–269.

Medaille, C., and A. Breind-Marchal. 2004. Comparison of amylase and lipase activities in serum and plasma of dogs. *Veterinary Clinical Pathology* 33:155–158.

Merkord, J., H. Weber, G. Kröning, and G. Henninghausen. 2001. Repeated administration of a mild acute toxic dose of di-*n*-butyltin dichloride at intervals of 3 weeks induces severe lesions in pancreas and liver of rats. *Human and Experimental Toxicology* 20:386–392.

Murtaugh, R. J., and R. M. Jacobs. 1985. Serum amylase and isoamylases and their organs in healthy dogs and dogs with experimentally induced acute pancreatitis. *American Journal of Veterinary Research* 46:742–747.

Parent, J. 1982. Effects of dexamethasone on pancreatic tissue and on serum amylase and lipase activities in dogs. *Journal of American Veterinary Medicine* 180:743–746.

Rajasingham, R., J. L. Bell, and D. N. Baron. 1971. A comparative study of the isoenzymes of mammalian alpha-amylase. *Enzyme* 12:180–186.

Ramos, O., O. R. Leitao, J. C. Repka, and S. G. Barros. 2005. Pancreatite aguada experimental induzida pela L-arginina: Avaliaao histologica e bioquimica. *Arquivos de Gastroenterologia* 42:55–59.

Robinovitch, M. R., and Sreebny, L. M. 1972. On the nature of molecular heterogeneity of rat parotid amylase. *Archives of Oral Biology* 17:595–600.

Seo, S. W. et al. 2005. Taraxacum officinale protects against cholecystokinin-induced acute pancreatitis. *World Journal of Gastroenterology* 11:597–599.

Sokolowski, A., H. Spormann, and G. Letko.1987. Influence of pancreatic edema and short-term ischemia of rat pancreas on lipase and alpha-amylase activities in the serum and in the pancreas. *Deutsche Zeitschrift für Verdauungs und Stoffwechsekrankheiten* 47:119–127.

Sparmann, G., J. Merkord, A. Jaschke, H. Nizze, L. Jonas, M. Lohr, S. Liebe, and J. Emmrich. 1997. Pancreatic fibrosis in experimental pancreatitis induced by dibutylin dichloride. *Gastroenterology* 112:1664–1672.

Steiner, J. M., G. M. Rutz, and D. A. Williams. 2006. Serum lipase and pancreatic lipase immunoreactivity concentrations in dogs treated with exocrine pancreatic insufficiency. *American Journal of Veterinary Research* 67:84–87.

Tormo, M. A., I. Gil-Exojo, A. Romero de Tejada, and J. E. Campillo. 2004. Hypoglycaemic and anorexigenic activities of an alpha-amylase inhibitor from white kidney beans (*Phaseolus vulgaris*) in Wistar rats. *British Journal of Nutrition* 92:785–790.

Wallig, M. A., A. M. Kore, J. Crawshaw, and E. H. Jeffery. 1992. Separation of the toxic and glutathione enhancing effects of the naturally occurring nitrile, cyanohydroxybutene. *Fundamental and Applied Toxicology* 19:598–606.

Walter, G. l., P. McGraw, and H. W. Tvedten. 1992. Serum lipase in the dog: A comparison of a titrimetric method with an automated method. *Veterinary Clinical Pathology* 21:23–27.

Trypsin and Trypsinogen

Archer, F. J., M. E. Kerr, and D. M. Houston. 1997. Evaluation for three pancreas-specific protein assays TLI (trypsin like immunoreactivity) PASP (pancreas specific protein) and CA19-9 (glycoprotein) for use in the diagnosis of pancreatitis. *Zentralblatt für Veterinarmedizin. Reihe A* 44:109–113.

Fletcher, T. S., H. Tsukamoto, and Largman C. 1986. Immunoenzymatic determination of trypsin/alpha 1-protease inhibitor complex in plasma of rats with experimental pancreatitis. *Clinical Chemistry* 32:1738–1741.

Geokas, M. C., C. Largman, P. R. Dune, J. W. Brodrick, and J. Vollmer. 1981. Immunoreactive forms of cationic trypsin in plasma and ascites of dogs in experimental pancreatitis. *American Journal of Pathology* 105:31–39.

Hedstrom, J. et al. 1996. Urine trypsinogen-2 as a marker of acute pancreatitis. *Clinical Chemistry* 42:685–690.

John-Baptiste, A., F. P. Sace, Z. Zong, R. Bell, A. Roth, D. Morton, and M. T. Rock. 2004. Biomarkers of pancreatic function. *Clinical Chemistry* 50:A35.

Reddy, S., N. J. Bibby, P. A. Smith, and R. B. Elliott. 1985. Rat trypsin: Purification radioimmunoassay and age related serum levels in normal and spontaneously diabetic BB Wistar rats. *Australian Journal of Experimental Biology and Medical Science* 63:667–681.

Schmidt, J., E. Ryschich, H. P. Sinn, S. Maksan, C. Herfarth, and E. Klar. 1999. Trypsinogen activation peptides (TAP) in peritoneal fluid as predictors of late histopathologic injury in necrotizing pancreatitis of the rat. *Digestive Diseases and Sciences* 44:823–829.

Waritani, T., Y. Okuno, Y. Ashida, M. Hisasue, R. Tsuchiya, K. Kobayashi, and T. Yamada. 2002. Development of a canine trypsin-like immunoreactivity assay system using monoclonal antibodies. *Veterinary Immunology and Immunopathology* 87:41–49.

Wilberg, M. E., A. K. Nurmi, and E. Westermarck. 1999. Serum trypsinlike immunoreactivity for the diagnosis of subclinical exocrine pancreatic insufficiency. *Journal of Veterinary Internal Medicine* 13:426–432.

Williams, D. A., and R. M. Batt. 1988. Sensitivity and specificity of radioimmunoassay of trypsin-like immunoreactivity for the diagnosis of canine exocrine pancreatic insufficiency. *Journal of the American Veterinary Medical Association* 192:195–201.

Other Enzymes

Ford, T. F., D. A. W. Grant, B. M. Austen, and J. Hermon-Taylor. 1985. Intramucosal activation of pepsinogens in the pathogenesis of acute gastric erosions and their prevention by the potent semisynthetic amphipathic inhibitor pepstatinyl-glycyl lysyl-lysine. *Clinica Chimica Acta* 145:37–47.

Lynch, K. M., D. Sellers, D. Ennulat, and L. Schwartz. 2004. Evaluation and use of a human ELISA method for measuring pepsinogen I in monkey serum. *Clinical Chemistry* 50 (Suppl.): A36.

Tani, S., A. Ishikawa, H. Yamazaki, and Y. Kudo. 1987. Serum pepsinogen levels in normal and experimental peptic ulcer rats measured by radioimmunoassay. *Chemical and Pharmaceutical Bulletin* (Tokyo) 35:1515–1522.

Will, P. C., W. E. Allbee, C. G. Witt, R. J. Bertko, and T. S. Gaginella. 1984. Quantification of pepsin A activity in canine and rat gastric juice with the chromogenic substrate Azocoll. *Clinical Chemistry* 30:707–711.

Glycated Hemoglobin, Fructosamine, and Ketones

Çakatay, U., and R. Kayali. 2006. The evaluation of altered redox status in plasma and mitochondria of acute and chronic diabetic rats. *Clinical Biochemistry* 39:907–912.

Cefalu, W. T., J. D. Wagner, and A. D. Bell-Farrow. 1993. Role of glycated proteins in monitoring diabetes in *Cynomolgus* monkeys. *Laboratory Animal Science* 43:73–77.

Dan, K., H. Fujita, Y. Seto, and R. Kato. 1997. Relation between stable glycated hemoglobin A_{1c} and plasma glucose in diabetes-model mice. *Experimental Animals* 46:135–140.

Hasegawa, S., T. Sako, N. Takemura, H. Koyama, and S. Motoyoshi. 1991. Glycated hemoglobin fractions in normal and diabetic dogs measured by high performance liquid chromatography. *Journal of Veterinary Medical Science* 53:65–68.

Higgins, P. J., R. L. Garlick, and H. F. Bunn. 1982. Glycosylated hemoglobin in human and animal red cells. Role of glucose permeability. *Diabetes* 31:743–748.

Hooghuis, M., M. Rodriguez, and M. Castano. 1994. Ion exchange microchromatography and thiobarbituric acid colorimetry for the measurement of canine glycated hemoglobin. *Veterinary Clinical Pathology* 23:110–116.

Johnson, R. N., R. W. Easdale, M. Tatnell, and J. R. Baker. 1991. Significance of variation in turnover of glycated albumin on indices of diabetic control. *Clinica Chimica Acta* 198:229–238.

Kondo, N., Y. Shibayama, Y. Toyomaki, M. Yamamoto, H. Ohara., K. Nakano, and K. Ienaga. 1989. Simple method for determination of A1c-type glycated hemoglobin(s) in rats using high performance liquid chromatography. *Journal of Pharmacology Methods* 21:211–221.

Laffel, L. 1999. Ketone bodies: A review of physiology, pathophysiology, and application of monitoring to diabetes. *Diabetes Research and Metabolism Reviews* 15:412–426.

Levi, B., and M. J. Werman. 1998. Long-term fructose consumption accelerates glycation and several age related variables in male rats. *Journal of Nutrition* 128:1442–1449.

Loste, A., and M. C. Marca. 2001. Fructosamine and glycated hemoglobin in the assessment of glycemic control in dogs. *Veterinary Research* 32:55–62.

Nagisa, Y., K. Kato, K. Watanabe, H. Murakoshi, H. Odaka, K. Yoshikawa, and Y. Sugiyama. 2003. Changes in glycated hemoglobin levels in diabetic rats measured with an automated affinity HPLC. *Clinical and Experimental Pharmacology and Physiology* 30:752–758.

Rendell, M., P. M. Stephen, R. Paulsen, J. L. Valentine, K. Rasbold, T. Hestorff, S. Eastberg, and D. C. Shint. 1985. An interspecies comparison of normal levels of glycosylated hemoglobin and glycosylated albumin. *Comparative Biochemistry and Physiology* 81B:819–822.

Srinivas, M., K. Ghosh, D. K. Shome, J. S. Virdi, S. Kumar, D. Mohanty, and K. C. Das. 1986. Glycosylated hemoglobin (HbA_1) in normal rhesus monkeys (*Macaca mulatta*). *Journal of Medical Primatology* 15:361–365.

Ukarapol, N., R. E. Begue, J. Hempe, H. Correa, R. Gomez, and A. Vargas. 2002. Association between *Helicobacter felis*-induced gastritis and elevated glycated hemoglobin levels in a mouse model of type 1 diabetes. *Journal of Infectious Diseases* 183:1463–1467.

Yue, D. K., S. McLennan, D. B. Church, and J. R. Turtle. 1992. The measurement of glycosylated hemoglobin in man and animals by aminophenylboronic acid affinity chromatography. *Diabetes* 31:701–705.

Fecal Occult Blood

Cook, A. K., S. D. Gilson, W. D. Fischer, and P. H. Kass. 1992. Effect of diet on results obtained by use of commercial test kits for detection of occult blood in feces of dogs. *American Journal of Veterinary Research* 18:1749–1751.

Dent, N. J. 1973. Occult blood detection in feces of various animal species. *Laboratory Practice* 22:674–676.

Jinbo, T., M. Shimizu, S. Hayashi, T. Shida, T. Sakamoto, S. Kitao, and S. Tyamamoto. 1998. Immunological determination of fecal hemoglobin concentrations in dogs. *Veterinary Research Communications* 22:193–201.

Johnson, D. A. 1989. Fecal occult blood testing. Problems, pitfalls and diagnostic concerns. *Postgraduate Medicine* 85:287–299.

Rice, J. E., and S. L. Ihle. 1994. Effects of diet on fecal occult blood testing in healthy dogs. *Canadian Journal of Veterinary Research* 5:134–137.

Hormones

Axelson, J., M. Kobari, J. F. Rehfeld, and I. Ihse. 1996. Changes in rat pancreas following gastric surgery are not correlated with basal levels of serum gastrin or plasma cholecystokinin. *Digestive Surgery* 13:6–11.

Cartañá, J., and L. Arola. 1992. Nickel-induced hyperglycemia: The role of insulin and glucagon. *Toxicology Letters* 71:181–192.

Chevenne, D., F. Trivin, and D. Porquet. 1999. Insulin assays and reference values. *Diabetes Metabolism* (Paris) 25:459–476.

Fletcher, H. P., W. J. Akbar, R. W. Peoples, and G. R. Spratto. 1988. Effect of acute soman on selected endocrine parameters and blood glucose in rats. *Fundamental and Applied Toxicology* 11:581–586.

Hagar, H. H., and A. H. Fahmy. 2002. A biochemical, histochemical and ultrastructural evaluation of the effect of dimethoate intoxication on rat pancreas. *Toxicology Letters* 133:161–170.

Ishikawa, H. et al. 1999. FR145715, a novel histamine H_2 receptor antagonist, with specific anti-*Helicobacter pylori* activities. *European Journal of Pharmacology* 378:299–310.

Jainu, M., C. Srinvasulu, and S. Devi. 2005. Anti-ulcerogenic and ulcer healing effects of *Solanum nigra* (L) on experimental ulcer model: Possible mechanism for the inhibition of acid formation. *Journal of Ethnopharmacology* 104:156–163.

Janssen, G. B., R. B. Beems, L. H. Elver, and E. Speijers. 2000. Subacute toxicity of α-ergocryptin in Sprague–Dawley rats. 2: Metabolic and hormonal changes. *Food Chemistry and Toxicology* 38:689–695.

Khayyal, M. T., M. Seif-El-Nasr, M. A. El Ghazlaly, S. N. Okpanyi, O. Kelber, and D. Weiser. 2006. Mechanisms involved in the gastro-protective effect of STW5 (Iberogast®) and its component against ulcers and rebound acidity. *Phytomedicine* 13 (Suppl. 1): 56–66.

Larsson, H. et al. 1986. Plasma gastrin and gastric enterochromaffin like cell activation and proliferation. *Gastroenterology* 90:391–399.

Mao, Y., X. Zhang, B. Yuan, and G. Lu. 2008. Subchronic toxicity and oxicolkeinetis of LZB, a new proton pump inhibitor, after 13 week repeat oral administration in dogs. *Regulatory Toxicology and Pharmacology* 50:75–86.

Morita, H. et al. 2001. Effects of Z-360, a novel CCK_B/gastrin (CCK_2) receptor antagonist on meals induced secretion and experimental ulcer models in dogs and rats. *Gastroenterology* 120:A311.

Obourn, J. D., S. R. Frame, R. H. Bell, D. S. Longnecker, G. S. Elliott, and J. C. Cook. 1997. Mechanism for pancreatic oncogenic effect of the peroxisome proliferator Wyeth-14,643. *Toxicology and Applied Pharmacology* 145:425–436.

Obourn, J. D., S. R. Frame, T. Chiu, T. E. Solomon, and J. C. Cook. 1997. Evidence that A8947 enhance pancreatic growth via a trypsin inhibitor mechanism. *Toxicology and Applied Pharmacology* 146:116–126.

O'Hagan, S., and A. Menzel. 2003. A subchronic rat toxicity study and in vitro genotoxicity studies with a conjugated linoleic product. *Food Chemistry and Toxicology* 41:1749–1760.

Rehfeld, J. F. 1998a. How to measure cholecystokinin in tissue, plasma and cerebrospinal fluid. *Regulatory Peptides* 78:31–39.

———. 1998b. Accurate measurement of cholecystokinin. *Clinical Chemistry* 44:991–1001.

Stockham, S. L., R. F. Nachreiner, and J. D. Krehbiel. 1983. Canine immunoreactive insulin quantitation using five commercial radioimmunoassay kits. *American Journal of Veterinary Research* 44:2179–2183.

Wang, Y., S. Naruse, M. Kitagawa, H. Ishiguro, Y. Nakae, T. Yoshikawa, and T. Hayakawa. 1998. Effects of a new cholecystokinin antagonist, TS-941, on experimental acute pancreatitis in rats. *Pancreas* 17:289–294.

Other Tests of Gastrointestinal and Pancreatic Function

Battersby, I. A., I. R. Peter, M. J. Day, A. J. German, and E. J. Hall. 2005. Effect of intestinal inflammation on fecal elastase in dogs. *Veterinary Clinical Pathology* 34:49–51.

Bjarnason, I., A. MacPherson, and D. Hollander. 1995. Intestinal permeability: An overview. *Gastroenterology* 108:1566–1581.

Domínguez-Muñoz, J. E., C. Heironymus, T. Sauerbruch, and P. Malfertheimer. 1995. Fecal elastase: Evaluation of a new noninvasive pancreatic function test. *American Journal of Gastroenterology* 90:1834–1837.

Ford, J., S. W. Martin, and J. B. Houston. 1995. Assessment of intestinal permeability changes induced by nonsteroidal anti-inflammatory drugs in the rat. *Journal of Pharmacological and Toxicological Methods* 34:9–16.

Goldberg, D. M. 2000. Proteases in the evaluation of pancreatic function and pancreatic disease. *Clinica Chimica Acta* 291:201–221.

Kristensson, J. et al. 1999. Granulocyte marker protein is increased in stools from rats with azoxymethane-induced colon cancer. *Scandinavian Journal of Gastroenterology* 34:1216–1223.

Roseth, A. G., M. K. Fagerhol, E. Aadland, and H. Schonsby. 1992. Assessment of the neutrophil dominating protein calprotectin in feces. A methodological study. *Scandinavian Journal of Gastroenterology* 27:793–798.

Schneider, A., B. Funk, W. Caspary, and J. Stein. 2005. Monoclonal versus polyclonal ELISA for assessment of fecal elastase concentration: Pitfalls of a new assay. *Clinical Chemistry* 51:1052–1054.

Searfoss, G. H. et al. 2003. Adipsin: A biomarker of gastrointestinal toxicity mediated by a functional gamma secretase inhibitor. *Journal of Biological Chemistry* 278:46107–46116.

Stein, J. G., M. Jung, A. Sziegoleit, S. Zeuzem, W. F. Caspary, and B. Lembcke. 1996. Immunoreactive elastase I: Clinical evaluation of a new noninvasive test of pancreatic function. *Clinical Chemistry* 42:222–226.

Walsh, C. T. 2001. Methods in gastrointestinal toxicology. In *Principles and methods of toxicology*. 4th ed., ed. A. W. Hayes. pp. 1215–1240. Philadelphia: Taylor and Francis.

Yanez, J. A., X. W. Tang, K. A. Roupe, M. W. Fariss, and N. M. Davies. 2003. Chemotherapy-induced gastrointestinal toxicity in rats: Involvement of mitochondrial DNA, gastrointestinal permeability and cyclooxygenase-2. *Journal of Pharmaceutical Science* 6:308–314.

6 Fluid Balance, Electrolytes, and Mineral Metabolism

6.1 GENERAL PHYSIOLOGY

The fluid spaces in the body occupy about 60% of the total body mass. The two main spaces are the intracellular fluid (ICF) and the extracellular fluid (ECF), with the ECF subdivided into the intravascular space (plasma), the interstitial space (lymph), and transcellular fluids such as pleural, cerebrospinal, pericardial, peritoneal, and gastrointestinal fluids. The ECF and ICF spaces are normally in an osmotic equilibrium in which body water moves under osmotic pressure between ICF and ECF, governed by the osmotically active molecules in each space. The electrolyte constituents of ICF and ECF are different, particularly for sodium, which is higher in ECF than ICF, and potassium, which is higher in ICF compared to ECF.

Oncotic pressure (or colloid osmotic pressure) is the osmotic pressure that results from the difference between the protein (mainly albumin) concentrations of plasma and the interstitial fluid. Water is lost from the body via feces, urine, salivation, insensible respiration, and through the skin, with sensible perspiration of sweat occurring in a few species. Although the movement of proteins between spaces is restricted, water and small ions can move across permeable membranes between the spaces. The volume of ECF is highly dependent on its sodium concentration and, under physiological conditions, the sodium ion concentrations of plasma and interstitial fluids are similar.

The overviews of the metabolism of the electrolytes presented here are highly simplified for the purposes of this chapter. In the last decade, our knowledge has grown about cellular transport systems and how ions and water are moved up and down electrical or concentration gradients by channel or transporter proteins through channels in the cellular membranes. Uniporters move ions down concentration gradients, antiporters move ions against the gradient, and symporters (or cotransporters) transport ions down one gradient and link this to the transport of other ions in the opposite direction (Berndt and Kumar 2007; Esteva-Font, Torra Balcells, and Férnandez-Llama 2007; Schmitz, Deason, and Perraud 2007; El-Sheikk, Masereeuw, and Russel 2008; Suketa 2008). Pharmacology, proteomics, and toxicogenomics may help in identifying which of these molecules will be helpful in understanding the toxic mechanisms that affect electrolyte metabolism, but for the present we are left with the currently available plasma and urine determinations for toxicology studies.

Some general references (not cited in the text) are provided in sections at the end of this chapter.

The electrolytes—both anions and cations—perform a number of vital roles in maintaining fluid balance and acid–base balance, membrane potentials, muscular functions, and nervous conduction. They act as cofactors in many enzyme-mediated reactions. In addition, calcium and phosphate are the main mineral constituents of the skeleton.

6.2 POTASSIUM, SODIUM, AND CHLORIDE

6.2.1 POTASSIUM

Approximately 98% of the body's potassium is present in the ICF, and the levels of potassium are controlled by the total body potassium and its distribution between the ECF and ICF. Many factors influence the distribution of potassium, including osmolality, acid–base balance, hormones (e.g., insulin and catecholamines), and the cellular potassium content. The cellular potassium levels are dependent upon the uptake of potassium via membrane-bound Na^+/K^+-ATPase and the passive diffusion of potassium from the cells. Insulin promotes active uptake of potassium, probably via action on Na^+/K^+-ATPase. Catecholamines promote cellular uptake through beta-adrenergic actions, and alpha-adrenergic actions increase plasma potassium. In the kidneys, potassium is freely filtered though the glomeruli, and up to 95% is reabsorbed from the tubular fluid before reaching the renal distal tubules, where potassium is secreted into the tubule. There is also some degree of secretion into the descending limb of the loop of Henle. High plasma potassium increases the secretion of aldosterone from the adrenal glands; aldosterone secretion is reduced when plasma potassium is low. The effects of aldosterone are to facilitate the renal exchange of potassium and hydrogen ions for sodium ions.

6.2.2 SODIUM

The concentrations of sodium in body fluids are related to osmotic homeostasis, maintaining the balance between the ECF and ICF volumes, and neuromuscular excitability. The ECF volume is controlled by the presence of sodium and osmoregulation so that sodium deficit or excess will cause changes in the ECF. Under normal physiological conditions, sodium loss from the body is associated with loss of body water. Any excessive loss of sodium reduces the ECF volume, while any loss of body fluids other than from plasma results in proportionally less sodium than fluid being lost. Plasma sodium is freely filtered through the renal glomeruli, with about 65% reabsorbed in the proximal tubules and approximately 25% reabsorbed in the loop of Henle, together with chloride ions and water under physiological conditions.

The balance of sodium ion concentrations is governed by a number of mechanisms, including osmoreceptors in the hypothalamus and several volume receptors (e.g., intrathoracic, atrial stretch, and hepatic), and baroreceptors (e.g., intrarenal and arterial). These physiological mechanisms normally balance the plasma sodium and renal excretion of sodium, with approximately 80% of the sodium in the glomerular filtrate reabsorbed. Renal reabsorption of sodium occurs mainly in the distal tubules and collecting ducts, although some sodium reabsorption occurs in the proximal tubules. The actions of several hormones affect electrolyte and fluid balance; these hormones include the renin–angiotensin–aldosterone axis, natriuretic hormones, and vasopressin.

6.2.2.1 Renin–Angiotensin–Aldosterone Axis

The proteolytic enzyme renin is secreted by the juxta-glomerular apparatus of the glomerular afferent arterioles in response to reduced renal perfusion and excessive loss of sodium. Renin cleaves angiotensinogen—an α-2-globulin synthesized by the liver—to release angiotensin I, which is converted to a decapeptide angiotensin I in the circulation and in the nephrons. Angiotensin-converting enzyme (ACE), which is present in the pulmonary circulation, kidney, and vascular beds of several organs, converts angiotensin I to the octapeptide angiotensin II. Angiotensin II increases aldosterone secretion and glomerular filtration rate via its vasoconstrictive actions influencing the effective plasma volume. Angiotensin II also can affect the central nervous system and cardiac myocytes. Aldosterone is the primary mineralocorticoid; other mineralocorticoids influence electrolyte transport to a lesser extent by regulating renal reabsorption and excretion of sodium, chloride, hydrogen, and potassium ions, thereby affecting blood pressure homeostasis. The simplified relationships between the renin–angiotensin system and aldosterone and their effects on sodium and potassium are shown in Figure 6.1.

6.2.2.2 Natriuretic Hormones

At least three natriuretic peptides influence sodium balance: atrial natriuretic peptide (ANP or atriopeptin), brain natriuretic peptide (BNP, named thusly because it was first isolated from porcine brain), and cardiac natriuretic peptide (CNP). As the names imply, these peptides act to decrease sodium reabsorption in the distal convoluted tubules and collecting ducts of the kidney and to increase urinary sodium

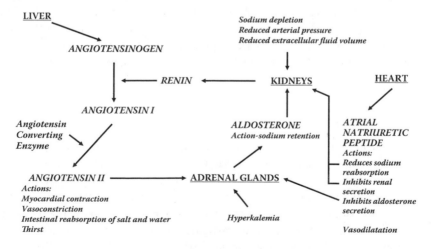

FIGURE 6.1 Renin–angiotensin–aldosterone axis.

(i.e., natriuretic effect). These are small peptides (fewer than 30 amino acid residues), although their precursors are larger (e.g., the precursor has 151 amino acid residues, which are shortened to the 28-amino-acid peptide ANP). These peptides are synthesized and secreted by cardiac myocytes, mainly in the right atrium, and they are highly conserved across species having similar actions. In response to increased atrial pressure (or stretch) following excessive sodium intake or volume expansion, ANP and BNP act to inhibit tubular sodium reabsorption, inhibit the renin–angiotensin aldosterone axis, and cause systemic vasodilatation (de Wardener and Clarkson 1985; Maack 1988). (Some of these peptides are used as biomarkers of congestive cardiac failure; see Chapter 7).

6.2.2.3   Vasopressin

Within the hypothalamus, osmoreceptor cells respond to increasing ECF osmolality by increasing the synthesis and release of the peptide hormone vasopressin (AVP—arginine vasopressin, which is also called antidiuretic hormone—ADH) in the hypothalamus and vice versa. Vasopressin is transported for storage in the posterior pituitary gland and then to the kidneys, where vasopressin regulates the reabsorption of water in the distal convoluted tubules. In these renal tubules, through a number of intermediary reactions, vasopressin acts on adenylate cyclase to convert adenosine triphosphate (ATP) to cyclic adenosine monophosphate (cAMP). There is a net movement of water from the tubular fluid into the cells, the excreted urine volume is reduced, and the urine concentration is higher (i.e., an antidiuretic effect).

6.2.3   CHLORIDE

This major extracellular anion plays an important role together with sodium in maintaining osmolality and acid–base balance, and in the central nervous system (e.g., where chloride facilitates the effects of some inhibitory compounds such as gamma aminobutyrate in neurons). After passing freely through the renal glomeruli, chloride is passively reabsorbed in the proximal convoluted tubules and actively reabsorbed in the loop of Henle by an active "chloride pump." It is also reabsorbed with sodium in the distal tubules. In most situations, plasma sodium and chloride tend to parallel each other.

6.2.4   BICARBONATE

The bicarbonate ion (HCO_3^-) is the second-largest anionic contributor to maintaining acid–base balance, and its secretion from the pancreas helps to neutralize the contents of the small intestine. Respiration controlling the carbon dioxide concentration of the blood ($PaCO_2$) and renal excretion of bicarbonate are the two main homeostatic influences on plasma bicarbonate. Within the renal tubular lumen, carbonic anhydrase converts carbonic acid into carbon dioxide, which diffuses into the epithelial cells and forms carbonic acid, which later dissociates to bicarbonate.

6.2.5 Acid–Base Balance

General body metabolism generates large amounts of acid, which are removed mainly either through the kidneys (where some acids are excreted and bicarbonate is retained) or the lungs where carbon dioxide is exhaled. Imbalances, which can affect the blood pH, may be due to alterations in metabolism or respiration, and pH may fall leading to acidosis or increase in alkalosis: the hydrogen ion concentration (or pH) of the ECF is normally maintained within narrow limits. In SI unitage, hydrogen ion concentration is expressed as nmol/l and replaces pH as a reporting unit but many investigators prefer and retain the pH unitage.

6.2.6 Calcium and Inorganic Phosphate (Phosphorus)

Calcium is the most abundant mineral in the body, with approximately 98% contained in the skeleton as hydroxyapatite—a combination of calcium and phosphate. There is a continual exchange of calcium between the bones and ECF. Approximately 40–50% of the plasma calcium is free or ionized; the remaining plasma fractions are bound to plasma proteins mainly with albumin and a smaller fraction containing calcium is associated with ligands such as phosphate sulfate citrate, bicarbonate, and anticoagulant proteins. In the kidney, about 75% of calcium is reabsorbed passively in the proximal tubule and another 20% in the thick ascending limb and distal convoluted tubule. The ionized calcium is the physiologically important fraction essential for excitation/contraction, signaling, coupling hormonal regulation, and energy metabolism where the intracellular calcium levels are very important for cell survival. Calcium is involved in neuromuscular transmissions, cardiac and skeletal muscular contraction and relaxation, coagulation, cell growth, membrane transport mechanisms, and enzymatic reactions.

Phosphate metabolism is governed by the same hormones as calcium, but inorganic phosphate (sometimes referred to as inorganic phosphorus) levels are more sensitive than calcium to dietary intake and the renal excretion rate. Inorganic phosphate takes mainly two forms: the monophosphate and a smaller proportion of dihydrogen phosphate; however, this balance is disturbed when the extracellular fluid pH alters. Phosphate is essential to many important endogenous molecules such as nucleic acids and nucleotides (e.g., adenosine diphosphate [ADP] and ATP). About 75% of the phosphate filtered through the glomerulus is reabsorbed in the proximal renal tubules with a further 10% absorbed in the distal tubules or collecting ducts.

6.2.7 PTH and Calcitonin

These two hormones, together with the vitamin calcitriol, regulate calcium homeostasis and thereby indirectly affect phosphate metabolism. Parathyroid hormone (parathormone; PTH) is secreted by the parathyroid glands as a polypeptide of 84 amino acid residues, and its action is to increase plasma calcium via parathyroid hormone receptors in bone, kidney, and a few other tissues. PTH secretion is increased in response to hypocalcemia and hyperphosphatemia; conversely, increased plasma calcium suppresses PTH secretion. The renal production of 1,25-dihydroxycholecalciferol is also

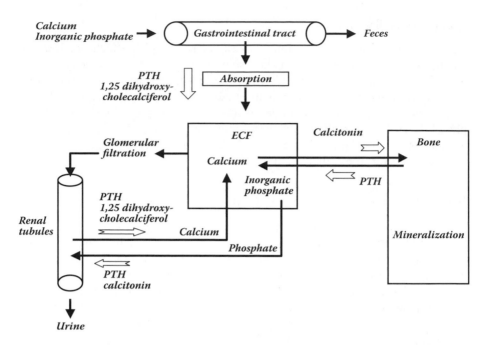

FIGURE 6.2 Simplified interrelationships of parathyroid hormone (PTH), calcitonin, and 1,25 dihydroxycholecalciferol. The open block arrows indicate increased movement due to hormones and vitamins.

stimulated by PTH. The peptide hormone calcitonin is produced in the parafollicular cells (C cells) of the thyroid and acts to decrease plasma calcium; it acts with opposite effects to those of PTH (Figure 6.2).

6.2.8 CALCITRIOL

This active vitamin D metabolite (1,25 dihydroxycholecalciferol) is an important cofactor for intestinal calcium absorption, which involves calbindins (calcium binding proteins) in the intestine and kidney. Calcitriol is produced in the kidneys by the conversion of 25-hydroxycholecalciferol (calcidiol) and its formation is stimulated by a reduction of plasma calcium and/or phosphate and increased production of parathyroid hormone and prolactin (Figure 6.3). Calcitriol also inhibits the release of calcitonin and, together with PTH, increases the absorption of calcium and phosphate from the gastrointestinal tract and the kidneys. Growth hormone, glucocorticoids, estrogens, testosterone, and the thyroid hormones also influence calcium metabolism.

6.2.9 MAGNESIUM

This cation is essential for many enzyme reactions, neuromuscular activity, and bone formation; it is the second most abundant intracellular cation. When compared

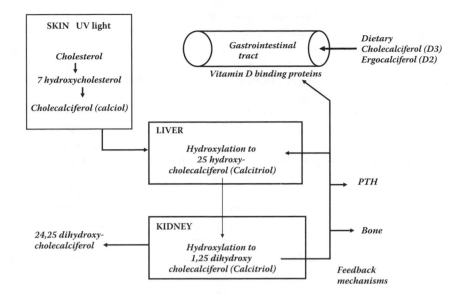

FIGURE 6.3 Simplified pathways for vitamin D metabolism.

with calcium, much less is known about homeostatic mechanisms for magnesium, although the normally narrow ranges for plasma magnesium imply close homeostatic control. About 50% of plasma magnesium is ionized; about 40% is bound to albumin, and the remainder is complexed with phosphate, citrate, and bicarbonate.

The physiology and pathology of calcium, magnesium, and phosphate are closely related in bone metabolism. Bone is metabolically active, with constant remodeling of the bone matrix deposition and resorption. Bone modeling describes the primary mechanism for bone growth to attain its ultimate structure (e.g., longitudinal growth occurring by endochondral ossification). The bone-resorbing cells–osteoclasts–digest the bone surface and create cavities for the bone-forming cells–osteoblasts–to fill by synthesizing and creating different types of collagen.

6.3 EFFECTS DUE TO TOXICITY

Fluid or water overloading may occur when excessive thirst is induced by a test compound, inappropriately high intravenous infusion rates, cardiac failure, or failure of renal excretion to act as a compensatory mechanism. This may cause reductions of plasma sodium, protein, albumin, and osmolality values. The osmolality of a test solution for intravenous administration may affect fluid balance when the injection volumes are relatively large compared to the ECF volume of the animal (Michel 1991). If the osmolality of the intravenous fluid is inappropriate, this may cause hemolysis, with subsequent changes to plasma electrolytes. Dehydration may occur when food and water intakes are severely reduced, and plasma sodium, total protein, albumin, and osmolality values tend to increase. In dehydration states, such as those associated with gastrointestinal toxicity, and diarrhea causing additional fluid loss, it is not uncommon for oliguria to occur until rehydration has taken place. Plasma osmolality is increased by a severe reduction of water intake and excessive water loss due to a loss of renal concentrating ability. Some xenobiotics and/or metabolites possess osmotic effects. Evidence of hemodilution or hemoconcentration may be found in the hematology data e.g., altered hematocrit [Hct]/packed cell volume [PCV]), although the relationship between Hct/PCV and plasma volume is not linear (Boyd, 1981).

Dietary requirements for electrolytes vary between species, and the general laboratory animal diets are more than sufficient to meet these requirements for both major and trace elements. Usually, animals will cope with slightly excessive amounts of minerals by normal physiological mechanisms; however, the scientific literature contains many examples of dietary manipulations used to investigate causations for both human and animal diseases (e.g., high-salt diets in cardiovascular studies). Discussion continues about the timings or the provision of nutrition to animals in studies, the need to balance the effects of feeding patterns with reductions of stress due to experimental procedures, and their effects on experimental measurements (Toth and Gardiner 2000; Rowland 2007). Prolonged and/or severe reductions of food and fluid intakes will have some effects on plasma electrolyte concentrations, particularly with xenobiotics, which have marked effects on the gastrointestinal tract.

Plasma electrolytes and fluid balance may be affected by toxicities in several tissues, including the gastrointestinal tract, kidneys, heart, lungs, and bone, although other organ toxicities can also affect these measurements. The main endocrine organs to affect electrolytes include the adrenals, thyroids, pancreas, and parathyroids. Cardiac output directly alters fluid balance and indirectly affects other organ functions (e.g., kidneys, because they receive approximately one quarter of the total cardiac output); altered fluid balance (e.g., with congestive cardiac failure) may be reflected by changes in plasma albumin (total protein) and osmolality. As reabsorption and exchange of electrolytes occur in various regions of the nephron and plasma electrolytes (and the urinary cations sodium and potassium), this may indicate renal dysfunction. The study observations made on water intake, food intake, body weight, urination patterns, and urine volumes are all relevant to data interpretation. Cationic changes are accompanied invariably by disturbances of plasma anionic concentrations and acid–base balance, and an extreme change in the ionic balance of one cation may influence the concentrations of the other cations.

Perturbations of the cations sodium, potassium, calcium, and magnesium may cause increased irritability of cardiac tissue and can be associated with arrhythmias; changes of these cations can also affect skeletal muscles. The interpretation of changing values for plasma electrolytes may be complex when cardiac output is a consequence of the failure of other organ functions (e.g., the kidneys) and, conversely, when impaired cardiac damage affects renal function. This interrelationship of organ functions is seen with several antitumor agents that may cause cardio- and nephrotoxicity.

6.3.1 POTASSIUM, SODIUM, AND CHLORIDE

Some causes of hyperkalemia and hypokalemia are listed in Table 6.1. Increases of plasma potassium may be observed following metabolic acidosis, severe tissue necrosis, and renal failure, and hyperkalemia is associated with respiratory acidosis. Potassium excess is rare and raised plasma potassium values are often due to artifacts. Hypokalemia is broadly associated with alkalosis and chronic fluid loss and can result in muscle weakness and respiratory failure when it is severe. Depending upon the total body potassium content, urine potassium values may take several days to show adaptation to changes of plasma potassium.

Hyper- or hyponatremia can occur due to various causes, and it is often strongly linked to changes of water/fluid balance, which is a major influence on several of these perturbations (see Table 6.2). Pseudohyponatremia occurs when there is a replacement of plasma water with lipid (e.g., with high content lipid vehicles used for dosing) or, less commonly, with protein. Although the sodium content for the plasma water remains normal, the plasma contains less water and the apparent plasma sodium is lower.

Changes in *plasma chloride* are generally paralleled by changes in plasma sodium and often show an inverse relationship to plasma bicarbonate. Hypochloridemia (or hypochloremia) is observed in conditions of severe dehydration, gastrointestinal fluid loss, and metabolic alkalosis. Hyperchloremia is associated with metabolic acidosis or respiratory alkalosis.

Tables 6.3–6.5 list some of the causes that affect plasma calcium, magnesium, and phosphate. Increased plasma calcium concentration may occur when the xenobiotic specifically targets calcium metabolism, behaves similarly to vitamin D, and causes hyperparathyroidism or renal disease. Lead and cadmium enter bone and inhibit bone growth, increase calcium release from bone, and inhibit renal tubular reabsorption of calcium salts; lead inhibits the renal bioactivation of 25-hydroxy-cholecalciferol (Sauk and Somerman 1991). In longer-term studies, increased plasma calcium may be associated with tumor burden. Because roughly half of circulating calcium is bound to plasma albumin, hypercalcemia can also arise from dehydration. Hypoparathyroidism, pancreatitis, and renal disease can reduce plasma calcium. Acidosis increases plasma-ionized calcium concentrations, whereas alkalosis causes a decrease due to the effects of pH in the ECF or on protein binding.

For both *calcium and magnesium,* which are partially bound to plasma proteins (particularly albumin), it is necessary to consider possible effects due to hypo- or hyperproteinemia on the proportions of ionized and bound cations. Xenobiotics bound to albumin may also decrease protein binding of divalent cations, which results in lower calcium values; reductions of plasma calcium and albumin tend to be correlated. Although calcium and magnesium play a pivotal role in the early stages of toxic injury leading to cell death including apoptosis (Trump and Berezesky 1995; Chang et al. 2000), these intracellular effects are not often mirrored by plasma calcium, unless tissue necrosis is severe.

Magnesium is less commonly measured in toxicological studies and clinical medicine despite several compounds, such as cyclosporin and cisplatin, which have marked effects on magnesium homeostasis (Borland et al. 1985; Evans 1988), and cisplatin (Magil et al. 1986; Yao et al. 2007). Hypomagnesemia is often associated with myopathies.

Changes of plasma inorganic phosphate can be indicative of renal injury and be associated with increases of urea (blood urea nitrogen, BUN) and creatinine

TABLE 6.1
Some Causes of Hyper- and Hypokalemia

Hyperkalemia

Increased intake via infusion solutions or use of potassium salts

Reduced potassium excretion due to:

Hormonal effects: hypoaldosteronism, adrenal toxicity

Renal effects: oliguria, chronic renal toxicity, diuresis

Metabolic and respiratory acidosis

Cellular necrosis, intravascular hemolysis

Hypertonic states

Artifactual:

Hemolysis

Release from leukocytes and platelets

Tissue injury during blood collection

Delayed sample separation

Use of potassium EDTA salts as anticoagulants

Example compounds causing hyperkalemia:

angiotensin converting enzyme inhibitors and antagonists of angiotensin II, cotrimoxazole

Hypokalemia

Decreased intake

Extrarenal loss:

Vomiting, diarrhea, increased fecal loss

Renal loss:

Increased mineralocorticoids

Hyperaldosteronism

Renal tubular acidosis and chronic alkalosis

Renal tubular injury

Redistribution of potassium between ECF and ICF—sometimes associated with alkalosis

Artifactual:

In hyperlipidemia and hyperproteinemia

Example compounds causing hypokalemia:

Increased gastrointestinal loss: laxatives

Altered renal excretion including aminoglycosides, antineoplastic agents, and diuretics

Reduced renal reabsorption of bicarbonate and increased potassium excretion

Carbonic anhydrase inhibitors

Alteration of ECF:ICF ratio

Beta-adrenergic agonists such as salbutamol, insulin, and folate

Reduced distal tubular reabsorption of sodium and chloride furosemide, loop diuretics, thiazide
diuretics

TABLE 6.2
Some Causes of Hyper- and Hyponatremia

Hypernatremia

With decreased body sodium:

Extra-renal loss:

Diarrhea, salivation, reduced ICF, and ECF

Shock, oliguria, hypotension, reduced ECF

With normal body sodium:

Insufficient fluid intake or increased water loss

With increased body sodium:

Excessive sodium intake or reduced renal excretion

Artifactual:

Sample evaporation, sample collection from limbs where hypertonic saline infusions have been administered

Example compounds causing hypernatremia:

Mineralocortioids and glucocorticoids: inhibition of AVP release—ethanol and phenytoin; reduction of AVP effect on renal tubules and diuresis—lithium

Hyponatremia

With low ECF volume (hypovolemia):

Extrarenal loss:

Vomiting, diarrhea, inflammatory exudate

Renal loss:

Adrenal insufficiency, mineralocorticoid deficiency, osmotic diuresis, renal tubular acidosis

With normal ECF volume (euvolemia):

In acute or chronic water retention, inappropriate AVP secretion, glucocorticoid deficiency, chronic renal injury, hypothyroidism

With increased ECF (hypervolemia):

Renal failure, nephrotic syndrome, congestive cardiac failure, hypoproteinemia

Dietary insufficiency

Artifactual:

Pseudohyponatremia

Hyperosmolar hyponatremia associated with hyperglycemia following mannitol infusion

Examples of compounds causing hyponatremia include diuretics, inhibitors, and antagonists of angiotensin converting enzymes: potentiation and increased production of AVP—acetoaminophen, barbiturates, carbamzepine, chlorpropamide; reduced reabsorption of sodium and chloride in the distal tubules and diuresis—furosemide, loop diuretics, thiazide diuretics

(Kempson and Dousa 1986). Severe depletion of phosphate may lead to altered erythrocytic metabolism and hemolysis, and dietary phosphate intake also has a major influence on the level of circulating phosphate.

Plasma levels of calcium and phosphate generally reflect periods of rapid bone growth, which occur in the neonatal and juvenile ages; they later show a gradual decline with age. Some age-related variations of sodium potassium and chloride in mice and rats have been reported (Nachbaur et al. 1977; Frith, Suber, and Umholtz

TABLE 6.3

Some Causes of Hyper- and Hypocalcemia

Hypercalcemia

Hyperparathyroidism

Malignancy

Other endocrine disorders

    Hyperthyroidism

    Hypoadrenalism

Dehydration

Hyperproteinemia, particularly hyperalbuminemia

Artifactual:

    Poor venepuncture technique

Example compounds causing hypercalcemia include thiazides, lithium, calciferol-containing
  rodenticides, estrogens, and glucocorticoids

Hypocalcemia

Renal injury associated with impaired hydroxylation of 25-hydroxycholecalciferol or acidosis

Inadequate nutritional intake of calcium, vitamin D, or both

Hypoparathyroidism

Acute pancreatitis

Hypoproteinemia, particularly hypoalbuminemia

Artifactual:

    EDTA, oxalate, and citrate anticoagulants

Example compounds causing hypocalcemia include calcitonin, diuretics, anticonvulsants, fluoride, and
  ethylene glycol; chelating agents—EDTA, metabolites of ethylene glycol

---

1980). Plasma alkaline phosphatase also changes during growth periods, but it is not a useful marker of bone metabolism in rats or nonhuman primates (see Chapter 2).

In contrast with some other clinical chemistry parameters, circulating mineral and electrolyte concentrations are regulated within relatively narrow limits, and small perturbations can be both biologically and statistically significant. Although the intake of fluids and urinary excretion may be highly variable in toxicological studies, the ionic concentrations in the body fluids often appear to be well controlled, with minimum perturbations of the common plasma electrolyte measurements. In some species (e.g., nonhuman primates, particularly marmosets), the plasma electrolyte concentrations may be more variable. However, it is not uncommon to find small but statistically significant changes for electrolyte measurements for either individuals or groups of animals that do not appear to dose related or to correlate with histopathological findings.

A number of preanalytical factors, including anesthetics, stress, dietary intakes, fluid intake, diurnal variation, and dark and light illumination cycles, are known to affect the electrolyte and related hormone measurement determinations. Therefore, these factors should be considered when interpreting these data. Plasma calcium and phosphate are subject to diurnal variation and may increase after feeding.

TABLE 6.4
Some Causes of Hyper- and Hypomagnesemia

Hypermagnesemia

Decreased excretion in acute and chronic renal failure
Increased intake (e.g., magnesium salts of test compounds)
Cellular necrosis
Adrenocortical hypofunction

Hypomagnesemia

Reduced nutritional intake
Malabsorption
Increased gastrointestinal fluid loss
Pancreatitis
Increased renal excretion
Hypoparathyroidism
Hyperthyroidism
Hyperkalemia
Example compounds causing hypomagnesemia include aminoglycosides, cisplatin, ciclosporin, and
  some diuretics

TABLE 6.5
Some Causes of Hyper- and Hypophosphatemia

Hyperphosphatemia

Increased dietary intake
Tissue necrosis
Acidosis
Altered bone metabolism
Decreased renal excretion
Artifactual: delayed sample separation or hemolysis
Example compounds causing hyperphosphatemia include anabolic steroids, furosemide, and thiazides

Hypophosphatemia

Redistribution of phosphate between ECF and ICF
Decreased nutritional intake
Hepatotoxicity
Hyperparathyroidism
Infection
Increased excretion
Example compounds causing hypophosphatemia include antacids, renal tubular toxins, ethanol,
  intravenous glucose, and insulin

Plasma proteins are amphoteric molecules having both positive and negative charges that contribute to the balance of plasma ions and osmolality, particularly albumin. In cardiotoxicity, plasma protein patterns may be altered with increases of total protein, albumin, and acute phase proteins (e.g., myoglobin, C-reactive protein, and fibrinogen; see Chapters 7 and 8). When proteins bind xenobiotics (or metabolites), their contributions to cation/anion balance may be altered.

Although acid–base balance perturbations may often accompany severe electrolyte changes, these measurements require controlled sampling conditions, particularly for small laboratory animals, and they are rarely included in toxicology studies. Although perturbations of acid–base balance may be respiratory or metabolic (Figure 6.4), often there is a mixture of these effects in severe toxicity. The effects may be of variable duration and severity within treatment groups and have differing compensatory and noncompensatory mechanisms. Evidence of ketoacidosis may be found from measurements of plasma and urinary ketones, and plasma lactate measurements can be used to demonstrate lactic acidosis.

6.4 LABORATORY INVESTIGATIONS

Electrolyte measurements in general toxicological studies are often confined to plasma sodium (Na^+), potassium (K^+), and calcium (Ca^{++}); see Chapter 1. Magnesium (Mg^{++}) and anions such as inorganic phosphate, chloride (Cl^-), bicarbonate (HCO_3^-), and lactate are measured less frequently; the use of combination triple-ion (sodium/potassium/chloride) selective electrodes leads to a tendency to include the

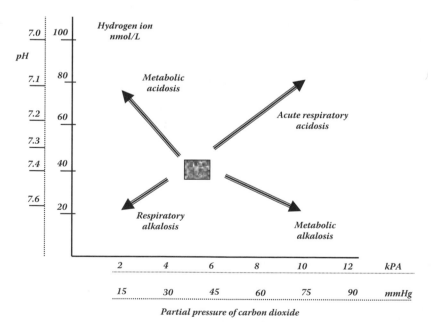

FIGURE 6.4   Relationships between arterial hydrogen ion concentration and partial pressure of carbon dioxide ($PaCO_2$). The shaded rectangle represents approximate reference ranges.

measurement of chloride (by default) in study requirements. Urinary sodium and potassium are also measured to meet some regulatory requirements where renal toxicity or marked alterations of fluid balance are suspected, as well as in safety pharmacology/renal physiology studies (ICH 2000; Emeigh-Hart 2005). The measurement of blood gases is largely confined to safety pharmacology studies and as efficacy biomarkers for compounds intended to alter the transport of blood gases and respiration. Occasionally, it is useful to analyze the constituents of some of the transcellular fluids such as pleural, peritoneal, and cerebrospinal fluids.

The ranges obtained for plasma electrolytes vary between species; in the smaller laboratory animals, these ranges are particularly dependent on the blood collection procedures (see Chapter 12 and Appendix C). There are very minor differences between serum and plasma. The use of plasma rather than serum reduces the times required for the blood separation procedures and may result in minor differences between serum and plasma. Plasma potassium (and inorganic phosphate) levels increase if the separation of whole blood is delayed and the values are higher where hemolysis is present. The effects of hemolysis on potassium are less marked in the dog, where the erythrocytic potassium concentration is lower (Holmgren, Palm, and Edqvist 1974). Marked thrombocytosis can cause factitious hyperkalemia in dog (Reimann, Knowlen, and Tvedten 1989). Tissue injury—particularly with cardiac sampling, which can occur during blood collection procedures—can lead to falsely high potassium values, and plasma potassium values are much higher when carbon dioxide is used for euthanasia.

Lithium heparinate is the anticoagulant of choice for plasma electrolyte measurements (except, of course, for plasma lithium). Falsely elevated potassium values occur when potassium sequestrenated (EDTA) samples are measured, and the anticoagulant sodium heparinate will give falsely elevated sodium values. Sodium fluoride is a suitable anticoagulant for plasma lactate measurements and is more convenient than iced perchloric acid (Evans 1987).

The majority of laboratories measure sodium or potassium ion-selective electrodes; older methods using flame photometry are largely obsolete and methods involving chromogenic or enzymatic procedures for these cations have not been widely used for laboratory animal samples. The antibiotic valinomycin can adversely affect potassium electrodes because it facilitates potassium transport. Chloride is measured by ion-selective electrodes or colorimetric methods. Halogenated test compounds may cause technical interferences in these measurements, which may also be affected by high chloride concentrations due to the test compound or vehicle. Hyperlipidemia may affect electrolyte measurements using ion-selective electrodes due to plasma displacement effects; the algorithms used by some analyzers do not compensate for effects due to marked hyperlipidemia and hyperproteinemia. Several examples of plasma electrolyte values altered by artifacts are given in Tables 6.1–6.5 (e.g., high plasma potassium values may be caused by hemolysis and thrombocytosis).

The *anion gap* (AG) is calculated by subtracting the sum of plasma chloride and bicarbonate concentrations from the sum of the sodium and potassium; it represents the balance between the plasma anions and cations (Feldman and Rosenberg 1981; Kraut and Madias 2007). The unmeasured anions that contribute to the anion gap include proteins, inorganic phosphate, lactate, pyruvate, sulfate, oxalate acetate, formate, and anions of other inorganic and organic acids, with proteins forming about 60% of the total anion gap. For plasma, the anion gap is approximately 10–20 mmol/L; in unanesthetized larger laboratory animals, the AG gap is occasionally useful as a check on the electrolyte balance, but it is markedly altered in samples collected under anesthesia. Anion gaps are dependent on the analytical technology—particularly the choice of method for determining bicarbonate. (The anion gap is increased in ketoacidosis, renal failure, and toxicities associated with methanol, salicylates, and ethylene glycol.)

6.4.1 Urinary Sodium, Potassium, and Chloride

The urinary concentrations of these cations are highly variable because they are dependent on diet, and samples are subject to the effects of fecal contamination. The data are also highly variable when urinary output is affected by dehydration or excessive fluid losses via the gastrointestinal tract. Urine electrolyte values vary in intravenous studies due to rate of administration, tonicity, and electrolyte concentration of the vehicle.

The fractional excretion (FE) of ions may be calculated as a measure of the urinary concentration of an analyte versus the amount of ion absorbed by the kidney. For example, the fractional excretion of sodium may be calculated by the formula:

$$\text{FE sodium} = \text{clearance}_{Na}/\text{glomerular filtration rate} \times 100$$

where

$$\text{Clearance}_{Na} = \frac{\text{Urine sodium}}{\text{Plasma sodium}} \times \text{Urine volume (ml/min)}$$

The use of these calculations is limited in toxicology (Lefebvre et al. 2008) but occasionally used when comparing the clearance of a xenobiotic that also affects electrolyte renal secretion and excretion rates.

Plasma and urine osmolalities are commonly determined by methods using depression of freezing point; some laboratories use a vapor pressure method. An approximation of plasma osmolality can be obtained by adding the concentrations of glucose, urea, and twice the sodium concentration when all are expressed as millimoles/L. Osmolality is the molal concentration of solute within a liter of water and is expressed as millimoles per kilogram of water; under physiological conditions, plasma osmolality equates to plasma osmotic pressure. Plasma osmolality values vary between species, mainly reflecting differences due to the plasma sodium concentrations. Plasma osmolality measurements are of value when some estimation of renal tubular function or free water clearance is required. Marked differences between the measured and calculated osmolality values may be caused by the test compound (e.g., ethylene glycol).

Urine osmolality measurements can be used as an alternative to specific gravity and urine creatinine as indicators of urine concentration. The maximal urine concentrating and diluting ability varies widely between species, with rats and dogs able to produce more concentrated urine (higher than 2500 mosmols/kg body water) than humans (see Chapter 4). Urinary electrolyte and osmolality values may appear to be falsely low when water is accidentally spilt from water bottles into the urine samples by animal movements. Such an event may be sometimes detected by measuring osmolality (specific gravity) and noting an unusually high urine volume together with a pale (water-like) appearance of the sample.

The osmolal clearance can be calculated using the formula:

$$\text{Clearance}_{\text{osmolal}} = \text{Urine volume (ml/min)} \times \frac{\text{Urine osmolality}}{\text{Plasma osmolality}}$$

where osmolality is measured in milliosmoles per kilogram of body water. When urine flow is greater than osmolal clearance, the urine is hypo-osmotic, and the urine is hyperosmotic when the osmolal clearance is higher than urine flow rate. Free water clearance represents the amount of water that is the plasma volume cleared of solute-free water per unit time, and this can be calculated using the following formula (Martinez-Maldonado and Opava-Stitzer 1978):

$$\text{Free water clearance} = \text{urine volume (mL/min)} - \text{clearance}_{\text{osmolal}}$$

Some published data are available for urinary values in dogs and rats (Shevlock, Khan, and Hackett 1993; Diez et al. 1996; Lane et al. 2000; Trevisan et al. 2001; Kulick et al. 2005). See also Appendix A for further references.

Colorimetric methods are generally used for plasma *total calcium, magnesium, and inorganic phosphate* measurements. Although ionized calcium and magnesium concentrations are more relevant to understand effects due to these ions, these measurements are not commonly used because they require analyzers with the appropriate selective ion electrodes. Sample collection and transport conditions must be carefully controlled to avoid pH changes, which affect these measurements (Szenci, Brydl, and Bajcsy 1991; Dewitte, Stock, and Theinpont 1999; CLSI 2001b; Rayana et al. 2008). The urinary sediments must be thoroughly mixed with the urine and dissolved if accurate measurements for urinary calcium, inorganic phosphate, and magnesium are required.

Plasma calcium and albumin do not show a linear relationship in hypo- and hyperalbuminemia (Schenck and Chew 2005). Although there are some formulae to correct plasma calcium for variations due to plasma proteins—particularly in hypoalbuminemia for humans—these often use a reference plasma albumin value of 40 g/L (White et al. 1986), which is inappropriate for many laboratory animals where the plasma protein reference values differ.

Acid–base balance measurements are affected by anesthesia and sedatives, and it is partly because of these effects that acid–base balance measurements are not included routinely in toxicological studies, although they may be used in safety pharmacology or inhalation studies. Measurement of oxygen (pO_2) can be important when testing compounds that bind with hemoglobin and therefore cause a shift in blood oxygenation. Acid–base measurements require carefully controlled conditions and sample collection and analytical procedures (Szenci et al. 1991; CLSI 2001b; Slaughter et al. 2002); the use of liquid anticoagulants with small samples can lead to errors (Hopper, Rezende, and Haskins 2005).

Some published but variable data are available for acid–base measurements in larger laboratory animals (Pickrell, Light, et al. 1973; Pickrell, Mauderley, et al. 1973; Cornelius and Rawlings 1981; Barzago et al. 1992), partly reflecting sample collection procedures and advances in blood gas analyzer technology. Although arterial sampling is the preferred procedure, some investigators have used capillary and mixed venous samples (Upton and Morgan 1975; Ilkiw, Rose, and Martin 1991); different methods of sampling produce variations in results.

Hormone measurements can be used selectively in mechanistic toxicological studies where the pharmacology/mode of action of the test compound suggests that the assays will be useful in determining the pathogenesis of renal or other changes. The measurement of hormones—PTH, calcitonin, renin, angiotensins, aldosterone, and atrial natriuretic hormone measurements—requires carefully controlled sampling procedures (Woodman 1997). The hormones and vitamins that govern electrolyte and fluid balance can be measured using radioimmunoassay, chemiluminescence, or enzyme immunoassays; these hormones are highly conserved and assays work in several species.

A downside in applying these assays is the relatively short half-lives of the hormones. Several of these hormones have very short half-lives (e.g., PTH < 10 min; calcitonin ~ 1–3 h; ANP < 5 min; and renin < 90 min). For hormones such as PTH, there were historic problems of specificity when second-generation assays cross-reacted with the large C-terminal fragment of PTH (7–84 amino acids). However, the third generation of PTH assays measured whole, intact PTH (1–84 amino acids; Kalu et al. 1983; Jara et al. 1994; Terry, Orrock, and Meilke 2003). Vitamin D and its metabolites may be measured by radioimmunoassay, chemiluminescence, or enzyme immunoassay (Glendenning et al. 2003; Zerwekh 2004). For aldosterone, there are circadian rhythms in the rat (Gomez-Sanchez et al. 1976; Kaplan 1976) and in the rabbit (Vernay, Marty, and Moalti 1984). Dietary sodium can also influence levels of plasma aldosterone (Kotchen et al. 1983). Urinary aldosterone measurements are of little value because less than 1% of secreted aldosterone is excreted.

Some molecules, such as *amino acids,* which are also ionized, are rarely measured in regulatory toxicology studies; however, the amino acids are some of the major metabolites measured by nuclear magnetic resonance spectroscopy for toxicological purposes (Lindon, Holmes, and Nicholson 2004).

During the last decade, commercially available kits have made available for plasma/serum and urinary biomarkers of bone formation and bone resorption. Some of the assays have been shown to be applicable in rats and dogs, but not all assays work across the species, and there is inherent variability with these markers. Some of the tests are listed in Table 6.6, and a number of references are provided. These tests will have a place in animal models, and they may be useful efficacy markers in the development of novel therapeutic agents.

TABLE 6.6
Some Biochemical Markers of Bone Resorption, Formation, and Turnover

Bone Formation

Bone alkaline phosphatase

N mid fragment osteocalcin (N-Mid)

Osteocalcin (or bone gla protein: OC or OCN)

Procollagen type I N telopeptide (PINP)

Procollagen type I C telopeptide (PICP)

Procollagen type III telopeptide (PIIINP or P3NP)

Soluble receptor activator for nuclear factor kappa beta-ligand (RANKL)

Bone Remodeling Biomarkers

Bone sialoprotein (BSP)

Glucosyl galactosyl hydroxylysine (Glc-Gal-Hyl)

N-terminal cross-linking telopeptide I collagen (NTX)

Osteoprotegerin (OPG)

Osteoprotegerin ligand (OPGL)

Urine deoxypyridinoline (UDPD)

Urine pyridinoline (UPYD)

Tartrate resistant acid phosphatase (TRAP5b or TRACP)

Cartilage Remodeling Markers

Aggrecan turnover CS-846, CTX-MMP, CI-2C

Cartilage oligomeric matrix protein (COMP)

Chondroitin sulfate

Cleavage assay for type II 3/4C (C2C)

Collagen type II C telopeptide

C propeptide of type II collagen (CPII)

N propeptide of type IIA procollagen (PIIANP)

Hyaluronic acid

Hydroxyproline

REFERENCES

Barzago, M. M., A. Bortolotti, D. Omarini, J. J. Aramayona, and M. Bonatti. 1992. Monitoring of blood gas parameters and acid–base balance of pregnant and nonpregnant rabbits (*Oryctolagus cuniculus*) in routine experimental conditions. *Laboratory Animals* 26:73–79.

Berndt, T., and R. Kumar. 2007. Phosphatonins and the regulation of phosphate homeostasis. *Annual Review of Physiology* 69:341–359.

Borland, I. A., J. R. Gosney, A. N. Hillis, E. P. M. Williamson, and R. A. Sells. 1985. Hypomagnesemia and cyclosporine toxicity. *Lancet* i:103–104.

Boyd, J. W. 1981. The relationships between blood haemoglobin concentrations, packed cell volume and plasma protein concentration in dehydration. *British Veterinary Journal* 137:166–172.

Chang, S. H., P. C. Phelps, M. Berezesky, M. L. Ebersberger, and B. F. Trump. 2000. Studies on the mechanisms and kinetics of apoptosis induced by microinjection of cytochrome C. *American Journal of Pathology* 156:637–649.

CLSI. 2001b. C46—*A blood gas and pH analysis and related measurements. Approved guideline,* 1st ed. Wayne, PA: Clinical and Laboratory Institute Standards.

Cornelius, I. M., and C. A. Rawlings.1981. Arterial blood gas and acid–base values in dogs with various diseases and signs of disease. *Journal of the American Veterinary Medical Association* 178:992–995.

de Wardener, H. E., and E. M. Clarkson. 1985. Concept of natiuretic hormone. *Physiological Reviews* 65:658–759.

Dewitte, K., I. D. Stock, and L. M. Theinpont. 1999. pH dependency of ionized calcium. *Lancet* 354:1793–1794.

Diez, I., C. C. Pérez, M. B. Garcia, M. J. Cano, and M. A. Rios. 1996. Twenty-four-hour urinary calcium and phosphorus excretion in beagle dogs. Preliminary report. *Scandinavian Journal of Laboratory Animal Science* 23:355–362.

El-Sheikk, A. A., R. Masereeuw, and F. G. Russel. 2008. Mechanisms of renal anionic transport. *European Journal of Pharmacology* 585:245–255.

Emeigh-Hart, S. G. 2005. Assessment of renal injury in vivo. *Journal of Pharmacological and Toxicological Methods* 52:30–45.

Esteva-Font, C., R. Torra Balcells, and P. Férnandez-Llama. 2007. Sodium transporters and aquaporins: Future renal biomarkers? *Medicina Clinica (Barcelona)* 129:433–437.

Evans, G. O. 1987. Plasma lactate measurements in healthy beagle dogs. *American Journal of Veterinary Research* 48:131–132.

———. 1988. Hypomagnesaemia, hypoalbuminaemia and plasma lipid changes in rats following the oral administration of ciclosporin. *Comparative Biochemistry and Physiology* 89C:375–376.

Feldman, B. P., and D. P. Rosenberg. 1981. Clinical use of anion and osmolal gaps in veterinary medicine. *Journal of the American Veterinary Medical Association* 178:396–398.

Frith, C. H., R. L. Suber, and R. Umholtz. 1980. Hematologic and clinical chemistry findings in control BALB/c and C57BL/6. *Laboratory Animal Science* 30:835–840.

Glendenning, P. et al. 2003. Issues of methodology, standardization and metabolite recognition of 25-hydroxyvitamin D when comparing the DiaSorin radioimmunoassay and the Nichols Advantage automated chemiluminescence protein binding assay in hip fracture cases. *Annals of Clinical Biochemistry* 40:546–551.

Gomez-Sanchez, C., O. B. Holland, J. R. Higgins, D. C. Kern, and N. M. Kaplan. 1976. Circadian rhythms of serum renin activity and serum corticosterone, prolactin and aldosterone concentrations in the male rat on normal and low-sodium diets. *Endocrinology* 99:567–572.

Holmgren, M-L., M. Palm, and L-E. Edqvist. 1974. Hemolysens inverkan på resultatet av några kliniskt-kemiska parametrar hos häst nötkreatur och hund. *Särtyck ur Svensk Veterinärtiding* 6:196–200.

Hopper, K., M. L. Rezende, and S. C. Haskins. 2005. Assessment of the effect of dilution of blood samples with sodium heparin on blood gas, electrolyte, and lactate measurements in dogs. *American Journal of Veterinary Research* 66:656–660.

ICH. 2000. *S7A Guideline: Safety pharmacology studies for human pharmaceuticals.* International Conference on Harmonization of Technical Requirements for Registration of Pharmaceuticals for Human Use.

Ilkiw, J. E., R. J. Rose, and I. C. Martin. 1991. A comparison of simultaneously collected arterial, mixed venous, jugular venous and cephalic venous blood samples in the assessment of blood–gas and acid–base status in the dog. *Journal of Veterinary Medicine* 5:294–298.

Jara, A., J. Bover, J. Lavigne, and A. Felsenfeld. 1994. Comparison of two parathyroid hormone assays for the rat: The new immunoradiometric and the older competitive binding assay. *Journal of Bone and Mineral Research* 1:1629–1633.

Kalu, D. N., R. Cockerman, B. P. Yu, and B. A. Roos. 1983. Lifelong dietary modulation of calcitonin levels in rats. *Endocrinology* 113:2010–2015.

Kaplan, N. M. 1976. Circadian rhythms of serum renin activity and serum corticosterone, prolactin and aldosterone concentrations in the male rat on normal and low-sodium diets. *Endocrinology* 99:567–572.

Kempson, S. A., and T. P. Dousa. 1986. Current concepts on regulation of phosphate transport in renal proximal tubules. *Biochemical Pharmacology* 35:721–726.

Kotchen, T. A., G. P. Guthrie, J. H. Galla, R. Luke, and W. J. Welch. 1983. Effects of NaCl on renin and aldosterone responses to potassium depletion. *American Journal of Physiology* 244:E164–169.

Kraut, J. A., and N. E. Madias. 2007. Serum anion gap: Its uses and limitations in clinical medicine. *Clinical Journal of the American Society of Nephrology* 2:162–174.

Kulick, L. J., D. J. Clemmons, R. L. Hall, and M. A. Koch. 2005. Refinement of the urine concentration test in rats. *Contemporary Topics in Laboratory Animal Science* 44:46–49.

Lane, I. F., D. H. Shaw, S. A. Burton, and A. W. Donald. 2000. Quantitative urinalysis in healthy beagle puppies from 9 to 27 weeks of age. *American Journal of Veterinary Research* 6:577–581.

Lefebvre, H. P., O. Dossin, C. Trumel, and J. P. Braun. 2008. Fractional excretion tests: A critical review of methods and applications in domestic animals. *Veterinary Clinical Pathology* 37:4–20.

Lindon, J. C., E. Holmes, and J. K. Nicholson. 2004. Metabonomics and its role in drug development and disease diagnosis. *Expert Reviews in Molecular Diagnosis* 4:189–199.

Maack, T. 1988. Functional properties of atrial natriuretic peptide and its receptors. In *Nephrology,* vol. 1, ed. A. M. Davidson, pp. 123–160. London: Bailliere Tindall.

Magil, A. B., V. Mavichak, N. L. Wong, G. A. Quamme, J. H. Dorks, and R. A. Surton. 1986. Long-term morphological and biochemical observations in cisplatin induced hypomagnesemia in rats. *Nephron* 43:223–230.

Martinez-Maldonado, M., and S. C. Opava-Stitzer. 1978. Free water clearance curves during saline, mannitol, glucose and urea diuresis in the rat. *Journal of Physiology* 280:487–498.

Michell, A. R. 1991. Regulation of salt and water balance. *Journal of Small Animal Practice* 32:135–145.

Nachbaur, J., M. R. Clarke, J-P. Provost, and J. L. Dancla. 1977. Variations of sodium, potassium and chloride plasma levels in the rat with age and sex. *Laboratory Animal Science* 27:972–975.

Pickrell, J. A., M. E. Light, J. L. Mauderley, P. B. Beckley, B. A. Muggenburg, and U. C. Luft. 1973. Certain effects of sampling and storage on canine blood of different oxygen tensions. *American Journal of Veterinary Research* 34:241–244.

Pickrell, J. A., J. L. Mauderley, B. A. Muggenburg, and U. C. Luft. 1973. Influence of fasting on blood gas tension, pH and related values in dogs. *American Journal of Veterinary Research* 34:805–808.

Rayana, M. C. et al. 2008. IFCC guideline for sampling, measuring and reporting ionized magnesium in plasma. *Clinical Chemistry and Laboratory Medicine* 46:21–26.

Reimann, K. A., G. G. Knowlen, and H. W. Tvedten. 1989. Factitious hyperkalemia in dogs with thrombocytosis. The effect of platelets on serum potassium concentration. *Journal of Veterinary Internal Medicine* 3:47–52.

Rowland, N. E. 2007. Food or fluid restriction in common laboratory animals: Balancing welfare with scientific inquiry. *Comparative Medicine* 57:149–160.

Sauk, J. J., and M. J. Somerman. 1991. Physiology of bone: Mineral compartment proteins as candidates for environmental perturbation by lead. *Environmental Health Perspectives* 91:9–16.

Schenck, P. A., and D. J. Chew. 2005. Prediction of serum ionized calcium concentration by use of serum total calcium in dogs. *American Journal of Veterinary Research* 66:1330–1336.

Schmitz, C., F. Deason, and A. L. Perraud. 2007. Molecular components of vertebrate Mg2+ homeostasis regulation. *Magnesium Research* 20:6–18.

Shevlock, P. N., S. R. Khan, and R. L. Hackett. 1993. Urinary chemistry of the normal Sprague–Dawley rat. *Urology Research* 21:309–312.

Slaughter, M. R., J. M. Birmingham, B. Patel, G. A. Whelan, A. J. Krebs-Brown, P. D. Hockings, and J. A. Osborne. 2002. Extended acclimatization is required to eliminate effects of periodic blood-sampling procedures on vasoactive hormones and blood volume in beagle dogs. *Laboratory Animals* 36:403–410.

Suketa, Y. 2008. Expression and regulation of renal sodium cotransporters and antiporters, and related transport proteins. *Yakugaku Zasshi* 128:901–917.

Szenci, O., E. Brydl, and C. A. Bajcsy. 1991. Effect of storage on measured ionized calcium and acid–base variables in equine, ovine, and canine venous blood. *Journal of the American Veterinary Medical Association* 199:1167–1169.

Terry, A. H., J. Orrock, and A. W. Meilke. 2003. Comparison of two third-generation parathyroid hormone assays. *Clinical Chemistry* 49:336–337.

Toth, L. A., and T. W. Gardiner. 2000. Food and water restriction protocols: Physiological and behavioral considerations. *Contemporary Topics in Laboratory Animal Science* 39:9–17.

Trevisan, A., M. Giraldo, M. Borella, and S. Maso. 2001. Historical control data on urinary and renal tissue biomarkers in naive Wistar rats. *Journal of Applied Toxicology* 21:409–413.

Trump, B. F., and I. Berezesky. 1995. Calcium-mediated cell injury and cell death. *FASEB Journal* 9:219–228.

Upton, P. K., and D. J. Morgan. 1975. The effect of sampling technique on some blood parameters in the rat. *Laboratory Animals* 9:85–91.

Vernay, M., J. Marty, and J. Moalti. 1984. Absorption of electrolytes and volatile fatty acid in the hind-gut of the rabbit. Circadian rhythm of hind-gut electrolytes and plasma aldosterone. *British Journal of Nutrition* 52:419–428.

White, T. F., J. R. Farndon, S. C. Conceicao, M. F. Laker, M. K. Ward, and D. N. Kerr. 1986. Serum calcium in health and disease: A comparison of measured and derived parameters. *Clinica Chimica Acta* 157:199–214.

Woodman, D. D. 1997. *Laboratory animal endocrinology: Hormonal action, control mechanisms and interactions with drugs.* Chichester, England: John Wiley & Sons.

Yao, X., K. Panichpisal, N. Kurztman, and K. Nugent. 2007. Cisplatin nephrotoxicity: A review. *American Journal of Medical Science* 334:115–124.

Zerwekh, J. E. 2004. The measurement of vitamin D: Analytical aspects. *Annals of Clinical Biochemistry* 41:272–281.

GENERAL REFERENCES*

Fluid Balance

Boyd, J. W. 1981. The relationships between blood hemoglobin concentrations, packed cell volume and plasma protein concentration in dehydration. *British Veterinary Journal* 137:166–172.

Kempson, S. A., and T. P. Dousa. 1986. Current concepts on regulation of phosphate transport in renal proximal tubules. *Biochemical Pharmacology* 35:721–726.

Kulpmann, W. R., H-K. Stummvoll, and P. Lehmann. 2007. *Electrolytes, acid–base balance and blood gases,* 2nd ed. New York: Springer.

Maack, T. 1988. Functional properties of atrial natriuretic peptide and its receptors. In *Nephrology,* Vol. 1, ed. A. M. Davidson, pp. 123–160. London: Bailliere Tindall.

McCormick, S. D., and D. Bradshaw. 2006. Hormonal control and water balance in vertebrates. *General and Comparative Endocrinology* 147:3–8.

Michell, A. R. 1991. Regulation of salt and water balance. *Journal of Small Animal Practice* 32:135–145.

Rose, B. D., and T. W. Post. 2001. *Clinical physiology of acid–base and electrolyte disorders,* 5th ed. New York: McGraw–Hill Professional.

Rowland, N. E. 2007. Food or fluid restriction in common laboratory animals: Balancing welfare with scientific inquiry. *Comparative Medicine* 57:149–160.

Toth, L. A., and T. W. Gardiner. 2000. Food and water restriction protocols: Physiological and behavioral considerations. *Contemporary Topics in Laboratory Animal Science* 39:9–17.

Willard, M. D. 2003. Electrolyte and acid–base disorders. In *Small animal clinical diagnosis by laboratory methods,* 4th ed., ed. M. D. Willard and H. Tvedten, pp. 117–135. Philadelphia: W. B. Saunders.

Examples of Transporters

Berndt, T., and R. Kumar. 2007. Phosphatonins and the regulation of phosphate homeostasis. *Annual Review of Physiology* 69:341–359.

El-Sheikk, A. A., R. Masereeuw, and F. G. Russel. 2008. Mechanisms of renal anionic transport. *European Journal of Pharmacology* 585:245–255.

Esteva-Font, C., R. Torra Balcells, and P. Férnandez-Llama. 2007. Sodium transporters and aquaporins: Future renal biomarkers? *Medicina Clinica (Barcelona)* 129:433–437.

Schmitz, C., F. Deason, and A. L. Perraud. 2007. Molecular components of vertebrate Mg2+ homeostasis regulation. *Magnesium Research* 20:6–18.

Suketa, Y. 2008. Expression and regulation of renal sodium cotransporters and antiporters, and related transport proteins. *Yakugaku Zasshi* 128:901–917.

Potassium, Sodium, and Chloride

Biondo, A. W., and H. A. de Morais. 2008. Chloride: A quick reference. *Veterinary Clinics of North America Small Animal Practice* 38:459–465.

DiBartola, S. P. 1998. Hyponatremia. *Veterinary Clinics of North America Small Animal Practice* 28:515–532.

Liamis, G., H. Milionis, and M. Elisfa. 2008. A review of drug-induced hyponatremia. *American Journal of Kidney Disease* 52:144–153.

Velazquez, H., and F. S. Wright. 1986. Control by drugs of renal potassium handling. *Annual Review of Pharmacology and Toxicology* 26:293–309.

Wingo, C. A., and B. D. Cain. 1993. The renal H-K-ATPase. Physiological significance and role in potassium homeostasis. *Annual Review of Physiology* 55:323–347.

---

* General references not cited in the text are included for background reading.

Hormones

Akashi, Y. J., J. Springer, M. Lainscak, and S. D. Anker. 2007. Atrial natriuretic peptide and related peptides. *Clinical Chemistry and Laboratory Medicine* 45:1259–1267.

Ball, S. G. 2007. Vasopressin and disorders of water balance: The physiology and pathophysiology of vasopressin. *Annals of Clinical Biochemistry* 44:417–431.

Capen, C. C. 1998. Correlation of mechanistic data and histopathology in the evaluation of selected toxic endpoints of the endocrine system. *Toxicology Letters* 28:102–110.

Capen, C. C., and T. J. Rosol. 1989. Recent advances in the structure and function of the parathyroid gland in animals and the effect of xenobiotics. *Toxicologic Pathology* 17:333–356.

Ceo, L. B. 2005. Natriuretic peptide family: New aspects. *Current Medical Chemistry Cardiovascular Hematology Agents* 3:87–98.

Cholewa, B. C., C. J. Meister, and D. L. Mattson. 2005. Importance of the renin–angiotensin system in the regulation of arterial blood pressure in conscious mice and rats. *Acta Physiologica Scandinavica* 183:309–320.

Crass, M. F., and L. V. Avioli, eds. 1994. *Calcium-regulating hormones and cardiovascular function.* Boca Raton, FL: CRC Press.

Eckermann-Ross, C. 2008. Hormonal regulation and calcium metabolism in rabbits. *Veterinary Clinics of North America Exotic Animal Practice* 11:139–152.

Funder, J. W. 1993. Aldosterone action. *Annual Review of Physiology* 55:115–130.

Giacchetti, G., L. A. Sechi, S. Rilli, and R. M. Carey. 2005. The renin–angiotensin–aldosterone system, glucose metabolism and diabetes. *Trends in Endocrinology and Metabolism* 16:120–126.

Hall, C. 2004. Essential biochemistry and physiology of (NT-pro) BNP. *European Journal of Heart Failure* 6:257–260.

Husain, A., and R. M. Graham. 2000. *Drugs, enzymes and receptors of the renin–angiotensin system: Celebrating a century of discovery.* Boca Raton, FL: CRC Press.

Kjolby, M. J., E. Kompanowska-Jezeirska, S. Wamberg, and P. Bie. 2005. Effects of sodium intake on plasma potassium and renin angiotensin aldosterone sytem in conscious dogs. *Acta Physiologica Scandinavica* 184:225–234.

McCormick, S. D., and D. Bradshaw. 2006. Hormonal control and water balance in vertebrates. *General and Comparative Endocrinology* 147:3–8.

Mohr, E., and D. Richter. 1994. Vasopressin in the regulation of body fluids. *Journal of Hypertension* 12:345–348.

Pagliaro, P., and C. Penna. 2005. Rethinking the renin–angiotensin system and its role in cardiovascular regulation. *Cardiovascular Drugs and Therapy* 19:77–87.

Rosenweig, A., and C. E. Seidman. 1991. Atrial natriuretic factor and related peptide hormones. *Annual Review of Biochemistry* 60:229–255.

Rowland, N. E., B. E. Goldstein, and K. L. Robertson. 2003. Role of angiotensin in body fluid homeostasis of mice: Fluid intake, plasma hormones and brain Fos. *American Journal of Physiology Regulatory Integrative and Comparative Physiology* 284:R1380–1381.

Silveira, P. F., J. Gil, L. Casis, and J. Irazusta. 2004. Peptide metabolism and the control of body fluid homeostasis. *Current Medicinal Chemistry and Cardiovascular Hematology Agents* 2:219–238.

Takei, Y., and N. Hazon. 2007. Endocrinology of salt and water balance. *General and Comparative Endocrinology* 152:339–351.

Treschan, T. A., and J. Peters. 2006. The vasopressin system: Physiology and clinical strategies. *Anesthesiology* 105:599–612.

Wells, T., R. J. Windle, K. Peysner, and M. L. Forsling. 1993. Intercolony variation in fluid balance and its relationship to vasopressin secretion in male Sprague–Dawley rats. *Laboratory Animals* 27:40–46.

White, P. C. 1994. Disorders of aldosterone biosynthesis and action. *New England Journal of Medicine* 331:250–258.

Woodman, D. D. 1997. *Laboratory animal endocrinology: Hormonal action, control mechanisms and interactions with drugs.* Chichester, England: John Wiley & Sons.

Acid–Base

Barzago, M. M., A. Bortolotti, D. Omarini, J. J. Aramayona, and M. Bonatti. 1992. Monitoring of blood gas parameters and acid–base balance of pregnant and nonpregnant rabbits (*Oryctolagus cuniculus*) in routine experimental conditions. *Laboratory Animals* 26:73–79.

CLSI. 2001b. C46—*A blood gas and pH analysis and related measurements. Approved guideline,* 1st ed. Wayne, PA: Clinical and Laboratory Institute Standards.

Constable, P. D. 1999. Clinical assessment of acid–base status. Strong ion difference theory. *Veterinary Clinics of North American Animal Practice* 15:447–471.

Cornelius, I. M., and C. A. Rawlings. 1981. Arterial blood gas and acid–base values in dogs with various diseases and signs of disease. *Journal of the American Veterinary Medical Association* 178:992–995.

Gluck, S. L. 1998. Acid–base. *Lancet* 352:474–479.

Hopper, K., M. L. Rezende, and S. C. Haskins. 2005. Assessment of the effect of dilution of blood samples with sodium heparin on blood gas, electrolyte, and lactate measurements in dogs. *American Journal of Veterinary Research* 66:656–660.

Ilkiw, J. E., R. J. Rose, and I. C. Martin. 1991. A comparison of simultaneously collected arterial, mixed venous, jugular venous and cephalic venous blood samples in the assessment of blood–gas and acid–base status in the dog. *Journal of Veterinary Medicine* 5:294–298.

Kellum, J. A. 2007. Disorders of acid–base balance. *Critical Care Medicine* 35:2630–2663.

Pickrell, J. A., M. E. Light, J. L. Mauderley, P. B. Beckley, B. A. Muggenburg, and U. C. Luft. 1973. Certain effects of sampling and storage on canine blood of different oxygen tensions. *American Journal of Veterinary Research* 34:241–244.

Pickrell, J. A., J. L. Mauderley, B. A. Muggenburg, and U. C. Luft. 1973. Influence of fasting on blood gas tension, pH and related values in dogs. *American Journal of Veterinary Research* 34:805–808.

Slaughter, M. R., J. M. Birmingham, B. Patel, G. A. Whelan, A. J. Krebs-Brown, P. D. Hockings, and J. A. Osborne. 2002. Extended acclimatization is required to eliminate effects of periodic blood-sampling procedures on vasoactive hormones and blood volume in beagle dogs. *Laboratory Animals* 36:403–410.

Szenci, O., E. Brydl, and C. A. Bajcsy. 1991. Effect of storage on measured ionized calcium and acid–base variables in equine, ovine, and canine venous blood. *Journal of the American Veterinary Medical Association* 199:1167–1169.

Thomson, W. S., J. F. Adams, and R. A. Cowan. 1997. *Understanding acid–base disorders. Clinical acid–base balance.* Oxford: Oxford University Press.

Upton, P. K., and D. J. Morgan. 1975. The effect of sampling technique on some blood parameters in the rat. *Laboratory Animals* 9:85–91.

Whitehair, K. J., S. C. Haskins, J. G. Whitehair, and P. J. Pascoe. 1995. Clinical applications of quantitative acid–base chemistry. *Journal of Veterinary Internal Medicine* 9:1–11.

Willard, M. D. 2003. Electrolyte and acid–base disorders. In *Small animal clinical diagnosis by laboratory methods,* 4th ed., ed. M. D. Willard and H. Tvedten, pp. 115–117. Philadelphia: W. B. Saunders.

Calcium, Magnesium, Inorganic Phosphate, and Vitamin D

Anderson, P. H., P. D. O'Loughlin, B. K. May, and H. A. Morris. 2004. Determinants of circulating 1,25-dihydroxyvitamin D3 levels: The role of renal synthesis and catabolism of vitamin D. *Journal of Steroid Biochemistry and Molecular Biology* 89–90:111–113.

Anderson, P. H., R. K. Sawyer, B. K. May, P. D. O'Loughlin, and H. A. Morris. 2007. 25-Hydroxyvitamin D requirement for maintaining skeletal health utilizing a Sprague–Dawley rat model. *Journal of Steroid Biochemistry and Molecular Biology* 103:592–595.

Arakawa, Y., M. Moriyama, and Y. Arakawa. 2004. Magnesium. *Nippon Rinsho* 62 (Suppl. 12): 261–266.

Barry, M. A., C. A. Behnke, and A. Eastman. 1990. Activation of programmed cell death (apoptosis) by cisplatin, other anticancer drugs, toxins and hyperthermia. *Biochemical Pharmacology* 40:2353–2362.

Bateman, S. W. 2008. Magnesium: A quick reference. *Veterinary Clinics of North America Small Animal Practice* 38:467–470.

Boden, S. D., and F. S. Kaplan. 1990. Calcium homeostasis. *Orthopedic Clinics of North America* 21:31–42.

Bushinsky, D. A., and R. D. Monk. 1998. Electrolyte quintet: Calcium. *Lancet* 352:306–311.

Chang, S. H., P. C. Phelps, M. Berezesky, M. L. Ebersberger, and B. F. Trump. 2000. Studies on the mechanisms and kinetics of apoptosis induced by microinjection of cytochrome C. *American Journal of Pathology* 156:637–649.

Dusso, A. S., A. J. Brown, and E. Slatopolsky. 2005. Vitamin D. *American Journal of Physiology and Renal Physiology* 289:F8–28.

Elin, R. J. 1987. Assessment of magnesium status. *Clinica Chemistry* 33:1965–1970.

Evans, G. O. 1988. Hypomagnesemia, hypoalbuminemia and plasma lipid changes in rats following the oral administration of cyclosporin. *Comparative Biochemistry and Physiology* 89C:375–376.

Fukuda, S., and H. Iida. 1994. Changes in histomorphometric values of iliac trabecular bone and serum biochemical constituents related to bone metabolism in beagle dogs during growth. *Experimental Animals* 43:159–165.

Jurutka, P. W. et al. 2007. Vitamin D receptor: Key roles in bone mineral pathophysiology, molecular mechanism of action, and novel nutritional ligands. *Journal of Bone and Mineral Research* 22 (Suppl. 2): V2–10.

Kalu, D. N., R. Cockerman, B. P. Yu, and B. A. Roos. 1983. Lifelong dietary modulation of calcitonin levels in rats. *Endocrinology* 113:2010–2015.

Konrad, M., K. P. Schlingmann, and T. Gudermann. 2004. Insights into the molecular nature of magnesium homeostasis. *American Journal of Physiology and Renal Physiology* 286:F599–605.

Kurokawa, K. 1994. The kidney and calcium homeostasis. *Kidney International* 45 (Suppl. 44): S97–105.

Lips, P. 2006. Vitamin D physiology. *Progress in Biophysics and Molecular Biology* 92:4–8.

Magil, A. B., V. Mavichak, N. L. Wong, G. A. Quamme, J. H. Dorks, and R. A. Surton. 1986. Long-term morphological and biochemical observations in cisplatin induced hypomagnesemia in rats. *Nephron* 43:223–230.

Mundy, G. R., and T. A. Guise. 1999. Hormonal control of calcium homeostasis. *Clinical Chemistry* 45B:1347–1352.

Murer, H., and J. Biber. 1997. A molecular view of proximal tubular inorganic phosphate (Pi) reabsoprtion and its regulation. *European Journal of Physiology* 433:379–389.

Ramasamy, I. 2006. Recent advances in physiological calcium homeostasis. *Clinical Chemistry and Laboratory Medicine* 44:237–273.

Renkema, N. Y., R. T. Alexander, R. J. Bindels, and J. G. Hoenderop. 2008. Calcium and phosphate homeostasis: Concerted interplay of new regulators. *Annals of Medicine* 40:82–91.

Sauk, J. J., and M. J. Somerman. 1991. Physiology of bone: Mineral compartment proteins as candidates for environmental perturbation by lead. *Environmental Health Perspectives* 91:9–16.

Schoenmakers, I., R. C. Nap, J. A. Mol, and H. A. Hazewinkel. 1999. Calcium metabolism: An overview of its hormonal regulation and interrelation with skeletal integrity. *Veterinary Quarterly* 21:147–153.

Selby, P. P., and P. H. Adams. 1994. The investigation of hypercalcemia. *Journal of Clinical Pathology* 47:579–584.

St-Arnaud, R. 2008. The direct role of vitamin D on bone homeostasis. *Archives of Biochemistry and Biophysics* 473:225–230.

Tenenhouse, H. S. 2007. Phosphate transport: Molecular basis, regulation and pathophysiology. *Journal of Steroid Biochemistry and Molecular Biology* 103:572–577.

Trump, B. F., and I. Berezesky. 1995. Calcium-mediated cell injury and cell death. *FASEB Journal* 9:219–228.

Wagner, C. A. 2007. Disorders of renal magnesium handling explain renal magnesium transport. *Journal of Nephrology* 20:507–510.

Yao, X., K. Panichpisal, N. Kurztman, and K. Nugent. 2007. Cisplatin nephrotoxicity: A review. *American Journal of Medical Science* 334:115–124.

Yasuda, S., K. Ono, and S. Wada. 2005. Calcitonin actions on kidney. *Nippon Rinsho* 63 (Suppl. 10): 207–210.

Age

Frith, C. H., R. L. Suber, and R. Umholtz. 1980. Hematologic and clinical chemistry findings in control BALB/c and C57BL/6. *Laboratory Animal Science* 30:835–840.

Nachbaur, J., M. R. Clarke, J-P. Provost, and J. L. Dancla. 1977. Variations of sodium, potassium and chloride plasma levels in the rat with age and sex. *Laboratory Animal Science* 27:972–975.

Laboratory Investigations

Emeigh-Hart, S. G. 2005. Assessment of renal injury in vivo. *Journal of Pharmacological and Toxicological Methods* 52:30–45.

Evans, G. O. 1987. Plasma lactate measurements in healthy beagle dogs. *American Journal of Veterinary Research* 48:131–132.

Feldman, B. P., and D. P. Rosenberg. 1981. Clinical use of anion and osmolal gaps in veterinary medicine. *Journal of the American Veterinary Medical Association* 178:396–398.

Holmgren, M-L., M. Palm, and L-E. Edqvist. 1974. Hemolysens inverkan på resultatet av några kliniskt-kemiska parametrar hos häst nötkreatur och hund. *Särtyck ur Svensk Veterinärtiding* 6:196–200.

ICH. 2000. *S7A Guideline: Safety pharmacology studies for human pharmaceuticals.* International Conference on Harmonization of Technical Requirements for Registration of Pharmaceuticals for Human Use.

Kraut, J. A., and N. E. Madias. 2007. Serum anion gap: Its uses and limitations in clinical medicine. *Clinical Journal of the American Society of Nephrology* 2:162–174.

Lefebvre, H. P., O. Dossin, C. Trumel, and J. P. Braun. 2008. Fractional excretion tests: A critical review of methods and applications in domestic animals. *Veterinary Clinical Pathology* 37:4–20.

Martinez-Maldonado, M., and S. C. Opava-Stitzer. 1978. Free water clearance curves during saline, mannitol, glucose and urea diuresis in the rat. *Journal of Physiology* 280:487–498.

Reimann, K. A., G. G. Knowlen, and H. W. Tvedten. 1989. Factitious hyperkalemia in dogs with thrombocytosis. The effect of platelets on serum potassium concentration. *Journal of Veterinary Internal Medicine* 3:47–52.

Urine Data

Diez, I., C. C. Pérez, M. B. Garcia, M. J. Cano, and M. A. Rios. 1996. Twenty-four-hour urinary calcium and phosphorus excretion in beagle dogs. Preliminary report. *Scandinavian Journal of Laboratory Animal Science* 23:355–362.

Kulick, L. J., D. J. Clemmons, R. L. Hall, and M. A. Koch. 2005. Refinement of the urine concentration test in rats. *Contemporary Topics in Laboratory Animal Science* 44:46–49.

Lane, I. F., D. H. Shaw, S. A. Burton, and A. W. Donald. 2000. Quantitative urinalysis in healthy beagle puppies from 9 to 27 weeks of age. *American Journal of Veterinary Research* 6:577–581.

Shevlock, P. N., S. R. Khan, and R. L. Hackett. 1993. Urinary chemistry of the normal Sprague–Dawley rat. *Urology Research* 21:309–312.

Trevisan, A., M. Giraldo, M. Borella, and S. Maso. 2001. Historical control data on urinary and renal tissue biomarkers in naive Wistar rats. *Journal of Applied Toxicology* 21:409–413.

Waldrop, J. E. 2008. Urinary electrolytes, solutes and osmolality. *Veterinary Clinics of North America Small Animal Practice* 38:503–512.

Calcium and Magnesium

CLSI. 2001a. C31-A2. *Ionized calcium determinations: Precollection variables, specimen choice, collection and handling. Approved guideline,* 2nd ed. Wayne, PA: Clinical and Laboratory Institute Standards.

Dewitte, K., I. D. Stock, and L. M. Theinpont. 1999. pH dependency of ionized calcium. *Lancet* 354:1793–1794.

Rayana, M. C. et al. 2008. IFCC guideline for sampling, measuring and reporting ionized magnesium in plasma. *Clinical Chemistry and Laboratory Medicine* 46:21–26.

Schenck, P. A., and D. J. Chew. 2005. Prediction of serum ionized calcium concentration by use of serum total calcium in dogs. *American Journal of Veterinary Research* 66:1330–1336.

White, T. F., J. R. Farndon, S. C. Conceicao, M. F. Laker, M. K. Ward, and D. N. Kerr. 1986. Serum calcium in health and disease: A comparison of measured and derived parameters. *Clinica Chimica Acta* 157:199–214.

Hormones

Woodman, D. D. 1997. *Laboratory animal endocrinology: Hormonal action, control mechanisms and interactions with drugs.* Chichester, England: John Wiley & Sons.

Aldosterone

Gomez-Sanchez, C., O. B. Holland, J. R. Higgins, D. C. Kern, and N. M. Kaplan. 1976. Circadian rhythms of serum renin activity and serum corticosterone, prolactin and aldosterone concentrations in the male rat on normal and low-sodium diets. *Endocrinology* 99:567–572.

Kaplan, N. M. 1976. Circadian rhythms of serum renin activity and serum corticosterone, prolactin and aldosterone concentrations in the male rat on normal and low-sodium diets. *Endocrinology* 99:567–572.

Kotchen, T. A., G. P. Guthrie, J. H. Galla, R. Luke, and W. J. Welch. 1983. Effects of NaCl on renin and aldosterone responses to potassium depletion. *American Journal of Physiology* 244:E164–169.

Vernay, M., J. Marty, and J. Moalti. 1984. Absorption of electrolytes and volatile fatty acid in the hind-gut of the rabbit. Circadian rhythm of hind-gut electrolytes and plasma aldosterone. *British Journal of Nutrition* 52:419–428.

PTH

Jara, A., J. Bover, J. Lavigne, and A. Felsenfeld. 1994. Comparison of two parathyroid hormone assays for the rat: The new immunoradiometric and the older competitive binding assay. *Journal of Bone and Mineral Research* 1:1629–1633.
Kalu, D. N., and R. H. Hardin. 1984. Age, strain and species differences in circulating parathyroid hormone. *Hormone and Metabolic Research* 16:654–657.
Terry, A. H., J. Orrock, and A. W. Meilke. 2003. Comparison of two third-generation parathyroid hormone assays. *Clinical Chemistry* 49:336–337.

Vitamin D

Glendenning, P. et al. 2003. Issues of methodology, standardization and metabolite recognition of 25-hydroxyvitamin D when comparing the DiaSorin radioimmunoassay and the Nichols Advantage automated chemiluminescence protein binding assay in hip fracture cases. *Annals of Clinical Biochemistry* 40:546–551.
Zerwekh, J. E. 2004. The measurement of vitamin D: Analytical aspects. *Annals of Clinical Biochemistry* 41:272–281.

Amino Acids

Lindon, J. C., E. Holmes, and J. K. Nicholson. 2004. Metabonomics and its role in drug development and disease diagnosis. *Expert Reviews in Molecular Diagnosis* 4:189–199.

Bone Biomarkers

Allen, M. J. 2003. Biochemical markers of bone metabolism in animals: Uses and limitations. *Veterinary Clinical Pathology* 32:101–113.
Allen, M. J., L. C. Allen, W. E. Hoffmann, D. C. Richardson, and G. J. Breur. 2000. Urinary markers of type I collagen degradation in the dog. *Research in Veterinary Science* 69:123–127.
Allen, M. J., W. E. Hoffmann, D. C. Richardson, and G. J. Breur. 1998. Serum bone markers of bone metabolism in dogs. *American Journal of Veterinary Research* 59:250–253.
Bernardi, D., M. Zaninotto, and M. Plebani. 2004. Requirement for improving quality in the measurements of bone markers. *Clinica Chimica Acta* 346:79–86.
Bilke, D. D. 1997. Biochemical markers in the assessment of bone disease. *American Journal of Medicine* 103:427–436.
Bonnet, J. 1994. Evaluation and comparison of urinary pyridinium cross-links in two rat models of bone loss—Ovariectomy and adjuvant polyarthritis. *Bone and Mineral* 26:155–167.
Christenson, R. H. 1997. Biochemical markers of bone metabolism: An overview. *Clinical Biochemistry* 30:573–593.
Delmas, P. D. 2001. Standardization of bone marker nomenclature. *Clinical Chemistry* 47:1497.
Delmas, P. D., R. Eastell, P. Garnero, M. J. Seibel, and J. Stepan. 2000. The use of biochemical markers of bone turnover in osteoporosis. *Osteoporosis International* 11 (Suppl. 6): S2–17.
Egger, C. D., R. C. Mühlbauer, R. Felix, P. D. Delmas, S. C. Marks, and H. Fleisch. 1994. Evaluation of using urinary pyridinium cross-link excretion as a marker of bone resorption in the rat. *Journal of Bone and Mineral Research* 9:1211–1219.
Gaumet, N., M. J. Seibel, V. Coxam, M. J. Davicco, P. Lebecque, and J. P. Barlet.1997. Influence of ovariectomy and estradiol treatment on calcium homeostasis during aging in rats. *Archives of Physiology and Biochemistry* 105:435–444.

Hannon, R., and R. Eastell. 2000. Preanalytical variability of biochemical markers of bone turnover. *Osteoporosis International* 6:30–44.

Herrmann, M. et al. 2007. Experimental hyperhomocysteinemia reduces bone quality in rats. *Clinical Chemistry* 53:1455–1461.

Ladlow, J. F., W. E. Hoffman, G. J. Breur, D. C. Richardson, and M.J. Allen. 2002. Biological variability in serum and urinary indices of bone formation and resorption in dogs. *Calcified Tissue International* 70:186–193.

Liesegang, A., R. Reutter, M.-L. Sassi, J. Risteli, M. Kraenzlin, J.-L. Riond, and M. Wanner. 1999. Diurnal variation in concentration of various markers of bone metabolism in dogs. *American Journal of Veterinary Research* 60:949–953.

Muhlnauer, R. C., and H. Fleisch. 1995. The diurnal rhythm of bone resorption in the rat: Effect of feeding habits and pharmacological inhibitors. *Journal of Clinical Investigation* 95:1933–1940.

Plebani, M., D. Bernardi, M. F. Meneghetti, F. Ujka, and M. Zaninotto. 2000. Biological variability in assessing biochemical markers of bone turnover. *Clinica Chimica Acta* 299:77–86.

Tordjman, C., A. Lhumeau, P. Pastoureau, F. Meunier, B. Serkiz, J. P. Volland, and J. Bonnet. 1994. Evaluation and comparison of urinary pyridinium cross-links in two rat models of bone loss—Ovariectomy and adjuvant polyarthritis. *Bone and Mineral* 26:155–167.

Vanderschueren, D., I. Jans, E. van Herck, K. Moermans, J. Verhaeghe, and R. Bouillon. 1994. Time-related increase of biochemical markers of bone turnover in androgen-deficient male rats. *Bone and Mineral* 26:123–131.

7 Assessment of Cardiotoxicity and Myotoxicity

P. J. O'Brien

7.1 CARDIOTOXICITY

Cardiotoxic effects may be broadly categorized as (1) functional changes that may or may not be accompanied by histopathological change, and (2) structural injury with or without functional change. Serious functional disturbances may occur without any structural alterations. For example, electrophysiological effects of drugs are typically mediated by their direct interaction with cardiac ion channels, which are involved in the transmission of cardiac impulses as action potentials that ensure normal cardiac function. Perturbations of these ion channels can lead to a prolongation of cardiac QT interval and/or to an arrhythmia and a myocardial event such as Torsades de Pointe, which is a variant of ventricular tachycardia that has distinct characteristics on the electrocardiogram. However, in these events, there typically is no obvious loss of structural integrity or release of cellular constituents into the plasma. Adverse functional effects may occur secondarily, due to excessive neuroendocrine alterations or chronically increased cardiac workload that overwhelms the heart's adaptive capacity and leads to failure. Degenerative structural effects that release intracellular constituents are mediated by direct myocardial toxic injury. These events may arise from adverse subcellular effects such as on mitochondria, calcium homeostasis, membrane permeability, and redox status.

Adverse cardiotoxic effects were responsible for the withdrawal of 9% of prescription drugs from the market from 1960 to 1999 (Fung et al. 2001). Cardiotoxicity occurred with 17% of pharmaceuticals in a survey of 150 compounds entered into clinical trials (Olson et al. 2000). Also, cardiotoxicity is a limiting factor in the use of a wide variety of drugs, such as those used for the treatment of cancer and retroviral diseases (Lewis 2004; Yeh 2006). Some specific examples of drug classes with known cardiotoxicity include (O'Brien 2008):

- anticancer drugs such as
  - alkylating compounds (e.g., cyclophosphamide)
  - antibiotic anthracyclines (e.g., doxorubicin)
  - antibiotic anthraquinones (e.g., mitoxantrone)

- antimetabolites (e.g., fluorouracil)
- interleukin-2
- antiretroviral compounds such as the nucleoside reverse transcriptase inhibitors (e.g., zidovudine)
- antipsychotics (e.g., clozapine)
- sympathomimetics such as
  - alpha-adrenergics (e.g., phenylpropanolamine)
  - beta-1 adrenergics (e.g., dolbutamine)
  - beta-2 (e.g., clenbuterol) and nonselective (e.g., isoproterenol) adrenergics
  - inhibitors of phosphodiesterase type 3 (e.g., milrinone) and 4 (rolipram); and
- peroxisome proliferator receptor agonists (e.g., fibrates)

7.1.1 PLASMA MEASUREMENTS IN CARDIAC TOXICITY

Although a large number of tissue proteins, enzymes, and metabolites are released into the plasma following tissue injury, only a few of these are used commonly for the diagnosis of cardiotoxicity. Of these measurements, the troponins now offer a significant improvement on the use of enzymes such as creatine kinase and lactate dehydrogenase for the detection of myocardial injury.

7.1.1.1 Cardiac Troponins

Troponin regulates the interaction of thin and thick contractile muscle filaments, which are composed of actin and myosin, respectively. It was first discovered by Ebashi and Ebashi in 1964. Troponin (Tn) is a complex of three small globular proteins: C, which binds calcium (TnC—calcium binding); I, which inhibits actin and myosin interaction (TnI—inhibits); and T, which binds tropomyosin (TnT). These proteins have molecular weights of approximately 23, 18, and 37 kDa, respectively. The binding of calcium binding to TnC causes a change in conformation that transfers to TnI and tropomyosin, causing TnI to detach from actin and tropomyosin and to roll out of the way of the myosin cross-bridges that pull on the actin filaments to contract muscle (Metzger and Westfall 2004).

Introduction of cardiac troponin (cTn) in the early nineties for assessment of myocardial infarct in humans demonstrated that cardiac injury could be monitored with high sensitivity, high specificity, and high practicality—in contrast to all previous biomarkers (Babuin and Jaffe 2005). It is now the preferred biomarker for myocardial infarctions in humans (Alpert et al. 2000) because it stratifies risk, increasing with severity of disease and with life expectancy. In human myocardial infarct, cTn concentration peaks at 18–24 hours and correlates highly with scintigraphic measurements of infarct size made at 72 hours following injury. The increase in blood cTn may persist for a couple of weeks.

Clinical diagnostic use of cTn has been extended to other cardiac diseases (Gupta and de Lemos 2007), and applications include monitoring acute injury from exacerbation of congestive heart failure, pulmonary embolism, sepsis, hypertensive emergency, cardiac trauma, myocarditis, and pericarditis. Also included are chronic conditions with ongoing injury such as congestive heart failure or left ventricular systolic dysfunction, left ventricular hypertrophy, chronic kidney disease, and diabetes mellitus. Of greater relevance to preclinical toxicology is the effective clinical use of cTn since 2002 to detect and monitor cardiotoxicity, especially with the anthracyclines used extensively in cancer treatment (Cardinale et al. 2002; Kilickap et al. 2005).

7.1.1.1.1 Preclinical Application of Cardiac Troponin

Animal models of human cardiac disease have been widely used to validate and develop understanding of cTn as a cardiac injury biomarker. Such studies have shown correlation of increases in blood cTn with loss from myocardium, compromised cardiac function, and structural injury to myocardium. The value of cTn in clinical assessment of cardiotoxicity from anticancer drugs was first demonstrated in mice (O'Brien et al. 1997a), rats (Herman et al. 1998), and dogs (Christiansen et al. 2002) with doxorubicin.

Since then, approximately 70 studies have been reported in the literature, and far more have been conducted internally within pharmaceutical companies, documenting the effectiveness of cTn as a biomarker to identify, assess, and monitor preclinical cardiac toxicity (O'Brien 2008). This has been demonstrated for several classes of drugs, including adrenergic agents, agonists of peroxisome proliferator-activated receptors (PPAR; especially for alpha-PPARs), anthracyclines and other anticancer drugs, and phosphodiesterase inhibitors.

7.1.1.1.2 Measurement of Cardiac Troponin

In healthy animals, cTn is found in only trace amounts in the blood. Individual values are considered to be increased when they are higher than the 99th percentile (mean plus three standard deviations) for a healthy population. The kinetics of myocardial release appear to be similar across species, in contrast to those for blood clearance, which appears to be faster in laboratory animals than in humans. Within minutes of myocardial injury, cTn is released and peaks as early as 2–6 hours, depending on the duration of the cardiac injury. Rat and dog studies of isoproterenol toxicity and ischemic injury have demonstrated blood cTn concentration peaks within 2–6 hours and highly correlate with severity of histopathological lesion (O'Brien et al. 1997a, 2006; York et al. 2007). cTn is cleared from blood within a few days.

Numerous commercially available assays and suitable analyzers for measurement of human cTnI are available. However, because of patent restrictions, there are only two cTnT assays: one for clinical use (Roche Diagnostics, Basel, Switzerland) and one for research and preclinical use (MesoScale Discovery, Gaithersburg, Maryland). Many cTn assays have good cross-species reactivity because of the high degree of conservation of cTn structure (O'Brien, Landt, and Ladenson 1997b), although some assays are species restricted because their antibodies target epitopes that are not well conserved (O'Brien et al. 2006). Thus, it is critical that an assay be validated for the species studied. Both cTnI and cTnT assays have similar tissue specificities, with negligible reactivity with skeletal Tn. The minimum detectable concentration is frequently an order of magnitude lower for cTnT than cTnI, although the values are typically an order of magnitude higher for the latter (O'Brien 2008). Several reports indicate that cTnT may be more sensitive immediately after injury, possibly because the cytoplasmic pool of cTnT is approximately 7%, which is twice that of cTnI, and the cytoplasmic Tn pool is thought to be released earlier than the myofibrillar pool. Also, cTn is released as a ternary complex, as binary complexes of cTnI and cTnC and as free cTnT.

False negative results for cTn may occur if the assay is insufficiently sensitive, especially in enzyme-linked immunosorbent assay (ELISA) methods where colorimetry rather than fluorescence or chemiluminescence is used as the detection method, and in those assays with poor cross-species reactivity. False negative results may also occur in samples that have deteriorated. Serum cTn is stable at –70°C, but it deteriorates several percent per day at 4°C and by 10% per week at –20°C. Rare false positive results may occur with circulating heterophilic antibodies, fibrin clots, or incomplete serum separation (or in the presence of rheumatoid factor). Hemolysis produces negligible interference.

There are several sources of increased background serum cTn in controls for animal studies. These sources include tissue contamination where samples are collected by cardiac puncture (O'Brien et al. 1997a); sample collection after ischemic injury during euthanasia may increase background levels, as may excessive stress, restraint, or exertion, or trauma during handling (O'Brien 2008). Spontaneous cardiomyopathy, such as typically occurs in Sprague–Dawley rats (especially in males and with age), also increases background levels of cTn (O'Brien et al. 2006). Lower blood levels of cTn may occur after injury if myocardial cTn content is decreased, such as with inanition, heart failure, or prior myocardial injury.

Analytical sensitivity may be significantly improved for samples from preclinical toxicology studies where samples are analyzed in batches with concurrent controls, in comparison with samples submitted for individual animals. This batch analysis reduces interassay variation due to differences in reagents, calibrators, controls, analyzers, and analysts.

In summary, cTnI and cTnT are specific and sensitive biomarkers of cardiac injury that correlate with the extent of myocardial cell injury, returning to baseline following cessation of active cell injury, although histological evidence persists. Plasma troponins and enzyme measurements are not biomarkers for all forms of drug-induced cardiac injury. For example, if the permeability of cardiac muscles does not change, then troponins will not increase. Similarly troponins will frequently not increase in drug-induced dysrhythmias, alterations of ion exchange channels, or contractile dysfunction.

7.1.1.2 Creatine Kinase (CK) and Lactate Dehydrogenase (LD) Isozymes

Historically, measurements of the isozymes of creatine kinase (CK) and lactate dehydrogenase (LD) have been used for the detection of myocardial injury. These are enzymes of intermediary metabolism found in both cardiac and skeletal muscle, although in different forms reflecting the different metabolic and functional properties of these tissues. There are also significant amounts of CK in nervous tissue and smooth muscle, whereas LD is expressed in most tissues (Aktas et al. 1993).

Two genes for both CK and LD are differentially expressed in tissues to produce subunits that spontaneously assemble: 43-kDa monomers form dimers for CK, and 36.5-kDa monomers form tetramers for LD. The three CK dimers formed from the B and M subunits are the "muscle" type dimer, CK-MM, the "brain" type dimer, CK-BB, and the mixed dimer CK-MB. In muscle and heart, most CK is MM. However, some expression of B subunit results in increased formation of MB in the heart and slow-twitch muscle, compared to fast-twitch skeletal muscle. However, this increased MB in the heart is generally minor, unless there is an underlying cardiomyopathy, which is known to cause a mild increase in B gene expression. For LD, expression of the M and H subunits results in increased formation of H_4 and H_3M_1 (LD1 and LD2, respectively) in the heart and M_3H_1 and M_4 in muscle (LD4 and LD5).

Although it is less likely, cross-species differences in tissue distribution of isoenzymes could also potentially limit use of CK and LD injury (O'Brien et al. 1997a). The distribution of tissue LDH isozymes differs with the various species of laboratory animals. For example, release of liver LD1 and LD2 may occur with hepatopathy in some species (e.g., demonstrated in pigs, horses, bovines) and could confound interpretation of increases in blood LD. Similarly, interpretation of increased blood CK may be confounded by release of CK-MB by injury to other tissues such as slow-twitch skeletal muscle, nervous tissue, and uterine smooth muscle (e.g., parturition). Hemolysis could also potentially cause mild increases in these enzymes in certain species.

Whereas CK and LD isozymes have been quite successful as cardiac biomarkers in humans, their use in animals has been limited by the need to exclude muscle injury (O'Brien et al. 1997a). This is clearly more difficult in animals because symptoms of myopathy are more difficult to detect and because of a greater background incidence of effects on skeletal muscle associated with handling and stress. The mildly greater concentration of specific isoenzymes in cardiac versus skeletal muscle that confers diagnostic relevance may be offset by the much larger amount of muscle mass.

7.1.1.2.1 CK and LDH Isozyme Measurements

The CK isozymes may be separated by electrophoresis and detected by stains for their enzyme activity. CK-MB immunoassays have also been developed for use in humans that occasionally cross-react with some animal species, although these must first be shown to have appropriate cross-reactivity for the species tested. The LD isozymes have been commonly and readily separated by electrophoresis and stained by their enzymatic activity. For both CK and LD isozymes, their absolute activity is inferred from their relative staining on electrophoretograms and determination of total plasma enzyme activity, typically using an automated chemistry analyzer.

7.1.1.3 Myoglobin

Another major cardiac injury biomarker is myoglobin, the cytoplasmic protein storing and shuttling oxygen from the cell surface to the mitochondria. This small protein can be easily measured by species-specific immunoassays (Spangenthal and Ellis 1995) or after separating it from hemoglobin and staining for peroxidase activity of the heme prosthetic group (O'Brien et al. 1992). Because of its small size, it is released early in cardiomyocyte injury and readily passes through the glomerular filter into the urine. Marked myoglobinuria imparts a mahogany brown color to the urine.

7.1.1.4   Fatty Acid Binding Proteins (FABPs)

Fatty acid binding protein (FABP3) is a cytosolic protein recently reported to be more sensitive for detection of cardiac injury in humans with myocardial infarct or congestive heart failure (Mion et al. 2007; Niizeki et al. 2007). However, FABP3 is also found, although in much lower concentrations, in muscle, brain, and kidney. As for CK and LD, its occurrence in skeletal muscle substantially diminishes its value as a cardiac biomarker because of the higher and variable background of mild skeletal muscle injury in laboratory animals. Its use as a cardiac biomarker would require exclusion of muscle injury and renal disease.

7.1.1.5   Timings of Sample Collections

For biomarkers such as the troponins and enzymes, timing and sample collection are particularly critical for the detection of cardiac injury, and consideration must be given to the half-life of the molecule and its mass. Although some data are available for humans, data are sparse for the same measurements in laboratory animals. In general, the half-lives of these molecules are less in smaller animals. The importance of sample times has been shown in several studies where myocardial lesions have been induced by the administration of toxic doses of sympathomimetics (O'Brien et al. 1997a, 2006; York et al. 2007).

7.1.2   BLOOD BIOMARKERS OF CARDIAC DYSFUNCTION

7.1.2.1   Natriuretic Peptides and Endothelin-1

Numerous neuroendocrine biomarkers correlate with severity of cardiac dysfunction. Heart failure is associated with increase in peripheral vascular resistance due to increases in sympathetic tone, norepinephrine, renin, angiotensin II, arginine vasopressin, and endothelin-1. The increased venous pressure causes atrial distension that stimulates production and release of atrial and brain natriuretic peptides (ANP, BNP) from the atria and ventricles, respectively. ANP inhibits the renin–angiotensin–aldosterone system. In humans and mammals, BNP has been found to be an early biomarker of left ventricular hypertrophy developing with doxorubicin cardiotoxicity, congestive heart failure, or occult dilated cardiomyopathy (Erkus et al. 2006; Walker 2006; Oyama, Sisson, and Solter 2007).

7.1.3   OTHER MEASUREMENTS

Other clinical pathology changes in cardiotoxicity are typically nonspecific and relate to the impairment in cardiac performance and activation of the neuroendocrine system. Other plasma measurements that may be altered by cardiotoxic compounds include electrolytes, proteins other than enzymes, lipids, and other enzymes with less tissue specificity, such as aspartate aminotransferase.

For example, in cobalt-induced cardiotoxicity, there were mild serum increases in cardiac enzymes along with a moderate hyperkalemia, hyperchloremia metabolic acidosis, and a characteristic polycythemia (O'Brien 2006). With marked cardiac dysfunction, blood volume expansion may be seen with hyponatremia and hypoalbuminemia, and serum increases in hepatocellular enzymes due to passive congestion and anoxia. Often, mild renal effects are indicated by mildly decreased glomerular filtration rate and hyposthenuria (urine of dilute concentration). Moderate lactic aciduria is characteristic. Decreases in circulating thyroid hormones occur along with increases in norepinephrine (O'Brien et al. 1993) and natriuretic peptides (Oyama et al. 2007).

Although hemoglobinuria, proteinuria, and enzymuria may occur following myocardial infarction or damage to pulmonary arteries, urine tests are generally not helpful in the detection of cardiotoxicity. Other biomarkers proposed for evaluating human cardiac diseases (e.g., homocysteine, myeloperoxidase, C-reactive protein, dimethylarginine, and ischemic albumin) have not found application in preclinical studies. Potential markers such as low molecular weight peptides and protein fragments identified by proteomic studies have yet to be translated into sufficiently robust assays for wider evaluation (Van Eyk and Dunn 2003; Petricoin et al. 2004).

7.2 MYOTOXICITY

Drug-induced myopathy has become increasingly recognized (Guis, Mattéi, and Lioté 2003; Mastaglia 2006; Scola et al. 2007), especially due to corticosteroids, propoxyphene, neuroleptics, zidovudine, and drug-induced hypokalemia. Probably the best-described myopathies are produced by lipid-lowering drugs such as ezetimibe, niacin, fibrates (PPAR agonists), and statins. Clinical myopathy occurs in more than 5% of human patients on statin therapy, where the cholesterol biosynthetic pathway step involving 3-hydroxy-3-methylglutaryl coenzyme A reductase (HMG-CoA reductase) is inhibited by statins. The myopathy is characterized by myalgia, myasthenia, muscle cramping, exacerbation by exertion, and elevations of CK to more than 10-fold the upper limit of normal. Mild ultrastructural changes in muscle and mild symptoms are present in a much higher proportion of patients. Rarely (fewer than 0.4 cases per 10,000 person years of treatment), there may be severe cases with marked muscle breakdown (i.e., rhabdomyolysis) that leads to renal failure or disseminated intravascular coagulation. Whereas the pathogenesis of these drug effects is not clearly known, impairment of intracellular calcium homeostasis, mitochondrial oxidative phosphorylation, production of selenoproteins, activation of apoptosis, and, especially, involvement of fast-twitch glycolytic fibers have been incriminated (Moosmann and Behl 2004; Westwood et al. 2005; Arora, Liebo, and Maldonado 2006; Dirks and Jones 2006; Liantonio et al. 2007).

Numerous other drugs have a myotoxic effect by various mechanisms, including
- antipsychotic and antidepressant drugs (e.g., olanzapine, clozapine) and drugs of abuse (e.g., cocaine, heroin, methamphetamine) that affect CNS and muscle dopamine and serotonin receptors;
- fluoroquinolones;
- glucocorticoids;
- certain cationic amphiphilic drugs that produce lysosomal phospholipid accumulation (e.g., perhexiline, amiodarone, chloroquine) (Vonderfecht et al. 2004);

antimicrotubule drugs (e.g., colchicine and vincristine);
alcohol; and
autoimmunogenic drugs (e.g., D-penicillamine and interferon-alpha) (Guis
   et al. 2003; Mastaglia 2006).

Myotoxicity and cardiotoxicity frequently occur together (Guis et al. 2003; Tan
et al. 2003) for a number of classes of drugs, such as with nucleoside reverse transcriptase inhibitors (NRTIs) used for treatment of retroviral disease, adrenergic
agents, anticancer drugs such as doxorubicin, and the PPAR-alpha agonists. Beta-
adrenergic agonists at low concentrations induce apoptosis and at high concentrations produce necrosis in both cardiac and muscle fibers, especially in slow-twitch
muscle (Burniston et al. 2006). PPAR-alpha activation leads to increased cardiac
and slow-twitch muscle fatty acid oxidation and subsequent accumulation of oxidative stress intermediates, resulting in myocyte necrosis (De Sousa et al. 2006;
Pruimboom-Brees et al. 2006). Zidovudine and other NRTIs inhibit mitochondrial
DNA polymerase in both cardiac and skeletal muscle, as well as in other tissues, and
thereby inhibit mitochondrial turnover and metabolism (Dagan et al. 2002).

7.2.1 Laboratory Investigations

7.2.1.1 Creatine Kinase, Lactate Dehydrogenase, and Other Enzymes

Although CK and LD isozymes and myoglobin are sensitive biomarkers of skeletal
muscle injury, they are also found in cardiac muscle and thus are not tissue specific. Cardiotoxicity must be excluded in order to use them effectively as biomarkers. Injured muscle releases other enzymes in significant amounts, such as alanine
aminotransferase (ALT), aspartate aminotransferase (AST), and aldolase; however,
these also lack tissue specificity.

Following injury, the different enzymes are released from muscle and cleared
from the blood at different rates (Aktas, Lefebvre, et al. 1995; O'Brien et al. 1997a).
Serum CK and AST peak after 12–24 hours and return to normal within 3–4 days,
whereas serum LD peaks after 24–48 hours and returns to normal within 7–10 days.
Thus, acute serial samples (e.g., taken every 12 hours for 36 hours after injury) are
likely to have the greatest diagnostic value. Clearance rates for LD are species and
isozyme specific. For example, the half-life of human H4 is 113 hours; however,
M4 half-life is considerably shorter: in the dog, 3.3 hours; human, 10 hours; pig, 40
hours; and sheep, 50 hours. H4 is considerably more heat stable. Nucleotide binding
sites are recognized by macrophages of liver, spleen, and bone marrow, resulting
in endocytosis of LD and CK. Plasma carboxypeptidases may partially cleave CK
isozymes to generate isoforms that reflect the timing of the injury (Aktas, Vinclair,
et al. 1995).

Numerous false positives for myotoxicity may occur because of background injury
associated with handling or restraint, especially with nonhuman primates; fighting;
biting; trauma; bumps and bruises; fever; unaccustomed or excessive exertion; injections; catheterization; surgery; and muscle puncture during sampling procedures
(O'Brien et al. 1997a; O'Brien 2008).

7.2.1.2 Skeletal Muscle Troponin

Skeletal muscle may be affected by cardiotoxic drugs because of its similar contractile, metabolic, and regulatory characteristics, such as with nucleoside reverse transcriptase inhibitors, doxorubicin, and adrenergic agonists (Guis et al. 2003; Tan et al. 2003). Similarly, cardiomyopathy is associated with myopathy, such as in vitamin E and selenium deficiency, mitochondrial myopathy, Duchenne's muscular dystrophy, and congestive heart failure. Furthermore, biomarkers of injury to heart and muscle are similar, such as creatine kinase, lactate dehydrogenase, myoglobin, and troponin (O'Brien et al. 1997a; O'Brien 2008). Because cTnI has been shown to be the gold-standard biomarker of cardiac injury, similar characteristics of skeletal muscle skTnI should likewise enable it to become a more highly specific and sensitive biomarker than current biomarkers (Takahashi et al. 1996). Several studies confirm it to be a more sensitive, persistent, and specific biomarker than CK, myosin, or myoglobin (Sorichter, Mair, and Koller 1997; Kiely et al. 2000; Simpson, Van Eyk, and Iscoe 2003).

7.2.1.3 Parvalbumin

Parvalbumin is a small (12 kDa), cytoplasmic, high-affinity, calcium-binding protein that has structural similarity to TnC and calmodulin. It is found especially in striated muscles in an amount proportional to their speed of relaxation. It acts as a calcium buffer, facilitating muscle relaxation by transferring calcium ions from TnC to the Ca-pump that sequesters calcium within the sarcoplasmic reticulum. Parvalbumin concentration in urine has been found to be increased with myotoxicity (Dare et al. 2002).

7.2.1.4 Fatty Acid-Binding Protein (FABP3)

FABP3 could be used as a biomarker if cardiotoxicity and renal disease are excluded (Pritt et al. 2008). It is found in highest concentration in heart and slow-twitch skeletal muscle. As a skeletal muscle biomarker, it has been shown to outperform CK-MM and AST with PPAR-alpha myotoxicity.

7.2.1.5 Other Plasma Measurements and Effects

Several other biochemical changes may occur with moderate to marked muscle toxicity. Lactic acidosis occurs if there is compromised mitochondrial activity, such as with NRTIs. If muscle injury is severe enough to cause serum CK to increase to several thousand, then serum calcium may decrease due to dystrophic calcification. Serum potassium increases (peracutely) with acidosis, rhabdomyolysis, and myoglobinuric nephrosis. Hemoconcentration occurs with hypermetabolic states (Guis et al. 2005). Whereas creatinine does not significantly increase with rhabdomyolysis due to release of cellular contents, it may increase dramatically with urea due to myoglobinuric nephrosis.

Hypocalcemia occurring with calcium chelators, magnesium antagonism, or certain loop diuretics may produce muscle spasm and tetanic contractions in most species by increasing cell membrane excitability of motor neurons with resultant increased neuromuscular transmission. Interestingly, flaccid paralysis and recumbency in ruminants is more common in hypocalcemia because of a failure of neuromuscular transmission (Cooper and Gittoes 2008). Hypocalcemia has a negative inotropic effect, leading to a compensatory, secondary positive chronotropic effect.

In contrast to the typical effects of hypocalcemia, hypokalemia may cause myasthenia and flaccid paralysis of muscle because potassium is a critical activator of intermediary metabolism. Potassium is also critical for vasodilation in muscle during exercise, so hypokalemia may cause exertional rhabdomyolysis. Hypokalemia may be produced by potassium-losing diuretics and secondary to hypomagnesemia (Scola et al. 2007).

Hypomagnesemia has been associated with more than 50 drugs, especially those that are nephrotoxic, including cisplatin, aminoglycoside antibiotics, cyclosporine, and amphotericin B. Secondary hypocalcemia and hypokalemia may result with myasthenia and tetany (Swaminathan 2003).

7.3   ARTERITIS AND VASCULITIS

Drug-induced vascular injury, arteritis, and phlebitis are some of the terms used to describe vascular injuries that are sometimes induced in preclinical toxicology studies (Greaves 2000; Louden and Morgan 2001). These lesions may be observed within a few hours of drug administration; the lesions occur more frequently in canine coronary vasculature and the mesenteric vasculature of rats. Although this animal vasculitis is seen in toxicology studies, these lesions remain undetectable in humans; however, this may a question of a lack of suitable monitoring methods. To enable risk assessments to be made, approximately 15 potential biomarkers have been suggested (Brott et al. 2004; Kerns et al. 2005). These biomarkers include endothelial markers (e.g., von Willebrand factor; Newsholme et al. 2000), E selectin, thrombomodulin, tissue plasminogen activator, markers of smooth muscle injury (e.g., alpha-actin), calveolin, some acute phase proteins, and several interleukins. Investigations are continuing to evaluate these potential markers in preclinical studies.

REFERENCES

Aktas, M., D. Auguste, H. P. Lefebvre, P. L. Toutain, and J. P. Braun. 1993. Creatine kinase in the dog: A review. *Veterinary Research* 17:353–369.

Aktas, M., H. P. Lefebvre, P. L. Toutain, and J. P. Braun. 1995. Disposition of creatine kinase activity in dog plasma following intravenous and intramuscular injection of skeletal muscle homogenates. *Journal of Veterinary Pharmacology and Therapeutics* 18:1–6.

Aktas, M., P. Vinclair, H. P. Lefebvre, P. L. Toutain, and J. P. Braun. 1995. In vivo quantification of muscle damage in dogs after intramuscular administration of drugs. *British Veterinary Journal* 151:189–196.

Alpert, J. S., K. Thygesen, E. Antman, and J. P. Bassand. 2000. Myocardial infarction redefined—A consensus document of The Joint European Society of Cardiology/American College of Cardiology Committee for the Redefinition of Myocardial Infarction. *Journal of the American College of Cardiologists* 36:959–969 and *European Heart Journal* 21:1502–1513.

Arora, R., M. Liebo, and F. Maldonado. 2006. Statin-induced myopathy: The two faces of Janus. *Journal of Cardiovascular and Pharmacological Therapeutics* 11:105–112.

Babuin, L., and A. S. Jaffe. 2005. Troponin: The biomarker of choice for the detection of cardiac injury. *Canadian Medical Association Journal* 173:1191–1202.

Brott, D. A., H. B. Jones, S. Gould, J-P. Valentin, G. O. Evans, R. J. Richardson, and C. Louden. 2004. Current status and future directions for diagnostic markers of drug-induced vascular injury. *Disease Markers* 18:1–14.

Burniston, J. G., W. A. Clark, L. B. Tan, and D. F. Goldspink. 2006. Dose-dependent separation of the hypertrophic and myotoxic effects of the β2-adrenergic receptor agonist clenbuterol in rat striated muscles. *Muscle and Nerve* 33:655–663.

Cardinale, D. et al. 2002. Myocardial injury revealed by plasma troponin I in breast cancer treated with high-dose chemotherapy. *Annals of Oncology* 13:710–715.

Christiansen, S., K. Redman, H. H. Scheld., U. R. Jahn, J. Stypmann, M. Fobker, A. D. Gruber, and D. Hammel. 2002. Adriamycin-induced cardiomyopathy in the dog—An appropriate model for research on partial left ventriculectomy. *Journal of Heart and Lung Transplantation* 21:783–790.

Cooper, M. S., and N. J. Gittoes. 2008. Diagnosis and management of hypocalcemia. *British Medical Journal* 336:1298–1302.

Dagan T., C. Sable, J. Bray, and M. Gerschenson. 2002. Mitochondrial dysfunction and antiretroviral nucleoside analog toxicities: What is the evidence? *Mitochondrion* 1:397–412.

Dare, T. O., H. A. Davies, J. A. Turton, T. Lomas, T. C. Williams, and M. J. York. 2002. Application of surface-enhanced desorption/ionization technology to the detection and identification of urinary paravalbumin-α: A biomarker of compound induced skeletal muscle toxicity in the rat. *Electrophoresis* 23:3241–3251.

De Souza, A. T., P. D. Cornwell, X. Dai, M. J. Caguyong, and R. G. Ulrich. 2006. Agonists of the peroxisone proliferator–activated receptor alpha induced a fiber-type-selective transcriptional response in rat skeletal muscle. *Toxicological Sciences* 92:578–586.

Dirks, A. J., and K. M. Jones. 2006. Statin-induced apoptosis and skeletal myopathy. *American Journal of Physiology and Cellular Physiology* 291:C1208–1212.

Ebashi, S., and F. Ebashi. 1964. A new protein component participating in the superprecipitation of myosin B. *Journal of Biochemistry Tokyo* 55:604–613.

Erkus, B., S. Demirtas, A. A. Yarpuzlu, M. Can, Y. Genc, and L. Karaca. 2006. Early prediction of anthracycline induced cardiotoxicity. *Acta Paediatrica* 96:506–509.

Fung, M., A. Thornton, K. Mybeck, J. Hsiao-Hui, K. Hornbuckle, and E. Muniz. 2001. Evaluation of the characteristics of safety withdrawal of prescription drugs from worldwide pharmaceutical markets: 1960 to 1999. *Drug Information Journal* 35:293–317.

Greaves, P. 2000. Patterns of cardiovascular pathology induced by diverse cardioactive drugs. *Toxicology Letters* 112–113:547–552.

Guis, S., J-P. Mattéi, and F. Lioté. 2003. Drug-induced and toxic myopathies. *Best Practice in Research in Clinical Rheumatology* 17:877–907.

Guis, S., J.-P. Mattéi, P. J. Cozzone, and D. Bendahan. 2005. Pathophysiology and clinical presentations of rhabdomyolysis. *Joint Bone and Spine* 72:382–391.

Gupta, S., and J. A. de Lemos. 2007. Use and misuse of cardiac troponins in clinical practice. *Progress in Cardiovascular Disease* 50:151–165.

Herman, E. H., S. E. Lipshultz, N. Rifai, J. Zhang, T. Papoian, Z. X. Yu, K. Takeda, and V. J. Ferrans. 1998. Use of cardiac troponin T levels as an indicator of doxorubicin-induced cardiotoxicity. *Cancer Research* 58:195–197.

Kerns, W. et al. 2005. Drug-induced vascular injury—A quest for biomarkers. Expert working group on drug-induced vascular injury. *Toxicology and Applied Pharmacology* 203:62–87.

Kiely, P. D. W., F. E. Bruckner, J. A. Nisbet, and A. Daghir. 2000. Serum skeletal troponin I in inflammatory muscle disease: Relation to creatine kinase, CKMB and cardiac troponin I. *Annals of Rheumatic Diseases* 59:750–752.

Kilickap, S. et al. 2005. cTnT can be a useful marker for early detection of anthracycline cardiotoxicity. *Annals of Oncology* 16:798–804.

Lewis, W. 2004. Cardiomyopathy, nucleoside reverse transcriptase inhibitors and mitochondria are linked through AIDS and its therapy. *Mitochondrion* 4:141–152.

Liantonio, A., V. Giannuzzi, V. Cippone, G. M. Camerino, S. Pierno, and D. C. Camerino. 2007. Fluvastatin and atorvastatin affect calcium homeostasis of rat skeletal muscle fibers in vivo and in vitro by impairing the sarcoplasmic reticulum/mitochondria Ca2+-release system. *Journal of Pharmacology and Experimental Therapeutics* 321:626–634.

Louden, C., and D. G. Morgan. 2001. Pathology and pathophysiology of drug-induced arterial injury in laboratory animals and its implications on the evaluation of novel chemical entities for human clinical trials. *Pharmacology and Toxicology* 89:158–170.

Mastaglia, F. L. 2006. Drug-induced myopathies. *Practical Neurology* 6:4–13.

Metzger, J. M., and M. V. Westfall. 2004. Covalent and noncovalent modification of thin filament action. The essential role of troponins in cardiac muscle regulation. *Circulation Research* 94:146–158.

Mion, M. M., E. Novello, S. Altinier, S. Rocco., M. Zaninotto, and M. Plebani. 2007. Analytical and clinical performance of a fully automated cardiac multimarkers strategy based on protein biochip microarray technology. *Clinical Biochemistry* 40:1245–1251.

Moosmann, B., and Behl, C. 2004. Selenoproteins, cholesterol-lowering drugs, and the consequences revisiting of the mevalonate pathway. *Trends in Cardiovascular Medicine* 14:273–81.

Newsholme, S. J., D. T. Thudium, K. A. Gossett, E. S. Watson, and M. Schwartz. 2000. Evaluation of plasma von Willebrand factor as a biomarker for acute arterial damage in rats. *Toxicologic Pathology* 28:688–693.

Niizeki, T. et al. 2007. Heart-type fatty acid-binding protein is more sensitive than troponin T to detect the ongoing myocardial damage in chronic heart failure patients. *Journal of Cardiac Failure* 13:120–127.

O'Brien, P. J. 2006. Blood cardiac troponin in toxic myocardial injury: Archetype of a translational safety biomarker. *Expert Reviews in Molecular Diagnosis* 6:685–702.

———. 2008. Cardiac troponin is the most effective translational safety biomarker for myocardial injury in cardiotoxicity. *Toxicology* 245:206–218.

O'Brien, P. J., Y. Landt, and J. H. Ladenson. 1997b. Differential reactivity of cardiac and skeletal muscle from various species in a cardiac troponin I immunoassay. *Clinical Chemistry* 43:2333–2338.

O'Brien, P. J. et al. 1992. Rapid, simple and sensitive microassay for skeletal and cardiac muscle myoglobin and hemoglobin: Use in various animals indicates functional role of myohemoproteins. *Molecular and Cellular Biochemistry* 112:45–52.

———. 1993. Clinical pathology profiles of dogs and turkeys with congestive heart failure, either noninduced or induced by rapid ventricular pacing, and turkeys with furazolidone toxicosis. *American Journal of Veterinary Research* 54:60–68.

———. 1997a. Cardiac troponin-T is a sensitive and specific biomarker of cardiac injury in laboratory animals. *Laboratory Animal Science* 47:486–495.

———. 2006. Cardiac troponin I is a sensitive, specific biomarker of cardiac injury in laboratory animals. *Laboratory Animals* 40:153–171.

Olson, H. et al. 2000. Concordance of the toxicity of pharmaceuticals in humans and in animals. *Regulatory Toxicology and Pharmacology* 32:56–67.

Oyama, M. A., D. D. Sisson, and P. F. Solter. 2007. Prospective screening for occult cardiomyopathy in dogs by measurement of plasma atrial natriuretic peptide, B-type natriuretic peptide, and cardiac troponin-I concentrations. *American Journal of Veterinary Research* 68:42–47.

Petricoin, E. F. et al. 2004. Toxicoproteomics: Serum proteomic pattern diagnostics for early detection of drug induced cardiac toxicities and cardioprotection. *Toxicologic Pathology* 32: Suppl. 1:122–130.

Pritt, M. L., D. G. Hall, J. Recknor, K. M. Credille, D. D. Brown, N. P. Yumibe, A. E. Schultze, and D. E. Watson. 2008. FABP3 as a biomarker of skeletal muscle toxicity in the rat: Comparison with conventional biomarkers. *Toxicological Sciences* 103:382–396.

Pruimboom-Brees, I. et al. 2006. A critical role for peroxisomal proliferator-activated receptor-alpha nuclear receptors in the development of cardiomyocyte degeneration and necrosis. *American Journal of Pathology* 169:750–760.

Scola, R. H., E. R. Pereira., P. J. Lorenzoni, and L. C. Werneck. 2007. Toxic myopathies: Muscle biopsy features. *Arquivos de Neuro-Psiquiatria* 65:82–86.

Simpson, J. A., J. Van Eyk, and S. Iscoe. 2003. Respiratory muscle injury, fatigue and serum skeletal troponin I in rat. *Journal of Physiology* 554:891–903.

Sorichter, S., J. Mair, and A. Koller. 1997. Skeletal troponin I as a marker of exercise-induced muscle damage. *Journal of Applied Physiology* 83:1076–1082.

Spangenthal, E. J., and A. K. Ellis. 1995. Cardiac and skeletal muscle myoglobin release after reperfusion of injured myocardium in dogs with systemic hypotension. *Circulation* 91:2635–2641.

Swaminathan, R. 2003. Magnesium metabolism and its disorders. *Clinical Biochemistry Reviews* 24:47–66.

Takahashi, M., L. Lee, Q. Shi, Y. Gawad, and G. Jackowski. 1996. Use of enzyme immunoassay for measurement of skeletal troponin-I utilizing isoform-specific monoclonal antibodies. *Clinical Biochemistry* 29:301–308.

Tan, L.-B., J. G. Burniston, W. A. Clark, Y. L. Ng, and D. F. Goldspink. 2003. Characterization of adrenoceptor involvement in skeletal and cardiac myotoxicity induced by sympathomimetic agents: Toward a new bioassay for beta-blockers. *Journal of Cardiovascular Pharmacology* 41:518–525.

Van Eyk, J. E., and M. J. Dunn, eds. 2003. *Proteomic and genomic analysis of cardiovascular disease.* Weinheim, Germany: Wiley VCH Verlag GmbH & Co.

Vonderfecht, S. L., M. L. Stone., R. R. Eversole, M. F. Yancey, M. R. Schuette, B. A. Duncan, and J. A. Ware. 2004. Myopathy related to administration of a cationic amphiphilic drug and use of multidose drug distribution analysis to predict occurrence. *Toxicologic Pathology* 32:318–325.

Walker, D. B. 2006. Serum chemical biomarkers of cardiac injury for nonclinical safety testing. *Toxicologic Pathology* 34:94–104.

Westwood, R., A. Bigley, K. Randall, A. Marsden, and R. Scott. 2005. Statin-induced muscle necrosis in the rat: Distribution, development, and fiber selectivity. *Toxicologic Pathology* 33:246–257.

Yeh, E. T. 2006. Cardiotoxicity induced by chemotherapy and antibody therapy. *Annual Review of Medicine* 57:485–498.

York, M. et al. 2007. Characterization of troponin responses in isoproterenol-induced cardiac injury in the Hanover Wistar rat. *Toxicologic Pathology* 35:606–607.

8 Proteins

Claire L. Watterson

8.1 INTRODUCTION

Although there are more than 3,000 distinct proteins, measurements in toxicology studies are often confined to total protein, albumin, calculated globulin, and albumin; globulin ratios in plasma or serum; and urinary total protein measured by either qualitative test strips (dipsticks) or quantitative methods as recommended in regulatory documents (see Chapter 1). Due to recent technological developments and the increasing number of commercially available assays, laboratories can now measure a variety of specific proteins and use several analytical systems for protein pattern recognition. Occasionally, protein measurements in other body fluids such as cerebrospinal fluid, peritoneal fluids, and saliva may be useful.

Many plasma proteins, including albumin and many of the globulins, are synthesized in the liver, while the immunoglobulins are synthesized in the plasma cells and B-lymphocytes of the spleen, bone marrow, and lymph nodes. Protein synthesis is influenced significantly by nutritional status, feedback mechanisms, and genetic and hormonal factors. Degradation of plasma proteins takes place mainly in the liver, although some proteins are eliminated via the kidneys (e.g., microalbumin). Once taken up by the hepatocytes (endocytosis), the plasma proteins are deglycosylated and then cleaved into amino acids by proteinases and peptidases; these processes occur in the lysosomes and in the cytosol.

The molecular masses of proteins range up to 2,750 kDa for the beta-lipoproteins, and the dynamic ranges for the plasma proteins range from millimoles per liter for albumin to femtomoles for the proteins in lower abundance. The molecular size of the individual protein is an important factor in determining its distribution and transport by the active and passive mechanisms of the body. Some proteins move freely in the extracellular and intravascular spaces, while other intracellular proteins are released only after cell damage. Some of the major plasma proteins are listed in Table 8.1, together with the broad protein fractions designated by their simple electrophoretic mobilities.

Collectively, plasma proteins perform a nutritive function; they exert colloidal osmotic pressure and aid in the maintenance of acid–base homeostasis. Individual proteins serve as enzymes, antibodies, coagulation factors, and hormones and in the transport of other molecules. The enzymatic roles of proteins are discussed in other chapters (see Chapter 2). On the basis of their metabolic roles, proteins can also be divided into several broad categories; several have more than one function. These categories are acute phase (reactant) proteins, immunoproteins, complement

TABLE 8.1
Some Plasma Proteins of Interest Listed
According to Their Electrophoretic
Mobility

Transthyretin (prealbumin)
Albumin
Alpha₁-globulins
   Alpha₁-antitrypsin
   Alpha₁-acid glycoprotein (orosomucoid)
   Alpha-lipoproteins
   Thiostatin
Alpha₂-globulins
   Alpha₂-macroglobulin
   Ceruloplasmin
   Haptoglobin
Beta-globulins
   C-reactive protein
   Amyloid A
   Complement, C3 and C4
   Transferrin
   Ferritin
   Beta-lipoprotein
   Beta₂-microglobulin
Fibrinogen
Gamma-globulins
   Immunoglobulins

proteins, coagulation proteins, and transport proteins. The metabolic rates for individual proteins vary in the different laboratory species, with generally faster rates in smaller laboratory animals (Table 8.2), so proteinic changes due to xenobiotics (as with enzymes) can occur more rapidly in smaller animals.

Plasma protein concentrations are dynamic parameters that depend on the biosynthesis, distribution between intravascular and extravascular fluid compartments, and elimination (degradation, catabolism, and loss) of the proteins. Table 8.3 lists some of the common causes for changes of plasma protein and albumin concentrations. A rise in plasma albumin is often due to dehydration, and this can be confirmed by associated increases of plasma globulins, blood hemoglobin, and hematocrit (packed cell volume).

Hypoproteinemias are characterized by reductions in albumin and/or globulin fractions; reductions of albumin may be due to reduced hepatic synthesis or increased losses via the kidney or intestinal mucosa and several other tissues. Severe hypoproteinemia can be associated with edema and ascites due to the major osmotic influence of albumin. Some compounds, such as colchicines and cycloheximide, can

TABLE 8.2
Estimated Half-Lives[a] for Albumin and Immunoglobulins in Some Laboratory Species

Species	Albumin	Immunoglobulins
Mouse	2.0	5
Rat	2.5	5
Guinea pig	3.0	5–7
Rabbit	5.7	7–9
Dog	8.0	8

[a] $T^{1/2}$ in days.

TABLE 8.3
Some Causes of Hypo- or Hyperproteinemia

Hypoproteinemia

Overhydration
Hemodilution
    Excess administration of intravenous fluid
Edema (e.g., in congestive heart failure, cirrhosis, nephrotic syndrome)
    Excess secretion of antidiuretic hormone
Increased protein loss
    Hemorrhage
    Protein-losing nephropathy
    Protein-losing enteropathy
Decreased protein synthesis/increased protein catabolism
    Cachectic states: starvation, malnutrition, neoplasia, chronic diseases
    Hepatotoxicity
    Malabsorption: intestinal mucosal disease, pancreatic insufficiency

Hyperproteinemia

Dehydration/hemoconcentration
Increased protein synthesis
Inflammation
Infections: viral, bacterial, protozoal, and fungal
Immune mediated effects
Neoplasia
Hepatotoxicity
Nephrotoxicity

reduce protein synthesis. In plasma, the total protein varies from approximately 50 to 70 g/L, depending on the species; albumin is slightly more than half of the total plasma protein. Thus, any major change of plasma albumin will be reflected by the total protein values. Few protein changes are pathognomonic, and opposing changes in the other protein fractions often mask small changes of individual proteins of the globulin fractions.

8.2 ACUTE PHASE (REACTANT) PROTEINS

The acute phase proteins (APPs) are a group of proteins that change in concentration in animals subjected to external or internal challenges, such as infection, inflammation, surgical trauma, and stress (Figure 8.1). These APPs have a wide range of activities that contribute to host defense mechanisms by directly neutralizing inflammatory agents, helping to minimize the extent of local tissue damage, and participating in tissue repair and regeneration. The proteins participate in the killing of infectious agents and the clearance of foreign and host cellular debris. Coagulation proteins, including fibrinogen, play an essential role in promoting wound healing, and proteinase inhibitors neutralize the lysosomal hydrolases released following the infiltration of activated macrophages and neutrophils, thus controlling the activity of the pro-inflammatory enzyme cascades. Plasma levels of some metal-binding proteins increase to prevent iron loss during infection and injury, minimizing the levels of heme iron available for uptake by bacteria and acting as scavengers for potentially damaging free radicals. The APPs act as components of the nonspecific innate immune responses by restraining microbial growth before the animals can develop

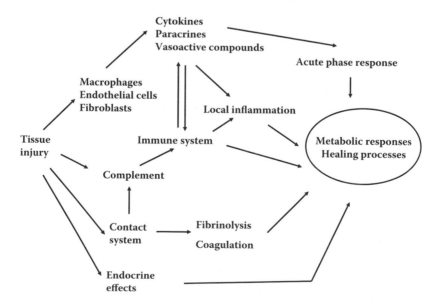

FIGURE 8.1   Mechanisms of the acute phase response.

acquired immunity to a challenge. Some general reviews of acute phase proteins are given in the references at the end of the chapter.

The production of APPs is strongly influenced by the actions of the cytokines. The majority of the members of the cytokine family—interleukins, tumor necrosis factor, chemokines, and transforming growth factor-beta—are polypeptides or glycoproteins with molecular masses of less than 30 kDa. The cytokines are produced by a variety of different cells and exert multiple actions on their target receptor cells. The range of actions of the cytokines is diverse, and some have similar actions; however, sometimes cytokines exhibit interactions and antagonistic actions with other cytokines. During inflammatory responses, primarily the increases of interleukin 6 (IL-6), interleukin 1 (IL-1), and tumor necrosis factor lead to the increased production of positive acute phase response proteins. Measurement of plasma cytokines can be difficult due to the temporal nature of the cytokine response compared to the longer responses observed with APPs (van Gool et al. 1990; Kimball 1991; Yamashita, Fujinaga, Hagio, et al. 1994; Yamashita, Fujinaga, Miyamoto, et al. 1994; Miyamoto et al. 1996; Banks 2000; Bienvenu et al. 2000; Fulop et al. 2001), and there is a lack of suitable reagents for some laboratory species such as the dog. The circulating concentrations of the APP are related to the severity and extent of the injury and tissue damage. Stress also may elevate the interleukin and APP responses by stimulating the hypothalamic–pituitary–adrenal axis and cause systemic or local cytokine production (van Gool et al. 1990; Murata, Shimada, and Yoshioka 2004). In the acute phase response, the increases of cytokines precede the changes of plasma proteins.

Acute phase response proteins (APPs) may be separated into three groups:

Positive acute phase response proteins are plasma APPs that are increased during the acute phase response within hours of the stimulus/injury and persist for the duration of the inflammatory response. Examples include C-reactive protein (CRP), alpha$_1$-acid glycoprotein (AAG), alpha$_2$-macroglobulin, fibrinogen, haptoglobin, and amyloid A (SAA) (Stockham and Scott 2002).

Delayed response proteins increase 1–3 weeks after the acute phase response (e.g., immunoglobulins and complement).

Negative acute phase proteins decrease during the acute phase response; albumin appears to be a negative APP in all laboratory species, and sometimes decreases of transferrin and retinol-binding protein are observed. Plasma albumin falls in the acute phase response due to hemodilution, transfer into the extravascular space due to increased vascular permeability, increased colloidal osmotic pressure, and decreased synthesis.

The major APPs may show a 10- to 100-fold increase in an acute response, and there are major differences among the major APPs in the laboratory animals. For example, C-reactive protein is the major APP in the dog and nonhuman primates, but not in the rat, where alpha$_2$-macroglobulin is the major APP. In reviews and comparative studies of the APPs, some of the major proteins in the different species have been identified (shown in Table 8.4).

TABLE 8.4

Examples of Interspecies Differences in Positive Acute Phase Proteins

Species	Major	Moderate	Minor
Dog	C-reactive protein	Alpha$_1$-acid glycoprotein Haptoglobin Fibrinogen	Alpha$_2$-macroglobulin
Mouse	Serum amyloid A	Alpha$_1$-acid glycoprotein Haptoglobin	Alpha$_2$-macroglobulin
Rat	Alpha$_2$-macroglobulin Thiostatin	Alpha$_1$-acid glycoprotein Haptoglobin Fibrinogen	Serum amyloid A

Some references to the application and methods for some of these major acute phase proteins are provided in the list of references at the end of the chapter.

8.2.1 ALPHA$_1$-ACID GLYCOPROTEIN (AGP, OROSOMUCOID)

This protein has a molecular mass of 41–43 kDa and in rats has an amino acid sequence that is 60% of the human protein. Antiserum to human alpha$_1$-AGP cannot be used for rats and mice because there are at least two forms of the protein. Alpha$_1$-AGP is synthesized primarily in the liver and the half-life is approximately 24 h. This protein transports hormones and cationic xenobiotics and may also act in nonspecific immunosuppression.

8.2.2 AMYLOID A

Often called serum amyloid A (SAA), this protein has a low molecular mass of about 12 kDa, and there are at least three isoforms in mice and four in hamsters. These proteins are primarily produced in the liver, but they are also produced in several extrahepatic tissues such as the spleen and testes. These proteins are involved with regulating lipid metabolism and accelerate the removal of high-density lipoproteins from the circulation. The concentrations of amyloid A increase in mice where it is the primary acute phase protein, dogs and to a lesser degree in rats, despite some evidence has suggesting that SAA is not an acute phase protein in rats. Amyloid A should not be confused with amyloid P, which has much larger molecular masses of 230–300 kDa and a much more complex structure of 10 subunits.

8.2.3 C-REACTIVE PROTEIN (CRP)

These are pentameric proteins with molecular masses of about 100–140 kDa; the proteins are primarily produced by the liver. The primary roles of CRP are in the initiation and immunomodulation of inflammatory responses and removal of cellular debris from the sites of tissue injury. CRP is a good marker of acute phase response in the dog. The general view that CRP is a very poor indicator of APR (Pepys et al. 1979; Giffen et al. 2003) in the rat is now being challenged, and the reasons for this disparity are unclear.

8.2.4   HAPTOGLOBINS

These are large proteins with molecular masses of about 85–100 kDa that are synthesized primarily in the liver, with half-lives of approximately 3 days. The primary role of haptoglobin is to bind free hemoglobin, particularly during episodes of intravascular hemolysis. Absence or low levels of haptoglobin are suggestive of hemolysis or severe acute/chronic hepatotoxicity. Conversely, plasma haptoglobin may be increased with some toxins that cause tissue inflammation, including hepatic tissue.

8.2.5   ALPHA$_2$-MACROGLOBULIN

These are large glycoproteins with four subunits and total molecular masses of approximately 780 kDa. Although there is a reported 80% homology between rat and human alpha$_2$-macroglobulins, very few of the antisera to the human protein react with the rat alpha$_2$-macroglobulin. Hepatocytes are the primary source of these proteins, and the alpha$_2$-globulin has a major role in host defense mechanisms.

8.2.6   THIOSTATIN

Also called alpha$_1$-major acute protein (alpha$_1$-MAP), thiostatin has a molecular mass of about 56 kDa. This protein exists in at least two forms and is primarily synthesized by the liver. The measurements of thiostatin have been investigated less than other acute phase proteins in the rat and therefore remain to be exploited.

Other proteins that in the future may prove to be useful in monitoring inflammation include *transforming growth factor-beta* (TGF-β) (Sasaki et al. 1992; Wahl 1992; Varedi et al. 2001) and *procalcitonin* (Rothenburger et al. 1999; Nijsten et al. 2000; Whicher, Bienvenu, and Monneret 2001).

Deliberate reductions of food intake have been shown to modify the responses of the APPs (Pickering and Pickering 1984; Maejima and Nagase 1991) and cytokines. There were mixed effects on alpha$_2$-macroglobulin in protein-deficient rats in turpentine- and lipopolysaccharide-induced acute phase response models (Jennings and Elia 1996; Lyoumi et al. 1998), but this may reflect the duration of protein deficiency and sampling times in relation to the induced injury. Such changes may occur in toxicology studies when there are marked reductions of food intake.

Several rat strains show differing APP responses to the same stimulus, and this may be important when studying animal disease models (Weimer et al. 1972; Strnad et al. 2000; Olofsson et al. 2002). In addition to the species differences for major APPs already described, there are several examples of species and gender differences for plasma proteins. These examples include a positive APP in hamsters that has a pentameric structure similar to that found in CRP (House, Pansky, and Jacobs 1961; Coe and Ross 1983) and mouse prealbumin (Reuter et al. 1968).

8.3 IMMUNOPROTEINS

8.3.1 IMMUNOGLOBULINS

The immune system can be subdivided into a nonspecific system involving factors such as lysozyme, complement and interferons, natural killer cells, and phagocytes. A second system involves the immunoglobulins and the T-lymphocytes. This system is triggered by the incomplete actions of nonspecific factors, with immunoglobulins having the functions of antigen recognition and subsequent initiation of effector mechanisms to destroy or nullify antigens. There are five primary immunoglobulin (Ig) isotypes (or classes): IgA, IgM, IgG, IgD, and IgE, and in laboratory animals they share some common structural features (Neoh et al. 1973; Bankert and Mazzaferro 1999). The immunoglobulins can be further divided into subclasses in several species, including the mouse, rat, and dog. They are composed of two different polypeptide chains (heavy and light); the genes encoding these polypeptides are highly segmented at the genetic level. In addition to any of the direct actions on the immune system, the levels of plasma immunoglobulins, lymph, and other body fluids may be altered by any general effect on the rate of protein synthesis or clearance, such as protein-losing enteropathy, nephrotoxicity, or hepatotoxicity. Specific classes or subclasses of immunoglobulins can be preferentially induced by different antigenic stimuli or disease states.

The expansion of immunology and the increasing recognition of immune responses to xenobiotics have led to immunotoxicology developing as a distinct discipline (Burrell, Flaherty, and Sauers 1992). Tiered approaches for evaluating the immune system have been proposed, and this includes the measurement of immunoglobulins, despite the lack of recognized, standardized, and validated procedures (Vos 1980; Luster et al. 1988). Xenobiotics may act as immunosuppressants, immunostimulants, or immunogens (i.e., the xenobiotic is coupled to a carrier protein or other molecule and induces antibody formation). Consequently, the application of immunoglobulin measurements in toxicology is becoming more common (Descotes and Mazue 1987; van Loveren and Vos 1989). The techniques available for the quantification of immunoglobulins rely on class- or subclass-specific antisera for detecting various isotypes. Thus, the ability to quantify immunoglobulins for various species is dependent upon the availability of species-specific antisera.

8.4 COMPLEMENT PROTEINS

These proteins constitute approximately 15% of the total globulin protein fraction, with differences occurring between species both in structure and concentration (Gigli and Austen 1971; Barta 1984). Thirty or more chemically and immunologically distinct proteins are capable of interacting with each other, antibodies, certain bacterial products, and cell membranes. These proteins are synthesized in the liver and their production can be affected by hepatotoxicity. The activating sequence for the complement cascade consists of four steps: triggering, amplification, a feedback loop, and lysis (Liszewski et al. 1996). The amplification is rapid, with the spread of this step affected by the feedback loop. Other regulating mechanisms of the complement system include the spontaneous decay of activated proteins, destabilization or inhibition of activation complexes, and proteolytic cleavage of activated components. Although total complement activity can be measured by hemolytic and antigenic assays, large reductions of complement proteins are required for this test to be abnormal, and complement proteins are not commonly measured in toxicology studies.

8.5   COAGULATION PROTEINS

Measurements of the coagulation proteins are generally the responsibility of the hematology laboratory and are usually confined to prothrombin time and activated partial thromboplastin time measurements, or some alternative measures of the performance of the intrinsic and extrinsic coagulation cascade pathways (Theus and Zbinden 1984). The coagulation proteins synthesized by the liver also can be used as markers of hepatotoxicity (Pritchard et al. 1987).

Fibrinogen has a central role in hemostasis and, in addition, acts as an acute phase protein in inflammatory and tissue repair processes. The increases of fibrinogen are often moderate two- to fourfold increases, unlike some of the other major APPs. An increased rate of liver fibrinogenesis represents a uniform response of the liver to hepatocyte damage induced by infectious, toxic, or metabolic agents. Coagulation protein measurements are of particular interest when testing compounds deliberately designed to affect fibrinolysis (Murata et al. 2004).

8.6   TRANSPORT PROTEINS

Major transport proteins include albumin, acid glycoprotein, hemopexin, haptoglobin, transferrin, transthyretin (prealbumin), ceruloplasmin, lipoproteins, thyroid hormone binding proteins, and corticosteroid binding globulin (the latter three groups of transport proteins are discussed in Chapters 9 and 10). Albumin binds and transports large organic anions that are normally insoluble in aqueous fluid—for example, bilirubin and long chain fatty acids, calcium, and magnesium (see the next section). Albumin and hemopexin together with haptoglobin are associated with the transport of circulating hemoglobin and heme. Transferrin and ferritin are important proteins in iron transport and storage.

8.7   PROTEIN BINDING OF XENOBIOTICS

Xenobiotics bind to plasma proteins in various ways, and this binding is an important factor in understanding the distribution, metabolism, and excretion of xenobiotics, particularly for drugs. Compounds that bind to proteins may be acidic or basic, and the degree of protein binding varies with each xenobiotic or metabolite. This protein binding also can be affected by competitive binding when two or more compounds are coadministered (Lindup and Orme 1981; Wilkinson 1983; Oracova, Bohs, and Lidner 1996; Proost, Wierda, and Meijer 1996; Kratochwil et al. 2004; Hernandez and Rathinavelu 2006). When plasma proteins are present in relatively high concentrations (e.g., albumin), the protein fraction acts as a depot for the xenobiotic as well as a transport protein. The binding of xenobiotics with albumin, which has at least six binding sites, occurs more frequently with other plasma proteins. Also, the binding of drugs with $alpha_1$-glycoprotein is common. The binding of xenobiotics with the individual proteins also differs between the animal species (Kosa, Maruyama, and Otagiri 1997; Colussi, Parisot, and Lefevre 1998; Son et al. 1998; Pahlman and Gozzi 1999). In summary, any alterations of the plasma proteins can change the available concentration of the xenobiotic, and this is particularly important for pharmaceuticals where the dynamics of drug/protein interactions are changed in either hypo- or hyperproteinemia.

The binding of a xenobiotic with proteins can have marked effects on other laboratory tests. This is exemplified by the effect on prothrombin time following the displacement of coagulation proteins by phenylbutazone and the action of drugs on thyroid hormones. Other compounds can bind with plasma proteins, and this includes metal cations such as iron and transferrin, copper, and ceruloplasmin. Lipoproteins can bind lipid-soluble compounds, and immunoglobulins act with antigens that may be biologicals or form drug haptens. It is perhaps surprising how few examples of interference by xenobiotics with albumin and total protein measurements have been reported.

8.8   URINE PROTEINS

The measurement of urinary proteins and their diagnostic value are discussed in Chapter 4. There are some important species differences, particularly for rodents: A family of prealbumins known as the major urinary protein (MUP) is found in the mouse (Finlayson and Baumann 1958), and $alpha_{2u}$-globulins are the major proteins in male rat urine. Generally, male rodents are more proteinuric (there are marked changes with age) and urinary albumin increases in the aged rat. An important side issue is the level of IgG antirat antibodies in some affected individuals when considering human allergy to laboratory animals (Botham et al. 1989).

Several test strips or dipsticks are commercially available and are commonly used to assess proteinuria, but there are several limitations to their use. Highly alkaline or buffered urines give false positive protein reactions, and the test strips are primarily sensitive to changes in albumin rather than globulin fractions (Evans and Parsons 1986). Allowances should be made for the urine volume and concentration when interpreting test strip results. The quantitative measurement of urine protein is being used more frequently in preclinical toxicological studies (see Chapter 4).

8.9   TRANSUDATES AND EXUDATES

The protein concentration of pleural fluid or abdominal ascites is occasionally measured to determine whether the sample is a transudate (fluid with a low protein content derived by filtration across the capillary endothelium) or an exudate (protein with a high protein content actively secreted in response to inflammation). Exudative pleural fluids generally have total protein concentrations approximately >30 g/L or a pleural fluid to plasma protein ratio of >0.5; however, the protein content of these fluids is variable (Light et al. 1972; Heffner, Brown, and Barbieri 1997). When a sample of fluid is analyzed, a critical question is whether the ascites/pleural fluid is infected or whether it is caused by malignancy; this can be determined by microbial and cytological examination. Simple protein electrophoresis may provide useful information on the nature and origin of these fluids.

8.10 ANALYSIS OF PROTEINS

For total plasma protein measurements, the majority of laboratories use the biuret method, which is based on the formation of a cupric ion–peptide complex in an alkaline solution. Other methods using Coomassie blue G-250, bicinchoninic acid, or the older Lowry reagents are generally reserved for measuring the lower protein levels found in body fluids other than plasma. The bromcresol (or BCG) green dye-binding method for plasma albumin appears to be suitable for most laboratory animal species, unlike some other albumin-binding dyes (Metz and Schutze 1975; Evans and Parsons 1988). An alternative dye, bromocresol purple, appears to be unsuitable for most laboratory species. The bromcresol green methods are said to overestimate values below 20 g/L, but this depends on the reagent constitution, reaction conditions, and, more importantly, the timing of absorbance measurements. Proteins other than albumin, such as alpha$_1$-globulins, may react with bromcresol green if the absorbance measurements are made more than 60 s after the reagent addition (Gustafsson 1976). Some investigators have reported problems when using bromcresol green to measure rabbit and canine plasma/serum albumin, but others have not confirmed this finding (Fox 1989; Hall 1992; Evans 1994; Kimball and Murray 1994; Stokol, Tarrant, and Scarlett 2001; Takano, Komiyama, and Nomura 2001). Refractometry is a quick and useful alternative for urine or plasma/serum total protein measurements in the diagnostic veterinary clinic, but the method is not commonly used in toxicology studies.

Measurements of plasma total protein and albumin may be supplemented by qualitative or quantitative separation of proteins by various electrophoretic techniques or specific protein determinations (Table 8.5). Plasma protein values are slightly higher (approximately 5%) than corresponding serum values due to the presence of fibrinogen, although cold storage can cause this fraction to precipitate. Globulin values are usually determined by subtracting albumin values from total protein, and the plasma globulin value will also include fibrinogen. Globulin measurements will be only as accurate as the measured total protein and albumin concentrations; methods exist for direct measurement of globulin (e.g., using glyoxylic acid) but are rarely used.

The calibration of total protein, albumin, and specific protein methods remains a problem when analyzing samples from laboratory animals. Many of the available protein calibration materials are bovine or human in origin, and there are international reference proteins for some human proteins (Whicher 1984; Price and Newman 1997; Tiffany 1999). However, because calibration standards for laboratory animals are not widely available, the values between methods may show wide variations due to differences in calibrators. When some protein fractions are available for laboratory animals, these materials are often less than 95% pure. The investigator therefore

TABLE 8.5

Qualitative and Quantitative Methods for Measuring Proteins[a]

Electrophoretic methods use various support media, buffers, voltage, amperage, and times. The media include agarose gel, cellulose acetate, starch gel, and polyacrylamide gel. Techniques include single dimensional electrophoresis, crossed immunoelectrophoresis, and immunoelectrophoretic fixation (IEF).

Methods for specific proteins:

    Enzyme-linked immunosorbent assay (ELISA)

    Radial immunodiffusion (RID)

    Laurell immunoelectrophoresis

    Chemiluminescence

    Fluorometry

    Immunoturbidimetry

    Immunonephelometry

    Radioimmunoassay

[a] See Section 8.11 for additional methods.

needs to consider reporting relative protein changes as a percentage of the control group or pretreatment value in absence of suitable calibration standards.

Simple electrophoretic techniques using cellulose acetate or agarose support media can be used to assess changes of albumin and globulin fractions, although the support media and electrophoretic conditions may affect the electrophoretograms and produce additional protein bands as the individual proteins separate (Scherer, Abd-El-Fattah, and Ruthenstroth-Bauer 1977; Allchin and Evans 1986; Watanabe 1995; Abate et al. 2000; Deschamps and Huard 2004). It is sometimes necessary to adjust the electrophoretic methods for particular species if satisfactory separations are to be obtained. Using serum rather than plasma avoids complications due to fibrinogen or fibrin. The commonest dyes used with these simple techniques are Amido black or Ponceau S; however, because neither of these dyes is uniformly bound by the various protein fractions, in most cases the results are semiquantitative. Scanning of the electrophoretograms to produce quantitative results can produce statistical differences that can be interpreted with consideration of the imprecision of electrophoretic methods—particularly for protein bands, which are less than 10% of the total plasma protein concentration.

The application of qualitative and quantitative immunochemical protein measurements has been limited by the lack of available antisera suitable for laboratory animals, although this situation is improving. Antisera against human proteins are often useful for closely related species, and some phylogenetically distant species have similar epitopes on their corresponding proteins, which then allows protein measurements in several species (Brun, Lingaas, and Larsen 1989; Hau et al. 1990; Pineiro, Alava, and Lampreave 2003). Some proteins require species-specific antisera (e.g., CRP; Balz et al. 1982; Eckersall, Conner, and Harvie 1991). When a suitable antiserum is available, it is still necessary to test that the concentrations of the antiserum and antigen are appropriate; inappropriate reagents may lead to over- or underestimation for the protein under examination. Immunochemical methods provide the advantages of good specificity and sensitivity; however, there is little doubt that specific antibodies and standards are essential to obtain reliable, accurate assays.

Quantitative immunoturbidometric and immunonephelometric methods using the precipitation of the antibody–antigen complex have been used for the measurement of haptoglobin and immunoglobulins; these methods are rapid and adaptable to many biochemical analyzers (Glickman et al. 1988; Ginel et al. 1997; German, Hall, and Day 1998). The sensitivity of immunoturbidometric assays is comparable to that of immunonephelometric assays, although nephelometry retains some advantages when measuring low-level antigen–antibody reactions. In addition, the performance of these methods can be improved significantly by the inclusion of water-soluble polymers, which enable the use of lower reactant concentrations and result in a more stable immune complex (Price and Newman 1997; Ullman 2001).

Solid phase immunoassays—as enzyme-linked immunosorbent assays (ELISA) (Schreiber et al. 1992; Salauze, Serre, and Perrin 1994; Jones, Offutt, and Longmore 2000) or as latex agglutination inhibition assays (Eckersall et al. 1999)—are being used more widely as species-specific antibodies become available. These methods are quicker than immunodiffusion agarose gel assays, which require 24 or 48 h for diffusion to be complete.

8.11 PROTEOMICS

The proteome describes the complete protein complement of a given genome, and proteomics is the analysis and study of these proteins (Haynes et al. 1998; Anderson and Anderson 2002; Conn 2003; Lundblad 2005; Hortin et al. 2006). Proteomic techniques have been used in studies of hepatic injury (Amacher et al. 2005), cardiotoxicity (van Eyk and Dunn 2003; Petricoin et al. 2004), renal injury (Hampel et al. 2001; Thongboonkerd and Klein 2003; Hewitt, Dear, and Star 2004), the central nervous system (Sironi et al. 2001), myotoxicity (Dare et al. 2002), neuromuscular diseases (van den Heuvel et al. 2003), and acute phase response (Higgins et al. 2003).

In the last decade, there has been considerable investment in this field with new technologies. These proteomic technologies include protein arrays, two-dimensional gel electrophoresis with or without mass spectrometry, high-performance liquid chromatography, and capillary electrophoresis, all of which can be applied to all biological fluids. Although plasma and serum are to be preferred for most investigations of organ toxicity, urine is probably a better sample for studies of nephrotoxicity. It is less complex than plasma, although its proteins are more subject to degradation. Two-dimensional gel electrophoresis can be used with a variety of staining procedures, immunoblotting, and imaging systems for the stained gel, which allow comparison between gels and samples. Proteins are separated by charge in one direction and then by mass in the second dimension. Following gel electrophoresis, proteins can be excised from the gel and subjected to matrix assisted laser desorption ionization and time-of-flight mass spectrometry analysis (MALDI TOF). Surface enhanced laser desorptive ionization (SELDI) offers an alternative technique in which protein samples are selectively adsorbed onto a hydrophobic metal chip; the molecules captured onto the metal are then treated with an energy absorber and a laser before transfer to a mass spectrometer. The other technologies of high-performance liquid chromatography and capillary electrophoresis have received less attention than SELDI- and MALDI-based technologies (Wijenen and van Dieijen-Visser 1996; Palfrey 1999).

Protein arrays with 10–500 antibodies printed onto an array use detection techniques, including fluorescence and multiple sandwich enzyme-linked immunosorbent assays, but the broad application of these assays is restricted by lack of suitable antibodies for laboratory animals and some potential cross-reactivities between antibodies with similar affinities. Calibration, reproducibility, and identification of proteins are common problems for all of these technologies. A number of databases are available to help investigators identify the numerous proteins found using these separation techniques, particularly for mass spectrometer data.

Given the wide range of protein concentrations in biological fluids and the presence of about 20 proteins (albumin, immunoglobulins, transferrin, etc.) in which the plasma concentrations are much higher than the other remaining proteins (which constitute less than 10–20% of plasma proteins), various methods for removing some of these abundant proteins have been used. These techniques include protein removal by immunoaffinity or immobilized dye removal, although it is now recognized that these depletion techniques may take out less abundant proteins (Duan et al. 2005). These protein removal procedures have also helped to reveal protein fragments (Eppel et al. 2000; Greive, Balazs, and Comper 2001) and peptides of potential interest, leading to the development of peptidomics (Hortin et al. 2006). Some protease inhibitors are used to prevent protease action on body fluids and tissues during sample handling. However, it must be recognized that many of these less abundant proteins have short half-lives, which might lessen their utility in toxicology except for studies of acute tissue injury.

Despite the investment in proteomics, the introduction of new protein tests in human medicine has not dramatically increased over the last decade and, to some extent, has been disappointing (Pognan 2004) except in animal clinical chemistry, where the number of available assays has improved due to availability of suitable antisera and commercial investment. If key proteins, which are highly diagnostic, are identified by proteomics, then commercially available reagent kits in suitable formats for liquid chemistry analyzers, enzyme-linked immunosorbent assays, or "chip" technology are required to ensure wider application of these potential biomarkers.

REFERENCES*

Acute Phase Proteins

Cerón, J. J., P. D. Eckersall, and S. Martýnez-Subiela. 2005. Acute phase proteins in dogs and cats: Current knowledge and future perspectives. *Veterinary Clinical Pathology* 34:85–89.
Eckersall, P. D. 2004. The time is right for acute phase protein assays. *Veterinary Journal* 168:3–5.

---

* Some references not cited in the text are included for background reading.

Ganrot, K. 1973. Plasma protein response in experimental inflammation in the dog. *Research in Experimental Medicine* 161:251–261.

Kushner, I., and A. Mackiewicz. 1987. Acute phase proteins as disease markers. *Disease Markers* 5:1–11.

Mackiewicz, A., I. Kushner, and H. Baumann, eds. 1993. *Acute phase proteins: Molecular biology, biochemistry and clinical applications.* Boca Raton, FL: CRC Press.

Murata, H., N. Shimada, and M. Yoshioka. 2004. Current research on acute phase proteins in veterinary diagnosis: An overview. *Veterinary Journal* 168:28–40.

Pineiro, M., M. A. Alava, and F. Lampreave. 2003. Acute phase proteins in different species: A review. *Animal welfare and acute phase proteins.* Invited papers from Fourth European Colloquium on Acute Phase Proteins, pp. 77–82.

Schreiber, G. et al. 1989. The acute phase response in the rodent. *Annals of the New York Academy of Sciences* 557:61–86.

Stockham, S. L., and M. A. Scott. 2002. Proteins. In *Fundamentals of veterinary clinical pathology,* 1st ed., pp. 251–278. Oxford, England: Blackwell Publishing.

Whicher, J. T. 1984. Functions of acute phase proteins in the inflammatory response. In *Marker proteins in inflammation,* vol. 2, ed. P. Arnaud, J. Bienvenu, and P. Laurent, pp. 90–98. New York: Walter de Gruyter.

Cytokines

Banks, R. E. 2000. Measurement of cytokines in clinical samples using immunoassays: Problems and pitfalls. *Critical Reviews in Clinical Laboratory Sciences* 37:131–182.

Bienvenu, J., G. Monneret, N. Fabien, and J. P. Revillard. 2000. The clinical usefulness of the measurement of cytokines. *Clinical Chemistry and Laboratory Medicine* 38:267–285.

Fulop, A. K. et al. 2001. Hepatic regeneration induces transient acute phase reaction: Systemic elevation of acute phase reactants and soluble cytokine receptors. *Cell Biology International* 25:585–592.

Kimball, E. S. 1991. *Cytokines and inflammation.* Boca Raton, FL: CRC Press.

Miyamoto, T., T. Fujinaga, K. Yamashita, and M. Hagio. 1996. Changes of serum cytokine activities and other parameters in dogs with experimentally induced endotoxic shock. *Japanese Journal of Veterinary Research* 44:107–118.

Murata, H., N. Shimada, and M. Yoshioka. 2004. Current research on acute phase proteins in veterinary diagnosis: An overview. *Veterinary Journal* 168:28–40.

van Gool, J., H. van Vugt, M. Helle, and L. A. Aarden. 1990. The relation among stress, adrenaline, interleukin 6 and acute phase proteins in the rat. *Clinical Immunology and Immunopathology* 57:200–210.

Yamashita, K., T. Fujinaga, M. Hagio, T. Miyamoto, Y. Izumisawa, and T. Kotani. 1994. Bioassay for interleukin-1, interleukin 6 and tumor necrosis factor-like activities in canine sera. *Journal of Veterinary Medical Science* 56:103–107.

Yamashita, K., T. Fujinaga, T. Miyamoto, M. Hagio, Y. Izumisawa, and T. Kotani. 1994. Canine acute phase response: Relationship between serum cytokine activity and acute phase protein in dogs. *Journal of Veterinary Medical Science* 56:487–492.

Amyloid A

Glojnaric, I., V. Erakovic, and M. J. Parnham. 2003. Inhibition of serum amyloid A (SAA) release by dexamethasone, azithromycin and clarithromycin during experimental inflammation in BALB/c mice. *Clinical Chemistry* 49 (Suppl.): A155.

Pepys, M. B., and M. L. Baltz. 1983. Acute phase proteins with special reference to C-reactive protein and related proteins (pentaxins) and serum amyloid A protein. *Advances in Immunology* 34:141–212.

Pepys, M. B., M. Baltz, K. Gomer, A. J. S. Davies, and M. Doenhoff. 1979. Serum amyloid
    P-component is an acute-phase reactant in the mouse. *Nature* 278:259–261.
Steel, D., and A. S. Whitehead. 1994. The major acute phase reactants: C-reactive protein,
    serum amyloid P and serum amyloid A protein. *Immunology Today* 15:81–88.

Alpha₁-Acid Glycoprotein

Fournier, T., N-N. Medjoubi, and D. Porquet. 2000. Alpha-1-acid glycoprotein. Review.
    Biochimica et Biophysica Acta 1482:157–171.
Kuribayashi, T., M. Shimizu, T. Shimada, T. Honjyo, Y. Yamamoto, K. Kuba, and S. Yamamoto.
    2003. Alpha 1-glycoprotein in healthy and pregnant beagle dogs. *Experimental Animals*
    52:377–381.
Metzger, J., M. Blobner, and P. B. Luppa. 2001. Sensitive chemiluminescence immunoas-
    say for the determination of rat serum α1-acid glycoprotein. *Clinical Chemistry and
    Laboratory Medicine* 39:514–518.
Schreiber, G., G. Howlett, M. Nagashima, A. Millership, H. Martin, J. Urban, and L. Kotler.
    1982. The acute phase response of plasma protein synthesis during experimental inflam-
    mation. *Journal of Biological Chemistry* 257:10271–10277

Alpha₁-Macroglobulin

Dolezalova, V., P. Stratil, M. Simickova, A. Kocent, and R. Nemecek. 1983. Alpha-fetoprotein
    (AFP) and α-2-macroglobulin (α2-M) as the markers of distinct responses of hepato-
    cytes to carcinogens in the rat: Carcinogenesis. *Annals of the New York Academy of
    Sciences* 417:294–307.
Kim, I. G., and S. Y. Park. 1997. Development of a competitive enzyme linked immunosor-
    bent assay to measure α-2-macroglobulin in irradiated rat serum. *Biochemistry and
    Molecular Biology International* 43:695–703.
Nakagawa, H., K. Watanabe, and S. Tsurufuji. 1984. Changes in serum and exudate levels of func-
    tional macroglobulins and anti-inflammatory effect of alpha-2-acute-phase-macroglobulin
    on carrageenin-induced inflammation in rats. *Biochemical Pharmacology* 33:1181–1186.
Stevenson, F. T., S. Greene, and G. A. Kaysen. 1998. Serum alpha-2-macroglobulin and alpha-
    1-inhibitor concentrations are increased in hypoalbuminemia by post-transcriptional
    mechanisms. *Kidney International* 53:67–75.
Strnad M., C. Radojicic, D. Marinkovic, and Z. Magic. 2000. Variability of haptoglobin and
    alpha-2-macroglobulin in albino Oxford and dark Augustin inbred strains of rats before
    and after trauma. *Vojnosanitetski Pregled* 57:381–386.

C-Reactive Protein

Balz, M. L. et al. 1982. Phylogenetic aspects of C-reactive protein and related proteins. *Annals
    of the New York Academy of Sciences* 389:49–73.
Burton, S. A., D. J. Honor, A. L. Mackenzie, P. D. Eckersall, R. J. F. Markham, and B.
    Horney. 1994. C-reactive protein concentrations in dogs with inflammatory leukograms.
    American Journal of Veterinary Research 55:613–618.
Eckersall, P. D., J. G. Conner, and J. Harvie. 1991. An immunoturbidometric method for
    C-reactive protein. *Veterinary Research Communications* 15:17–24.
Kuribayashi, T. et al. 2003. Determination of serum C-reactive protein in healthy beagle dogs
    of various ages and pregnant beagle dogs. *Experimental Animals* 52:387–390.
Otabe, K. et al. 1998. Physiological levels of C-reactive protein in normal canine sera.
    Veterinary Research Communications 22:77–85.
Parra, M. D., M. Tuomola, J. Cabezas-Herrera, and J. J. Cerón. 2005. Use of a time-resolved
    immunofluormetric assay for determination of canine C-reactive protein concentrations
    in whole blood. *American Journal of Veterinary Research* 66:62–66.

Pepys, M. B., and G. M. Hirschfield. 2003. C-reactive protein: A critical update. *Journal of Clinical Investigation* 111:1803–1812.

Riley, R. F., and M. K. Coleman. 1970. Isolation of C-reactive protein of man, monkey, rabbit and dog by affinity chromatography on phosphorylated cellulose. *Clinica Chimica Acta* 30:483–486.

Steel, D., and A. S. Whitehead. 1994. The major acute phase reactants: C-reactive protein, serum amyloid P and serum amyloid A protein. *Immunology Today* 15:81–88.

Wang, C-M., N. Y. Nguyen, K. Yonaha, F. Robey, and T-Y. Liu. 1982. Primary structure of rabbit C-reactive protein. *Journal of Biological Chemistry* 257:13610–13615.

Haptoglobin

Adams, D. F., N. Lee, K. Lynch, T. Sellers, D. Ennulat, and L. Schwartz. 2004. Automated measurement of serum haptoglobin in rats, dogs and monkeys using the Tridelta PHASE tm method on the Bayer Advia 1650 chemistry system. *Clinical Chemistry* 50 (Suppl.): A36.

Eckersall, P. D., S. Duthie, S. Safi, M. Moffatt, N. U. Horadagoda, S. Doyle, R. Parton, D. Bennett, and J. L. Fitzpatrick. 1999. An automated biochemical assay for haptoglobin: Prevention of interference from albumin. *Comparative Haematology International* 9:117–124.

Giffen, P. S. et al. 2003. Markers of experimental acute inflammation in the Wistar Han rat with particular reference to haptoglobin and C-reactive protein. *Archives of Toxicology* 77:392–402.

Harvey, J. W., and C. L. West. 1987. Prednisolone-induced increases of alpha-2-globulin and haptoglobin concentrations in dogs. *Veterinary Pathology* 24:90–92.

Katnik, I., M. Pupek, and T. Stefaniak. 1998. Cross reactivities among some mammalian haptoglobins studied by a monoclonal antibody. *Comparative Biochemistry and Physiology B* 119:335–340.

Lewis, E. J., J. Bishop, and C. H. Cashin. 1989. Automated quantification of rat plasma acute phase reactants in experimental inflammation. *Journal of Pharmacological Methods* 21:183–194.

Parra, M. D., V. Väisänen, and J. J. Cerón. 2005. Development of a time-resolved fluorometry based immunoassay for the determination of canine haptoglobin in various body fluids. *Veterinary Research* 36:117–129.

Solter, P. F., W. E. Hoffman, L. L. Hungerford, J. P. Siegel, S. H. St Denis, and J. L. Dorner. 1991. Haptoglobin and ceruloplasmin as determinant of inflammation in dogs. *American Journal of Veterinary Research* 52:1738–1742.

Walker, A. K., B. A. Ganney, and G. Brown. 1991. Haptoglobin measurements in a number of laboratory animal species. *Comparative Haematology International* 1:224–228.

Thiostatin

Cole, T., and G. Schreiber. 1989. Synthesis of thiostatins (major acute-phase alpha-1 proteins) in different strains of *Rattus norvigicus*. *Comparative Biochemistry and Physiology B* 93:813–818.

Fung, W-P., and G. Schreiber. 1987. Structure and expression of the genes for major acute α-1-protein and kininogen in the rat. *Journal of Biological Chemistry* 262:9298–9308.

Miller, I., P. Haynes, I. Eberini, M. Gemeiner, R. Aebersold, and E. Gianazza. 1999. Proteins of rat serum: III. Gender-related differences in protein concentration under baseline conditions and upon experimental inflammation as evaluated by two-dimensional electrophoresis. *Electrophoresis* 20:836–845.

Fibrinogen

Gardner, S. Y., J. R. Lehman, and D. L. Costa. 2000. Oil fly ash-induced elevation of plasma fibrinogen levels in rats. *Toxicological Sciences* 56:178–180.

Transforming Growth Factor-Beta (TGF-β)

Sasaki, H., R. B. Pollard, D. Schmitt, and F. Suzuki. 1992. Transforming growth factor-beta in the regulation of the immune system. *Clinical Immunology and Immunopathology* 65:1–9.

Varedi, M., M. G. Jeschke, E. W. Englander, D. N. Herdon, and R. E. Barrow. 2001. Serum TGF-β in thermally injured rats. *Shock* 16:380–382.

Wahl, S. M. 1992. Transforming growth factor beta (TGF-β) in inflammation: A cause and a cure. *Journal of Clinical Immunology* 12:61–74.

Procalcitonin

Nijsten, M. W. et al. 2000. Procalcitonin behaves as a fast responding acute phase protein in vivo and in vitro. *Critical Care Medicine* 28:458–461.

Rothenburger, M., A. Markewitz, T. Lenz, H. G. Kaulbach, K. Marohl, W. D. Kuhlmann, and C. Weinhold. 1999. Detection of acute phase response and infection. The role of procalcitonin and C-reactive protein. *Clinical Chemistry and Laboratory Medicine* 37:275–279.

Whicher, J., J. Bienvenu, and G. Monneret. 2001. Procalcitonin as an acute phase marker. *Annals of Clinical Biochemistry* 38:483–494.

Nutritional Effects

Jennings, G., and M. Elia. 1996. Changes in protein distribution in normal and protein-deficient rats during an acute-phase injury response. *British Journal of Nutrition* 76:123–132.

Lyoumi, S. et al. 1998. Induction and modulation of acute-phase response by protein malnutrition in rats: Comparative effects of systemic and localized inflammation on interleukin-6 and acute-phase synthesis. *Journal of Nutrition* 128:166–174.

Maejima, K., and S. Nagase. 1991. Effect of starvation and refeeding on the circadian rhythms of hematological and clinico-biochemical values and water intake of rats. *Experimental Animals* 40:389–393.

Pickering, R. G., and E. C. Pickering. 1984. The effects of reduced dietary intake on the body and organ weights, and some clinical chemistry and hematology of the young Wistar rat. *Toxicology Letters* 21:271–277.

Some Examples of Species and Strain Differences

Coe, J. E., and M. J. Ross. 1983. Hamster female protein. A divergent acute phase protein in male and female Syrian hamsters. *Journal of Experimental Medicine* 157:1421–1433.

House, E. L., B. Pansky, and M. S. Jacobs. 1961. Age changes in blood of golden hamster. *American Journal of Physiology* 200:1018–1022.

Olofsson, P., N. Nordquist, C. Vingsbo-Lundberg, A. Larsson, C. Falkenberg, U. Pettersson, B. Akerstrom, and R. Holmdahl. 2002. Genetic links between the acute phase response and arthritis development in rats. *Arthritis and Rheumatism* 46:259–268.

Reuter, A. M., F. Kennes, A. Leonard, and A. Sassen. 1968. Variations of the prealbumin in serum and urine of mice, according to strain and sex. *Comparative Biochemistry and Physiology* 25:921–928.

Strnad, M., C. Radojicic, D. Marinkovic, and Z. Magic. 2000. Variability of haptoglobin and alpha-2-macroglobulin in albino Oxford and dark Augustin inbred strains of rats before and after trauma. *Vojnosanitetski Pregled* 57:381–386.

Weimer, H. E., D. M. Roberts, P. Villanuevo, and H. G. Porter. 1972. Genetic differences in electrophoretic patterns during the phlogistic response in the albino rat. *Comparative Biochemistry and Physiology B* 43:965–973.

Immunoproteins and Immunotoxicology

Bankert, R. B., and P. K. Mazzaferro. 1999. Biochemistry of immunoglobulins. In *The clinical chemistry of laboratory animals,* 2nd ed., ed. W. F. Loeb and F. W. Quimby, pp. 231–266. Philadelphia: Taylor & Francis.

Burrell, R., D. K. Flaherty, and L. J. Sauers. 1992. *Toxicology of the immune system: A human approach.* New York: Van Nostrand Reinhold.

Descotes, G., and G. Mazue. 1987. Immunotoxicology. *Advances in Veterinary Science and Comparative Medicine* 31:95–119.

Luster, M. L. et al. 1988. Development of a testing battery to assess chemical-induced immunotoxicity: National Toxicology Program's guidelines for immunotoxicity evaluation in mice. *Fundamental and Applied Toxicology* 10:2–19.

Neoh, S. N., D. M. Jahoda, D. S. Rowe, and A. Voller. 1973. Immunoglobulin classes in mammalian species identified by cross reactivity with antisera to human immunoglobulins. *Immunochemistry* 10:805–813.

van Loveren, H., and J. G. Vos. 1989. Immunotoxicological considerations: A practical approach to immunotoxicity in the rat. In *Advances in applied toxicology,* ed. A. D. Dayan and A. J. Payne, pp. 143–163. London: Taylor & Francis.

Vos, J. G. 1980. Immunotoxicity assessment: Screening and function. *Archives of Toxicology* 4 (Suppl.): 95–108.

Complement

Barta, O. 1984. *Laboratory techniques of veterinary clinical immunology.* Springfield, IL: Charles C Thomas.

Gigli, I., and K. F. Austen. 1971. Phytogeny and function of the complement system. *Annual Review of Microbiology* 25:309–332.

Liszewski, M. K., T. C. Farries, D. M. Lubin, I. A. Rooney, and J. P. Atkinson. 1996. Control of the complement system. *Advances in Immunology* 16:201–283.

Quimby, F. W. 1999. Complement. In *The clinical chemistry of laboratory animals,* 2nd ed., ed. W. F. Loeb and F. W. Quimby, pp. 266–308. Boca Raton FL: Taylor & Francis.

Coagulation Proteins

Pritchard, D. H., M. G. Wright, S. Sulsh, and W. H. Butler. 1987. The assessment of chemically induced liver injury in rats. *Journal of Applied Toxicology* 7:229–236.

Theus, R., and G. Zbinden. 1984. Toxicological assessment of the hemostatic system, regulatory requirements, and industry practice. *Regulatory Toxicology and Pharmacology* 4:74–95.

Protein Binding with Xenobiotics

Colussi, D. M., C. Y. Parisot, and G. Y. Lefevre. 1998. Plasma protein binding of letrozole, a new nonsteroidal aromatase enzyme inhibitor. *Journal of Clinical Pharmacology* 38:727–735.

Hernandez, M. A., and A. Rathinavelu. 2006. *Basic pharmacology: Understanding drug actions and reactions.* Boca Raton, FL: CRC Press.

Kosa, T., T. Maruyama, and M. Otagiri. 1997. Species differences of serum albumins: I. Drug binding sites. *Pharmaceutical Research* 14:1607–1612.

Kratochwil, N. A., W. Huber, F. Muller, M. Kansy, and P. R. Gerber. 2004. Predicting plasma protein binding of drugs—Revisited. *Current Opinion in Drug Discovery and Development* 7:507–512.

Lindup, W. E., and M. C. Orme. 1981. Clinical pharmacology: Plasma protein binding of drugs. *British Medical Journal* 282:212–214.

Oracova, J., B. Bohs, and W. Lidner. 1996. Drug–protein binding studies. New trends in analytical and experimental methodology. *Journal of Chromatography B. Biomedical Applications* 677:1–28.

Pahlman, I., and P. Gozzi. 1999. Serum protein binding of tolterodine and its major metabolites. *Biopharmaceutics and Drug Disposition* 20:91–99.

Proost, J. H., J. M. K. H. Wierda, and D. K. F. Meijer. 1996. An extended pharmacokinetic/pharmacodynamic model describing quantitatively the influence of plasma protein binding, tissue binding and receptor binding on the potency and time course of action of drugs. *Journal of Pharmacokinetics and Biopharmaceutics* 24:45–77.

Son, D. S., M. Osabe, M. Shimoda, and E. Kokue. 1998. Contribution of alpha-1-acid glycoprotein to species difference in lincosamides-plasma protein binding kinetics. *Journal of Veterinary Pharmacology and Therapeutics* 21:34–40.

Wilkinson, G. R. 1983. Plasma and tissue binding considerations in drug disposition. *Drug Metabolism Reviews* 14:427–465.

Witiak, D. T., and M. W. Whitehouse. 1969. Species differences in the albumin binding of 2,4,6-trinitrobenzaldehyde, chlorophenoxy-acetic acids, 2-(4'-hydroxybenzeneazo) benzoic acid and some other acidic drugs—The unique behavior of plasma. *Biochemical Pharmacology* 18:971–977.

Urine Proteins (See Chapter 4)

Botham, J. W., J. C. McCall, E. L. Teasdale, and P. A. Botham. 1989. The relationship between exposure to rats and antibody production in man: IgG antibody levels to rat urinary protein. *Clinical and Experimental Allergy* 19:437–441.

Evans, G. O., and C. E. Parsons. 1986. Potential errors in the measurement of total protein in male rat urine using test strips. *Laboratory Animals* 20:27–31.

Finlayson, J. S., and C. A. Baumann. 1958. Mouse proteinuria. *American Journal of Physiology* 192:69–72.

Transudates and Exudates

Heffner, J. E., L. K. Brown, and C. A. Barbieri. 1997. Diagnostic value of tests that discriminate between exudative and transudative pleural effusions. *Chest* 111:970–980.

Light, R. W., M. I. Macgregor, P. C. Luchisinger, and W. C. Ball. 1972. Pleural effusions: The diagnostic separation of transudates and exudates. *Annals of Internal Medicine* 77:507–513.

Analysis of Proteins

Evans, G. O. 1994. Plasma albumin measurement in New Zealand white rabbits. *World Rabbit Science* 1:25–27.

Evans, G. O., and C. E. Parsons. 1988. A comparison of two dye binding methods for the determination of dog, rat and human plasma albumin. *Journal of Comparative Pathology* 98:453–460.

Fox, R. R. 1989. The rabbit. In *The clinical chemistry of laboratory animals,* ed. W. F. Loeb and F. W. Quimby, pp. 45–46. New York: Pergamon Press.

Gustafsson, J. E. C. 1976. Improved specificity of serum albumin and estimation of "acute phase reactants" by use of bromcresol green reaction. *Clinical Chemistry* 22:616–622.

Hall, R. E. 1992. Clinical pathology of laboratory animals. In *Animal models in toxicology,* ed. S. C. Gad and C. P. Chengelis. New York: Marcel Dekker.

Kimball, J. P., and P. M. Murray. 1994. Performance of bromcresol green (BCG) albumin reagents for laboratory animals on the Hitachi 717. *Clinical Chemistry* 40:990.

Metz, A., and A. Schutze. 1975. Vergleichende untersuchungen zur bestimmung von gesamt-protein und albumin im serum von mensch, affe, hund und ratte. *Zeitschrift für Klinische Chemie und Klinische Biochemie* 13:423–426.

Price, C. P., and D. J. Newman. 1997. Light scattering immunoassay. In *Principles and practice of immunoassay*, 2nd ed., ed. C. P. Price and D. J. Newman, pp. 443–480. London: Macmillan Reference Ltd.

Stokol T., J. M. Tarrant, and J. M. Scarlett. 2001. Overestimation of canine albumin with bromcresol green method in heparinized plasma samples. *Veterinary Clinical Pathology* 30:170–176.

Takano, S., H. Komiyama, and M. Nomura. 2001. A study of the correction of assay variation caused by the reagents in the measurement of rat albumin. *Japanese Journal of Clinical Chemistry* 30:164–167.

Tiffany, T. O. 1999. Fluorimetry, nephelometry and turbidimetry. In *Tietz textbook of clinical chemistry*, 3rd ed., ed. C. A. Burtis and E. R. Ashwood, pp. 94–112. Philadelphia: W. B. Saunders Company.

Whicher, J. T. et al. 1994. New international standard reference preparation for proteins in human serum (RPPHS). *Clinical Chemistry* 40:934–938.

Electrophoresis

Abate, O., R. Zanatta, T. Malisano, and U. Dotta. 2000. Canine serum proteins using high-resolution electrophoresis (HRE). *Veterinary Journal* 159:154–160.

Allchin, J. P., and G. O. Evans. 1986. Serum protein electrophoretic patterns of the marmoset, *Callithrix jacchus*. *Journal of Comparative Pathology* 96:349–352.

Deschamps, Y., and L. Huard. 2004. Evaluation of dog serum protein electrophoresis using the Sebia Hydrasys system. *Clinical Chemistry* 50:A37.

Scherer, R., M. Abd-El-Fattah, and G. Ruthenstroth-Bauer. 1977. Some applications of quantitative two-dimensional immunoelectrophoresis in the study of the systemic acute-phase reaction of the rat. In *Perspectives in inflammation, future trends and developments*, ed. D. A. Willoughby, J. P. Giroud, and G. P. Veto. Lancaster, England: MTP Press.

Watanabe, T. 1995. Analysis of a polyacrylamide gel electrophoretogram of beagle serum protein by laser densitometer. *Laboratory Animal Science* 45:295–298.

Immunoglobulin Assays

Brun, E., F. Lingaas, and H. J. Larsen. 1989. Turbidimetric measurement of immunoglobulin G in serum using an automatic centrifugal analyzer. *Research in Veterinary Science* 46:168–171.

Eckersall, P. D., J. G. Conner, and J. Harvie. 1991. An immunoturbidometric method for C-reactive protein. *Veterinary Research Communications* 15:17–24.

Eckersall, P. D., S. Duthie, M. J. M. Toussaint, E. Gruys, P. Heegaard, M. Alava, C. Lipperheide, and F. Madec. 1999. Standardization of diagnostic assays for animal acute phase proteins. *Advances in Veterinary Medicine* 41:643–655.

German, A. J., E. J. Hall, and M. J. Day. 1998. Measurement of IgG, IgM and IgA concentrations in canine serum, saliva, tears and bile. *Veterinary Immunology and Immunopathology* 64:107–121.

Ginel, P. J., J. M. Margarito, R. Lucena, and J. M. Molleda. 1997. Concentrations of plasma immunoglobulins in the dog as determined by laser nephelometry. Comparison with radial immunodiffusion and enzyme-linked immunosorbent assay. *European Journal of Clinical Biochemistry and Clinical Chemistry* 35:223–228.

Glickman, L. T., F. S. Shofer, A. J. Payton, L. L. Laster, and P. J. Felsburg. 1988. Survey of serum IgA, IgG and IgM concentrations in a large beagle population in which IgA deficiency had been identified. *American Journal of Veterinary Research* 49:1240–1245.

Hau, J., M. Nilsson, H. J. Skovgaard-Jensen, A. de Souza, E. Eriksen, and L. T. Wandall. 1990. Analysis of animal serum proteins using antisera against human analogous proteins. *Scandinavian Journal of Laboratory Animal Science* 17:3–7.

Hill, P. B., K. A. Moriello, and D. J. DeBoer. 1995. Concentrations of total serum IgE, IgA and IgG in atopic and parasitized dogs. *Veterinary Immunology and Immunopathology* 44:105–113.

Jones, R. D., D. Offutt, and B. A. Longmore. 2000. Capture ELISA and flow cytometry methods for the toxicologic assessment following immunization and cyclophosphamide challenges in beagles. *Toxicology Letters* 115:33–44.

Provost, J-P., K. Nahas, and B. Geffray. 2003. Normal values for blood immunoglobulins in the beagle dog. *Comparative Clinical Pathology* 12:17–20.

Salauze, D., V. Serre, and C. Perrin. 1994. Quantification of total IgM and IgG in rat sera by a sandwich ELISA technique. *Comparative Haematology International* 4:30–33.

Schreiber, M., D. Kantimm, D. Kirchhoff, G. Heimann, and A. S. Bhargava. 1992. Concentrations in serum IgG, IgM and IgA and their age-dependence in beagle dogs as determined by a newly developed enzyme-linked immunosorbent assay ELISA. *European Journal of Clinical Biochemistry and Clinical Chemistry* 30:775–778.

Ullman, E. F. 2001. Homogeneous immunoassays. In *The immunoassay handbook,* 2nd ed., ed. D. Wild, pp. 177–194. London: Nature Publishing Group.

Proteomics

Albala, J. S., and I. Humphery-Smith. 2003. *Protein arrays, biochips and proteomics: The next phase of genomic discovery.* Boca Raton, FL: CRC Press.

Albrethsen, J. 2007. Reproducibility in protein profiling by MALDI TOF mass spectrometry. *Clinical Chemistry* 53:852–858.

Amacher, D. E., R. Adler, A. Herath, and R. R. Townsend. 2005. Use of proteomic methods to identify serum biomarkers associated with rat liver toxicity or hypertrophy. *Clinical Chemistry* 51:1796–1803.

Anderson, N. L., and N. G. Anderson. 2002. The human plasma proteome: History, character and diagnostic prospects. *Molecular and Cellular Proteomics* 1:845–867.

Conn, P. M., ed. 2003. *Handbook of proteomic methods.* Towata, NJ: Humana Press.

Dare, T. O., H. A. Davies, J. A. Turton, L. Lomas, T. C. Williams, and M. J. York. 2002. Application of surface-enhanced laser desorption/ionization technology to the detection and identification of urinary parvalbumin-alpha: A biomarker of compound-induced skeletal muscle toxicity in the rat. *Electrophoresis* 23:3241–3251.

Duan, X., D. Yarmush, F. Berthiaume, A. Jayaraman, and M. L. Yarmush. 2005. Immunodepletion of albumin for two-dimensional gel detection of new mouse acute-phase protein and other plasma proteins. *Proteomics* 5:3991–4000.

Eppel, G. A., S. Nagy, M. Jenkins, R. N. Tudball, M. Daskalalis, D. H. Balzacs, and W. D. Comper. 2000. Variability of standard clinical protein assays in the analysis of a model urine solution of fragmented albumin. *Clinical Biochemistry* 33:487–494.

Greive, K. A., D. H. Balazs, and W. D. Comper. 2001. Protein fragments in urine have been considerably underestimated by various protein assays. *Clinical Chemistry* 47:1717–1719.

Hampel, D. J., C. Sansome, M. Sha, S. Brodsky, W. E. Lawson, and M. S. Goligorsky. 2001. Towards proteomics in uroscopy: Urine protein profiles after radiocontrast medium administration. *Journal of the American Society of Nephrology* 12:1026–1035.

Haynes, P., I. Miller, R. Aebersold, M. Gemeiner, I. Eberini, M. R. Lovati, C. Manzoni, M. Vignati, and E. Gianazza. 1998. Proteins of rat serum: I. Establishing a reference two-dimensional electrophoresis map by immunodetection and microbore high-performance liquid chromatography-electrospray mass spectrometry. *Electrophoresis* 19:1484–1492.

Hewitt, S. M., J. Dear, and R. A. Star. 2004. Discovery of protein biomarkers for renal disease. *Journal of the American Society of Nephrology* 15:1667–1689.

Higgins, M. A., B. R. Berridge, B. J. Mills, A. E. Schultze, H. Gao, G. H. Searfoss, T. K. Baker, and T. P. Ryan. 2003. Gene expression analysis of the acute phase response using a canine microarray. *Toxicological Sciences* 74:470–484.

Hortin, G. L., B. Meilinger, and S. K. Drake. 2004. Size-selective extraction of peptides from urine for mass-spectrophotometric analysis. *Clinical Chemistry* 50:1092–1095.

Hortin, G. L., S. A. Jortani, J. C. Ritchie, R. Valdes, and D. W. Chan. 2006. Proteomics: A new diagnostic frontier. *Clinical Chemistry* 52:1218–1222.

Luigi, S. et al. 2001. Acute phase proteins before cerebral ischemia in stroke-prone rats: Identification by proteomics. *Stroke* 32:753–760.

Lundblad, R. L. 2005. *The evolution from protein chemistry to proteomics: Basic science to clinical application.* Boca Raton, FL: CRC Press.

Palfrey, S. M., ed. 1999. *Methods in molecular medicine: Clinical applications of capillary electrophoresis.* Towata, NJ: Humana Press Inc.

Petricoin, E. F. et al. 2004. Toxicoproteomics: Serum proteomic pattern diagnostics for early detection of drug-induced cardiac toxicities and cardioprotection. *Toxicologic Pathology* 32 (Suppl. 1): 122–130.

Pognan, F. 2004. Genomics, proteomics and metabonomics in toxicology hopefully not "fashionomics." *Pharmacogenomics* 5:879–893.

Sironi, L. et al. 2001. Acute-phase protein before cerebral ischemia in stroke-prone rats. Identification by proteomics. *Stroke* 32:753–760.

Thongboonkerd, V., and J. B. Klein, eds. 2003. *Proteomics in nephrology. Contributions to nephrology.* Basel, Switzerland: S. Karger AG.

van den Heuvel, L. P., M. H. Farhoud, R. A. Wevers, B. G. M. Van Engelen, and J. A. M. Smeitink. 2003. Proteomic and neuromuscular diseases: Theoretical concept and first results. *Annals of Clinical Biochemistry* 40:9–16.

van Eyk, J., and M. J. Dunn. 2003. *Proteomic and genomic analysis of cardiovascular disease.* Weinheim, Germany: Wiley–VCH Verlag GmbH and Co.

Wijenen, P. A., and M. P. van Dieijen-Visser. 1996. Capillary electrophoresis of serum proteins. Reproducibility, comparison with agarose gel electrophoresis and a review of the literature. *European Journal of Clinical Biochemistry and Clinical Chemistry* 34:535–545.

9 Lipids

9.1 BIOCHEMISTRY AND PHYSIOLOGY

The collective term *lipids* is used to describe molecules that have diverse chemical and functional relationships; they all have poor solubility in water but are soluble in organic solvents. They can be broadly divided into sterols, including cholesterol, fatty acids, or molecules containing fatty acids—for example, triglycerides and phospholipids, the fat-soluble vitamins, eicosanoids, and sphingolipids. A more recent comprehensive classification of lipids proposes that they are divided into eight categories: fatty acyls, glycerolipids, glycerophospholipids, sphingolipids, sterol lipids, prenol lipids, saccharolipids, and polyketides, based on the hydrophobic and hydrophilic properties of the lipids (Fahy et al. 2005). This classification should prove useful as the analytical approaches using liquid chromatography and mass spectrometry provide more information on lipids and their interactions in the field of lipidomics (Wenk 2005).

Cholesterol is the major sterol in the body and occurs mainly as the nonesterified free form, which is a fundamental component of cell membranes and the precursor for steroid hormones and bile acids. Cholesteryl esters present in the tissues and plasma are mainly formed by cholesterol esterification with long chain fatty acids; these cholesterol esters act as a storage pool. Most of the requirements for cholesterol are met by endogenous synthesis, mainly in the liver, with the exogenous supplementation from the diet.

Fatty acids have a basic structure, R-COOH, and the important fatty acids have long chains with an even number of carbon atoms (C12–C20), which may be described as saturated (e.g., stearic acid, C18:1), monounsaturated (e.g., oleic acid, C18:2), and polysaturated (e.g., linoleic, C18:2, and linolenic, C18:3, acids). These long chain fatty acids are used to provide energy by beta-oxidation, which shortens the fatty acid by two carbon atoms with the production of acetyl CoA (known as the fatty acid spiral).

Triacylglycerols (or triglycerides) serve mainly as a source of cellular metabolic energy, accumulating in adipose tissue from which triglycerides are mobilized and transported in response to energy demands of the body. Dietary triglycerides are hydrolyzed by pancreatic lipases to fatty acids and monoacylglycerols, which are later re-esterified. Endogenous triglyceride metabolism occurs mainly in the liver and adipose tissue.

Phospholipids have a glycerol backbone where one hydroxyl group is linked by a phosphodiester bond to an alcohol; the other two hydroxyl groups are esterified with fatty acids. These phospholipids are a structural component of cell membranes with both a hydrophobic fatty acid domain and the hydrophilic domain of the phosphate group.

Apolipoproteins are structural components of plasma lipoproteins, and they maintain the integrity of the lipoproteins through the interactions with the hydrophilic core and the surrounding aqueous environments. These apolipoproteins act as ligands for specific cell receptors and activators or inhibitors for enzymes involved in lipoprotein metabolism. There are at least 11 apolipoproteins, which differ in molecular mass (from 6.5 to 600 kDa) and amino-acid composition, and they form less than 2 g/L of "normal" plasma protein. The apolipoprotein classes are designated by letters of the alphabet—A, B, C, D, and E—and numerals for subclasses (e.g., apo C-II).

The lipoproteins are macromolecules with varying complexes of lipids where the hydrophobic lipid portions—cholesterol esters and triglycerides—are localized at the core of the molecules. The amphipathic surface layers surrounding the core contain the apolipoproteins and phospholipids. The lipoproteins vary in size, density, lipid composition, and apolipoprotein constituents, and they can be classified by size, the flotation rate determined by ultracentrifugation, or their electrophoretic mobilities. Put simply, the density of a lipoprotein particle is determined by the relative amounts of lipid and protein contained in the particle. Chylomicrons and very low density lipoproteins have the highest lipid content and the lowest protein content; thus, very excessive amounts of chylomicrons float on the surface of plasma. In descending order of size, the broad lipoprotein fractions (with their electrophoretic mobility) are

chylomicrons (do not migrate);
VLDL—very low density lipoproteins (pre-beta-lipoproteins);
IDL—intermediate density lipoproteins (slow pre-beta-lipoproteins);
LDL—low density lipoproteins (beta-lipoproteins); and
HDL—high density lipoproteins (alpha-1-lipoproteins).

These broad lipoprotein classes are heterogeneous, with particle fractions of differing size, density, and function; the subclasses are denoted by subscript numbers (e.g., HDL_2).

The apolipoproteins are broadly associated with lipoprotein fractions, and some of these associations include:

apo A-I: HDL and activator of lecithin cholesterol acyltransferase;
apo A-II: HDL;
apo A-IV: HDL and chylomicrons;
apo B-48: chylomicrons, remnants;
apo B-100: LDL, IDL, and VLDL: ligand for LDL receptor;
apo C-I: chylomicrons, VLDL, IDL, HDL: activator for lecithin cholesterol acyltransferase;
apo C-II: chylomicrons, VLDL, IDL, HDL: activator for lipoprotein lipase;
apo C-III: chylomicrons, VLDL, IDL, HDL: inhibitor of lipoprotein binding receptor; inhibitor of lipoprotein lipase;
apo D: VLDL, IDL, LDL, HDL;
apo E: VLDL, IDL, HDL, remnants: ligand for LDL, interacts with LDL and apo E receptors; and
apo (a): bridges with apo B-100 Lp(a).

Several enzymes are involved in lipid metabolism, including:

cholesterol ester transfer protein (CETP), which enables the transfer of cholesteryl esters from the HDL core to VLDL and chylomicron remnants;
further metabolism by VLDL allows the return of cholesteryl esters to the
liver via LDL (Tall 1993; Barter and Rye 1994);

lecithin-cholesterol acyltransferase (LCAT), which catalyses the esterification
of free cholesterol and the conversion of phospholipid to lysolecithin on
HDL particle surfaces, and these cholesteryl esters move into the core of
the particle, which then enables the HDL particles to acquire more free
cholesterol from other lipoproteins and cell membranes; this enzyme is synthesized by the liver (Hitz, Steinmetz, and Siest 1983);

hepatic triglyceride lipase, which acts on the endothelial surfaces of the hepatic
sinusoids and removes triglycerides and phospholipids from lipoproteins,
particularly from HDL (Zambon et al. 2003); and

lipoprotein lipase, which partially hydrolyzes triglyceride-rich lipoproteins
to monoglyceride and fatty acids in peripheral cells; the monoglyceride is
hydrolyzed to glycerol and fatty acid, and the fatty acids are taken into
tissues for storage by esterification or to meet energy requirements. This
extracellular enzyme is attached to capillary endothelial cells by proteogly-
cans (Wu, Olivecrona, and Olivecrona 2003).

Lipoprotein metabolism is shown in a simplified overview in Figure 9.1. For reviews
of lipid metabolism, see Levy 1981; Watson and Barrie 1993; Kreuzer and von
Hodenberg 1994; Bauer 1996; Rifai, Warnick, and Dominiczak 2000; and Moffatt
and Stamford 2005.

In an exogenous pathway, dietary cholesterol and triglycerides are absorbed by
the gut enterocytes in the form of free cholesterol, fatty acids, and monoacylglycerols. Subsequently, the cholesteryl esters and triglycerides are incorporated into the
triglyceride-rich chylomicrons and these processes involve several of the apolipoproteins. The chylomicrons pass into the intestinal lymph system and then into the vascular circulation via the thoracic duct. Lipoprotein lipase (LPL) enables the transfer
of fatty acids and triglycerides to the cells. Chylomicron "remnants" are transported
to hepatic receptor sites.

In the endogenous pathways, the liver synthesizes VLDL, IDL, and LDL, and the
LDL, which are then transported to nonhepatic tissues to undergo further metabolism. The HDL may be released directly from the liver as "nascent HDL" or may be
formed from HDL precursors and the chylomicrons in the small intestine or hepatic
VLDL fractions. Although the liver is the main site of uptake for chylomicrons, the
perisinusoidal bone marrow macrophages also account for a significant proportion
of the total uptake of chylomicrons in several species (Ross 1986; Hussain et al.
1989). A reverse transport mechanism involves the esterification of free cholesterol
catalyzed by LCAT. These esters are then incorporated into HDL before transferring
to LDL in exchange for triglyceride; this second step is catalyzed by CETP.

Thus, two lipoprotein fractions—VLDL from the liver and chylomicrons from the
intestinal tract—transport lipids to the peripheral tissues. As lipid is removed from these

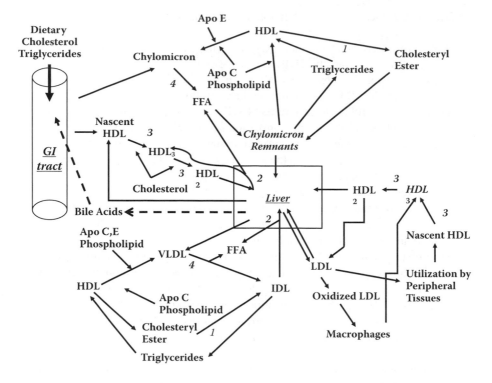

FIGURE 9.1 Simplified overview of lipid and lipoprotein metabolism with some key enzymes numbered: (1) cholesteryl ester transfer protein (CETP), (2) hepatic triglyceride lipase, (3) lecithin cholesterol acyl transferase (LCAT), and (4) lipoprotein lipase.

fractions, the density of each fraction increases: VLDL changes to IDL and then LDL and chylomicrons become chylomicron remnants. HDL is primarily involved in returning lipid to the liver in the reverse cholesterol transport process and, as the HDL cholesterol increases, the density of the particle decreases (Fielding and Fielding 1995).

9.1.1 Species Differences

There are marked differences between the species and strains for plasma cholesterol, triglycerides, and lipoproteins, and some of the lipoprotein metabolizing enzymes (Alexander and Day 1973; Chapman 1980; van Lenten and Roheim 1982; Aubert et al. 1988; Lehmann et al. 1993; Watson and Barrie 1993; Kulikov and Chirkin 2004; Fernandez and Volek 2006). The magnitude for plasma cholesterol and triglycerides varies across the species (Table 9.1). Differences also are observed in the rates of absorption, synthesis, and metabolism of lipids (Beynon 1988).

Some of these differences are reflected by the plasma lipoprotein patterns; for example, the major plasma lipoprotein fractions in mice, rats, hamsters, rabbits, and dogs are the HDL fractions, whereas in guinea pigs and Old World monkeys the LDL fraction is the dominant fraction (Alexander and Day 1973; Terpstra et al. 1981; Barrie, Nash, and Watson 1993; Terpstra and Beynen 1984; Hollanders et al. 1986;

TABLE 9.1

Relative Plasma Levels for Common Laboratory Animals in Descending Order of Magnitude

Total Cholesterol	Triglycerides
Monkey	Mouse
Dog	Rabbit
Hamster	Monkey
Mouse	Hamster
Rabbit	Rat
Rat	Dog
Guinea pig	Guinea pig

Barrie et al. 1993; Lehmann et al. 1993; Maldonado et al. 2001). Structural differences of the apolipoproteins are also found, but there are close similarities between some species; for example, several of the apolipoproteins in the common marmoset and man are similar (Crook et al. 1990). The apolipoprotein-E structure of the rat is similar to that of humans, but the plasma levels are 5 to 10 times higher (Leininger-Muller and Siest 1996).

Although most laboratory animals have LCAT activity, CETP is much lower in several species, including mouse, rat, and dog; guinea pigs have slightly higher activity and rabbits have higher activity. Higher levels of cholesteryl esters and apolipoprotein E in HDL particles are often associated with the low CETP levels. With little or low CETP levels, the HDL particles become enriched with cholesterol ester and apo E and develop into larger and less dense particles.

Fatty acid–binding proteins (FABPs) are a family of hydrophobic molecule transporters and play a pivotal role in cellular fatty acid transport in the cytosol and at the plasma membrane. At least nine FABPs have been identified and named after the tissues with which they were initially associated (Glatz and van der Vusse 1996; Glatz and Storch 2001; Zimmerman and Veerkamp 2002). Heart FABP (H-FABP) is found in cytoplasm of myocytes and these bind long chain fatty acids. These proteins may be markers of myocardial ischemia, but other FABPs are present in several other tissues. Liver FABP (L-FABP) occurs mainly in hepatocytes and also in smaller amounts in the kidney and small intestine (Bass et al. 1989).

9.1.2 Animal Models of Hyperlipidemia

The association between atherosclerosis in humans and plasma lipoproteins has led to the development and use of several animal models to help our understanding of familial hypercholesterolemias and atherosclerosis; however, the species differences in lipoproteins and their metabolism must be considered when developing models of atherosclerosis and novel therapeutic agents. Dietary manipulations in animals with dominant LDL-C fractions are perhaps more appropriate models for these studies than in animals where HDL is the dominant fraction (Cayen, Givner, and Kraml

1972; Beynon 1988; Gouache et al. 1991; Overturf and Loose-Mitchell 1992; Kris-Etherton and Dietschy 1997). Large amounts of data on the effects of dietary manipulations in several laboratory animal species have been published; examples include rats (Tabacchi and Kirksey 1973; Mahley and Holcombe 1977; van Zutphen and den Bieman 1981), hamsters (Weingand and Daggy 1991), gerbils (Temmerman et al. 1989), and marmosets (McIntosh et al. 1984). When atherosclerosis has been deliberately induced in laboratory animals, the testing of potential hypolipidemic agents may yield different responses from those obtained in healthy animals (Zimetbaum, Frishman, and Kahn 1991).

Several hyperlipidemic animal models have been extensively studied; these models include the Yoshida and Zucker rats and the heritable hyperlipidemic Watanabe rabbits (WHHL: Watanabe 1980; Havel et al. 1982; Lind et al. 1990; Mortensen and Frandsen 1997). More recently, a transgenic mouse has been developed that overexpresses human proteins or underexpresses murine proteins required for cholesterol metabolism. These animal models are not generally used for toxicology studies.

9.2   XENOBIOTICS' EFFECTS ON LIPID METABOLISM

Sometimes relatively small changes of plasma cholesterol (and triglycerides) occur in studies, but the reasons for these changes are not always identifiable. However, from our knowledge of lipid metabolism, the possible reasons for toxicological effects can include nutritional, intestinal, hepatic, hormonal, cardiac, and renal factors. Reduced food and energy intake resulting from toxicity will cause the body to release energy from the adipose and muscle tissues to compensate for these deficiencies, and these changes may be reflected by the plasma triglyceride and cholesterol levels. These effects on serum cholesterol and triglyceride concentrations are easier to detect in young rats than in older animals, which exhibit much more variability in these measurements.

Hepatotoxicity may cause perturbations of lipoprotein metabolism in several ways. In acute hepatic injury, the levels of hepatic enzymes may be reduced (e.g., triglyceride lipase), thus elevating plasma triglycerides with a concomitant decrease in cholesterol. The liver plays a major role in the maintenance of cholesterol levels, and biliary lipid secretion is an important part of these processes (Mazer and Carey 1984; Dietschy, Turley, and Spady 1993). Prolonged cholestasis will result in bile not reaching the duodenum, with consequential malabsorption of fat and fat-soluble vitamins (Hollander 1981). As the plasma bile acids increase during cholestasis, plasma cholesterol also tends to rise. Impaired hepatic protein metabolism will also affect lipoprotein synthesis, resulting in hypolipoproteinemia and hypotriglyceridemia.

"Fatty liver" is a description for the abnormal accumulation of fat (mainly triglycerides) in the hepatic parenchymal cells; this occurs with several xenobiotics, but fat accumulation does not always equate to liver damage. In the liver, smaller Ito (or fat-storing or stellate) cells differentiate into myofibroblastic cells and form collagen. Several mechanisms can be implicated in the development of fatty liver (Henderson 1963; Lombardi 1966; Shift, Roheim, and Eder 1971). These mechanisms include:

The release and utilization of hepatic triglycerides are blocked, although the
   hepatic synthesis of triglycerides is normal.
The rate of hepatic synthesis of triglycerides is increased, but utilization
   is impaired.
Hepatic synthesis is increased together with impaired utilization.
Additional cellular hepatic synthesis of triglycerides occurs other than in the
   endoplasmic reticulum.

If the synthesis of lipoprotein is reduced, then lipoprotein transport and utilization
are reduced.

Peroxisome proliferators can cause hypocholesterolemia in rodents (Reddy and
Lalwani 1987; Graham et al. 1996; Reddy and Chu 1994; Reddy and Hashimoto
2001). Induction of hepatic peroxisomal proliferation associated with hypolipidemia
occurs in some other species such as rhesus monkeys (Lalwani et al. 1985).

Acute phase responses are also associated with lipid changes, with the cytokine
mediators of inflammation causing disturbances in circulating and hepatic lipid
metabolism. This can lead to hypocholesterolemia (Cabana, Gerwurz, and Siegel
1983; Cabana, Siegel, and Sabesin 1989; Hardardottir et al. 1994; Cabana et al. 1996;
Feingold, Hardardottir, and Grunfeld 1998). Additionally, as part of the acute phase,
the resulting hypoalbuminemia can affect the transport of fatty acid proteins.

Several other conditions affect plasma lipids. In hypothyroidism, plasma cholesterol and triglyceride levels increase; however, the plasma cholesterol falls in hyperthyroidism with the associated increase of basal metabolic rate. These changes linked
to the thyroid may be driven by initial hepatic toxicity. Changes in plasma cholesterol
may occur secondarily to hormonal changes (e.g., during pregnancy, in diabetes mellitus, and in alterations of corticosteroid metabolism). Alternatively, gross changes
in lipid metabolism may affect hormonal patterns, particularly when cholesterol is
used for hormone synthesis (i.e., steroid hormones). With the current interest in anti-
obesity compounds, numerous studies have been conducted on the roles of leptin,
ghrelin, adiponectin, and resistin and their effects on lipid metabolism, as well as
investigation of agents capable of modulating their effects (Gil-Campos, Carlete, and
Gil 2004; Meier and Gressner 2004).

In cases when gastrointestinal or pancreatic toxicity is present, plasma lipids will
be affected. The nephrotic syndrome is characterized by hyperlipidemia, hypoproteinemia, and hyperproteinuria in several species, and lipid changes may also be
observed with chronic renal damage (Moestrup and Nielsen 2005).

When natural antioxidant defenses are overloaded by oxidative processes or
defenses are lowered, oxidative stress results. The oxidative damage caused by peroxidation with reactive oxygen species acts on both unsaturated fatty acids and cholesterol. Reactive oxygen species (ROS) target important biological molecules, which
include lipids; these subsequent reactions also can involve proteins, protein-bound
metal cations, radicals, and DNA. Some severe consequences result in cellular dysfunction, apoptosis, and necrosis with possible DNA damage (Horton and Fairhurst
1987; Moslen and Smith 1992; Eberhardt 2000; Berdeaux et al. 2005; Molgulkoc et
al. 2005; Roberts, Fessel, and Davies 2005; Tong et al. 2005).

9.2.1 Phospholipidosis

The term *phospholipidosis* describes an excessive accumulation of intracellular lipids that may be induced by the action of xenobiotics on the synthesis and metabolism of phospholipids; the accumulation of phospholipids in lysosomes becomes multilamellar in appearance (Halliwell 1997; Reasor and Kacew 2001; Nonoyama and Fukuda 2008). There is strong association between cationic amphiphilic xenobiotics (cationic amphiphilic drugs, CADs) and phospholipidosis. The excessive accumulation of phospholipids may occur in lung, liver, brain, kidneys, eyes, and many other tissues; the patterns of accumulating phospholipids differ between species and tissues. The CADs may bind directly to phospholipids and then accumulate, or CADs may inhibit some phospholipases, and this enzyme inhibition then leads to the accumulation of phospholipids. Most investigators have focused on blood leukocytes to demonstrate the development of phospholipidosis in the blood using electron microscopy or dyes such as Nile red (Xia et al. 1997; Halstead et al. 2006), although measurement of urinary docosahexenoyl (C22:6)-bis(monoacylglycerol) phosphate using liquid chromatography/mass spectrometry as a marker has been reported (Tengstrand Baronas et al. 2006).

9.2.2 Vehicles

Some vehicles used for the administration of test compounds or to maintain nutritional states in intravenous pharmacological studies may alter plasma lipids. Intralipid™ is a source of essential fatty acids—linoleic and linolenic acids—used for intravenous nutrition; in addition, it can be used to test methods for interference from lipemia. When it was given to rats, it increased plasma cholesterol, HDL, and LDL (Hajri, Ferezou, and Lutton 1990; Wasan, Grossie, and Lopez-Berestein 1994). Another vehicle, beta-cyclodextrin, also affects plasma lipids and can cause hypolipidemia (Trautwein et al. 1999).

9.3 LABORATORY INVESTIGATIONS

In toxicology studies, the lipids commonly assayed in plasma are total cholesterol (TC or CHOL) and triglycerides (triacylglycerides: TG), although triglycerides are not included in some regulatory documents. Plasma phospholipids, nonesterified fatty acids (NEFAs), and total lipids are measured less frequently. Measurements of lipids in urine are rare, although they have been utilized when renal papillary necrosis has been induced (Bach et al. 1991). Age-related changes have been reported in rats for cholesterol and lipoproteins (Carlson, Froberg, and Nye 1968; Uchida et al. 1978; van Lenten and Roheim 1982) and for triglycerides in the mouse (Wolford et al. 1986; Levine 1995). Standardization for assays of animal lipids, lipoproteins, and apolipoproteins remains a challenge due to the lack of available reference materials.

9.3.1 BLOOD SAMPLES

Although heparinized plasma (or serum) lipoproteins are relatively stable, some investigators use sequestrenated (EDTA) samples because they chelate heavy metals that promote the auto-oxidation of unsaturated fatty acids and cholesterol; EDTA inhibits phospholipase-C activity due to bacterial contamination. Given the effects of diet on plasma lipids (where determining effects on lipid metabolism are a primary objective of a study), blood samples should be collected after a period of fasting appropriate for the species, and lipoprotein measurements should be performed promptly with fresh samples to avoid problems due to lipoproteins denaturing during storage.

Recording the simple observation of a creamy layer or dispersed opalescence in the plasma indicating hyperchylomicronemia (associated with high triglyceride levels) can be important. This lipid layering may increase when plasma samples are stored overnight at 4°C, and lipemic samples should be thoroughly mixed prior to analysis. Lipemia can interfere with several routine photometric analyses and enhance the effects of interference due to hemolysis (Brady and O'Leary 1994; Sampson, Ruddel, and Elin 1994). Some reagents contain solubilizers, which act on the lipid micelles and reduce interference effects due to lipemia.

9.3.2 TOTAL AND FREE CHOLESTEROL

Enzymatic methods are commonly used for this measurement, and many of the current methods use a cholesterol esterase to hydrolyze lipoprotein–cholesteryl esters, followed by further reactions where cholesterol oxidase is linked to a peroxidase–chromogen system (Richmond 1992). Free cholesterol can be measured by omitting cholesterol esterase of the first reaction step, although many reagent formulations prevent this elimination of the esterase.

Some of the cholesterol esterases used in these analytical systems show varying degrees of specificity toward the different cholesterol esters, and problems have occurred when these reagents are used for several species. For example, in rats, where there is a fivefold-higher concentration of cholesteryl arachidonate ester compared to human plasma, plasma cholesterol may be underestimated with some reagents (Demacker et al. 1983; Noel, Dupras, and Fillion 1983; Wiebe and Bernert 1984; Evans 1986).

9.3.3 TRIGLYCERIDES (TRIACYLGLYCEROLS)

These can be measured with one of several enzymatic reagents (Klotzsch and McNamara 1990). Lipases are used to hydrolyze the triglycerides; the released glycerol is then linked by the actions of glycerol kinase and glycerol-3-phosphate oxidase to a peroxidase–chromogen system. Again, the effectiveness of some of the enzyme reagents appears to differ with the various species (e.g., underestimation of triglycerides in porcine sera using the lipase–glycerol method; Tuten, Robinson, and Sgoutas 1993). Many methods measure the plasma free glycerol together with triglycerides; ideally, a free glycerol blank should be carried out without glycerol kinase and/or with lipase containing reagents. Corrections for free glycerol are not commonly performed, although free glycerol may be sometimes increased (e.g., in diabetes) and result in falsely high triglyceride values. The contribution of free glycerol to total triglyceride values varies from species to species (Weingand and Hudson 1989).

9.3.4 PLASMA NONESTERIFIED FATTY ACIDS (NEFAS)

The terms *NEFA, unesterified fatty acids,* and *free fatty acids* have been used synonymously in the literature, although these fatty acids are mainly bound to plasma proteins. Enzymatic assays are convenient with NEFA in the presence of added acyl-coenzyme A (CoA) synthetase forming acyl CoA esters, which are then oxidized by acyl CoA oxidase to yield hydrogen peroxide. The hydrogen peroxide produced is measured by a peroxidase-linked colorimetric detection reaction. Plasma samples should be separated promptly and stored frozen to prevent in vitro lipolysis (Zambon, Hashimoto, and Brunzell 1993).

9.3.5 PHOSPHOLIPIDS

Again, there are several methods for measuring individual phospholipids; enzymatic assays for total phospholipids provide a convenient starting point. Because most plasma phospholipids contain choline, the enzyme phospholipase-D is used to release choline from phospholipids. The choline is then oxidized by added choline oxidase to yield betaine and hydrogen peroxide, which are then measured using a peroxidase-linked colorimetric detection method. In cases of phospholipidosis, it is essential to use cells (e.g., leukocytes) to demonstrate the accumulation of phospholipids.

9.3.6 LIPOPROTEINS AND APOLIPOPROTEINS

These are not commonly measured in toxicology studies but may be required to provide supporting data. Ultracentrifugation remains the reference method for studying lipoproteins (Hollanders et al. 1986), but few toxicology laboratories have direct access to this technology. Methods for lipoprotein testing have been reviewed by Rifai et al. (2000). Alternative techniques include affinity chromatography, fast protein liquid chromatography, and high-performance liquid chromatography. Apolipoproteins have been measured by immunoelectrophoretic and nephelometric assays in several species (Chirtel et al. 1989); these methods depend on the availability of suitable antisera and their cross-reactivity with the antigens.

Lipoprotein electrophoresis provides a relatively simple method to study gross changes of the major lipoproteins; various support media, buffers systems, and electrophoretic equipment and detection reagents have been employed (Groulade et al. 1981; Oppermann, Hubner, and Ehlers 1983). Electrophoresis may also be used to check the suitability of some methods for HDL and LDL. The Friedewald formula is used to determine LDL-cholesterol with human samples by measuring plasma cholesterol, triglycerides, and HDL-cholesterol (Friedewald, Levy, and Fredrickson

1972). This formula cannot be used to determine LDL-cholesterol for laboratory animals, where the proportions of the lipoprotein fractions are markedly different.

Direct methods for LDL-C have evolved from a first generation, which required the initial precipitation of LDL particles by various agents including dextran sulfate, polyvinylsulfate, and heparin; after separation of the precipitated LDL, the LDL-C was calculated by measuring the cholesterol in the supernatant and subtracting this value from the total cholesterol. Alternative later methods employed heparin-coated magnetic beads for the separation of LDL, and the next generation of assays uses various homogeneous methods to avoid the necessity of the separation steps (Rifai et al. 1992, 2000; Nauck, Warnick, and Rifai 2002; Ensign, Hill, and Howerd 2006).

For HDL-C measurements, similar developments have taken place with direct homogeneous assays, which eliminate the need for precipitation and separation steps (Okazaki et al. 1997; Reed 1997; Warnick, Nauck, and Rifai 2001). The differing proportions of lipoproteins (and their cholesterol content) in the plasmas of the various laboratory species mean that the suitability of these homogeneous and precipitation methods must be checked if meaningful results are to be obtained, particularly when lipoprotein antibodies are used (Warnick and Albers 1978; Hoffmann et al. 1985; Sjoblom and Eklund 1989; Tschantz and Sunahara 1993; Escola-Gil et al. 1999; Ensign et al. 2006).

9.3.7 KETONES

The liver is the main origin of ketones in laboratory animals, where the long chain fatty acids are released from plasma albumin and bound to fatty acid–binding proteins in the hepatocytes. The long chain fatty acids react with CoA and then can be used to synthesize triacylglycerol or undergo beta-oxidation to acetyl CoA. When the levels of plasma fatty acids are elevated, acetyl CoA can be metabolized to form acetoacetate and 3-hydroxybutyrate or enter the tricarboxylic acid cycle. In ketosis, the levels of acetone, acetoacetate, and 3-hydroxybutyrate (also known as beta-hydroxybutyrate) are increased in both plasma and urine; these three compounds historically were collectively called ketone bodies. Urine test strips can be used to test for ketonuria, and there are several enzymatic assays for 3-hydroxybutyrate and acetoacetate.

9.3.8 MEASUREMENTS FOR OXIDATIVE STRESS AND LIPID PEROXIDATION

These measurements include the F2 isoprostanes—the oxidation products of arachidonic acid—and methods require mass spectrometry or immunoassay. Other measures of lipid peroxidation include hydroperoxides by luminometry or colorimetric assays, or a third colorimetric measurement of aldehyde products (TBAR) with thiobarbituric acid where malondialdehyde is measured; malondialdehyde is an end-product derived from the breakdown of polyunsaturated fatty acids and esters.

Other measures for monitoring oxidative stress include superoxide dismutase, glutathione peroxidase, catalase, glutathione, glutathione disulphide, and glutathione reductase. The oxidation of LDL has been implicated in the development of cardiovascular diseases and diabetes. Oxidized LDL can be measured using enzyme-linked immunoassays or chemiluminescence, but this assay works better in species where LDL is the dominant lipoprotein. A number of measures of monitoring oxidative stress are emerging, including superoxide dismutase, glutathione peroxidase, catalase, glutathione reductase, myeloperoxidase, and total peroxidases. Impaired fatty acid metabolism can also be studied by more elegant techniques, such as nuclear magnetic resonance spectroscopy or mass spectrometry, although this is not common practice (Mortishire-Smith et al. 2004).

REFERENCES

Alexander, C., and C. E. Day. 1973. Distribution of serum lipoproteins of selected vertebrates. *Comparative Biochemistry and Physiology B* 46:295–312.

Aubert, R., D. Perdereau, M. Roubiscoul, J. Herzog, and D. Lemmonier. 1988. Genetic variations in serum lipid levels of inbred mice and response to hypercholesterolemic diet. *Lipids* 23:48–54.

Bach, P. H., D. J. Scholey, L. Delacruz, M. Moret, and S. Nichol. 1991. Renal and urinary lipid changes associated with an acutely induced renal papillary necrosis in rats. *Food Chemistry and Toxicology* 29:211–219.

Barrie, J., A. S. Nash, and T. D. G. Watson. 1993. Quantitative analysis of canine plasma lipoproteins. *Journal of Small Animal Practice* 34:226–231.

Barrie, J., T. G. Watson, M. J. Stear, and A. S. Nash. 1993. Plasma cholesterol and lipoprotein concentrations in the dog: The effects of age, gender and endocrine disease. *Journal of Small Animal Practice* 34:507–512.

Barter, P., and K-A. Rye. 1994. Cholesteryl ester transfer protein: Its role in plasma lipid transport. *Clinical and Experimental Pharmacology and Physiology* 21:663–672.

Bass, N. M., M. E. Barker, J. A. Manning, A. L. Jones, and R. K. Ockner. 1989. Acinar heterogeneity of fatty acid-binding proteins in the livers of male, female and clofibrate treated rats. *Hepatology* 9:12–21.

Bauer, J. 1996. Comparative lipid and lipoprotein metabolism. *Veterinary Clinical Pathology* 25:49–56.

Berdeaux, O., O. Scruel, T. Durand, and J. L. Cracowski. 2005. Isoprostanes, biomarkers of lipid peroxidation in humans. Part 2: Quantification methods. *Pathologie Biologie (Paris)* 53:356–363.

Beynen, A. C. 1988. Animal models in cholesterol metabolism studies. In *New developments in biosciences: Their implications for laboratory animal welfare,* ed. A. C. Beynen and H. A. Solleveld, pp. 279–288. Dordrecht, the Netherlands: Kluwer Academic Publishers.

Brady, J., and N. O'Leary. 1994. Interference due to lipemia in routine photometric analysis—Survey of an underrated problem. *Annals of Clinical Biochemistry* 31:281–288.

Cabana, V. G., H. Gerwurz, and J. N. Siegel. 1983. Inflammation-induced changes in rabbit CRP and plasma lipoproteins. *Journal of Immunology* 130:1736–1742.

Cabana, V. G., J. R. Lukens, K. S. Rice, T. J. Hawkins, and G. S. Getz. 1996. HDL content and composition in acute phase response in three species: Triglyceride enrichment in HDL, a factor in its decrease. *Journal of Lipid Research* 27:2662–2674.

Cabana, V. G., J. N. Siegel, and S. M. Sabesin. 1989. Effects of acute phase response on the concentration and density distribution of plasma lipids and apolipoproteins. *Journal of Lipid Research* 30:39–49.

Carlson, L. A., S. O. Froberg, and E. R. Nye. 1968. Effect of age on blood and tissue lipids in the male rat. *Gerontologia* 14:65–79.

Cayen, M. N., M. L. Givner, and M. Kraml. 1972. Effect of diurnal rhythm and food with-drawal on serum lipids in the rat. *Experientia* 28:502–503.

Chapman, M. J. 1980. Animal lipoproteins: Chemistry, structure and comparative aspects. *Journal of Lipid Research* 21:789–848.

Chirtel, S. J., P. J. Coutlakis, L. L. Chambers, and M. R. Lakshman. 1989. A novel use of end-point nephelometry to standardize the rate nephelometric assay of human and rat plasma apoprotein A. *Journal of Laboratory and Clinical Medicine* 113:632–641.

Crook, D., K. H. Weisgraber, S. C. Rall, and R. W. Mahley. 1990. Isolation and characteriza-tion of several plasma apolipoproteins of common marmoset monkey. *Arteriosclerosis* 10:625–632.

Demacker, P. N., G. J. Boerma, H. Baadenenhuijsen, R. van Strik, B. Leijnse, and A. P. Jansen. 1983. Evaluation of accuracy of 20 different test kits for the enzyme determination of cholesterol. *Clinical Chemistry* 29:1916–1922.

Dietschy, J. M., S. D. Turley, and D. K. Spady. 1993. Role of liver in the maintenance of cho-lesterol and low density lipoprotein homeostasis in different animal species. *Journal of Lipid Research* 34:1637–1659.

Eberhardt, M. K. 2000. *Reactive oxygen metabolites: Chemistry and medical consequences.* Boca Raton, FL: CRC Press Inc.

Ensign, W., N. Hill, and C. B. Howerd. 2006. Disparate LDL phenotypic classification among four different methods for assessing LDL particle characteristics. *Clinical Chemistry* 52:1722–1727.

Escolà-Gil, J. C., O. Jorba, J. Julve-Gil, F. González-Sastre, J. Ordónez-Llanos, and F. Blanco-Vaca. 1999. Pitfalls of direct HDL-cholesterol measurements in mouse models of hyper-lipidemia and atherosclerosis. *Clinical Chemistry* 45:1567–1569.

Evans, G. O. 1986. The use of three esterase kits to measure plasma cholesterol concentrations in the rat and three other species. *Journal of Comparative Pathology* 96:551–556.

Fahy, E. et al. 2005. A comprehensive classification system for lipids. *Journal of Lipid Research* 46:839–861.

Feingold, K. R., I. Hardardottir, and C. Grunfeld. 1998. Beneficial effects of cytokine induced hyperlipidemia. *Zeitschrift für Ernahrungswiss* 37 (Suppl. l): 66–74.

Fernandez, M. L., and J. S. Volek. 2006. Guinea pigs: A suitable animal model to study lipopro-tein metabolism, atherosclerosis and inflammation. *Nutrition and Metabolism* 3:17–23.

Fielding, C. J., and P. E. Fielding. 1995. Molecular physiology of reverse cholesterol transport. *Journal of Lipid Research* 36:211–228.

Friedewald, W. T., R. J. Levy, and D. S. Fredrickson. 1972. Estimation of the concentration of low-density lipoprotein cholesterol in plasma without the use of the preparative ultra-centrifuge. *Clinical Chemistry* 18:499–509.

Gil-Campos, M., R. Carlete, and A. Gil. 2004. Hormones regulating lipid metabolism and plasma lipids in childhood obesity. *International Journal of Obesity* 28:S75–80.

Glatz, J. F., and G. J. van der Vusse. 1996. Cellular fatty acid binding proteins: Their function and physiological significance. *Review of Progress in Lipid Research* 3:243–282.

Glatz, J. F. C., and J. Storch. 2001. Unraveling the significance of cellular fatty acid-binding proteins. *Current Opinions in Lipidology* 12:267–274.

Gouache, P., B. Le Moullac, F. Bleiberg-Daniel, R. Aubert, and C. Flament. 1991. Changes in rat plasma apolipoproteins and lipoproteins during moderate protein deficiency: Potential use in the assessment of nutritional status. *Journal of Nutrition* 121:653–662.

Graham, M. J., M. A. Winham, S. L. Old, and T. J. B. Gray. 1996. Comparative hypolipidemic and peroxisomal effects of ciprofibrate, clofibric acid, and their respective difluorocy-clopropyl and 4-fluoro-substituted analogues in rat. *Xenobiotica* 26:695–707.

Groulade, P., P. Groslambert, T. Foulon, and J. Groulade. 1981. Electrophorese des lipo-proteines seriques de l'homme et du chien adultes normaux. *Bulletin de l'Academie Nationale de Medecine* 165:1243–1250.

Hajri, T., J. Férézou, and C. Lutton. 1990. Effects of intravenous infusions of commercial fat emulsions (Intralipid 10 or 20%) on rat plasma lipoproteins: Phospholipids in excess are the main precursors of lipoprotein-X-like particles. *Biochimica et Biophysica Acta* 1047:121–130.

Halliwell, W. H. 1997. Cationic amphiphilic drug-induced phospholipidosis. *Toxicologic Pathology* 25:53–60.

Halstead, B. W., C. M. Zwicki, R. E. Morgan, D. K. Monteith, C. E. Thomas, R. K. Bowers, and B. R. Berridge. 2006. A clinical flow cytometric biomarker strategy: Validation of peripheral leukocyte phospholipidosis using Nile red. *Journal of Applied Toxicology* 26:169–177.

Hardardottir, I., A. H. Moser, R. R. Memom, C. Grunfeld, and K. R. Feingold. 1994. Effects of TNF, IL-1 and the combination of both cytokines on cholesterol metabolism in Syrian hamsters. *Lymphokine and Cytokine Research* 13:161–166.

Havel, R. J., T. Kita, L. Kotite, J. P. Kane, R. L. Hamilton, J. L. Goldstein, and M. S. Brown. 1982. Concentration and composition in blood plasma of the WHHL rabbit. An animal model of human familial hypercholesterolemia. *Arteriosclerosis* 2:467–474.

Henderson, J. F. 1963. Studies on fatty liver induction by 4-aminopyrazolopyrimidine. *Journal of Lipid Research* 34:68–74.

Hitz, J., J. Steinmetz, and G. Siest. 1983. Plasma lecithin:cholesterol acyltransferase—Reference values and effects of xenobiotics. *Clinica Chimica Acta* 133:85–96.

Hoffmann, G. E., R. Hiefinger, L. Weiss, and W. Poppe. 1985. Five methods for measuring low-density lipoprotein cholesterol concentration in serum compared. *Clinical Chemistry* 31:1729–1730.

Hollander, D. 1981. Intestinal absorption of vitamins A, E, D, and K. *Journal of Laboratory and Clinical Medicine* 97:449–462.

Hollanders, B., A. Mougin, F. N'Diaye, E. Hentz, X. Aude, and A. Girard. 1986. Comparison of the lipoprotein profiles obtained from rat, bovine, horse, dog, rabbit and pig serum by a new two-step ultracentrifugal gradient procedure. *Comparative Biochemistry and Physiology B* 84:83–89.

Horton, A. A., and S. Fairhurst. 1987. Lipid peroxidation and mechanisms of toxicity. CRC *Critical Reviews in Toxicology* 18:27–79.

Hussain, M. M., R. W. Mahley, J. R. Boyles, P. A. Lindquist, W. J. Brecht, and T. L. Innerarity. 1989. Chylomicron metabolism. Chylomicron uptake by bone marrow in different animal species. *Journal of Biological Chemistry* 264:17931–17938.

Klotzsch, S. G., and J. R. McNamara. 1990. Triglyceride measurements; a review of methods and interferences. *Clinical Chemistry* 36:1605–1613.

Kreuzer, J., and E. von Hodenberg. 1994. The role of apolipoproteins in lipid metabolism and atherogenesis: Aspects in man and mice. *Journal of Hypertension* 12:113–118.

Kris-Etherton, P. M., and J. Dietschy. 1997. Design criteria for studies examining individual fatty acid effects on cardiovascular disease risk factors; human and animal studies. *American Journal of Clinical Nutrition* 65 (Suppl. 5): 1590S–1596S.

Kulikov, V. A., and A. A. Chirkin. 2004. Specificity of the lipoproteins metabolism in rats. *Patologicheskaia Fiziologiia I Eksperimentalnaia Terapiia* 1:26–27.

Lalwani, N. D., M. K. Reddy, S. Ghosh, S. D. Barnard, J. A. Molello, and J. K. Reddy. 1985. Induction of fatty acid β-oxidation and peroxisome proliferation in the liver of rhesus monkeys by DL-040, a new hypolipidemic agent. *Biochemical Pharmacology* 34:3473–3482.

Lehmann, R., A. S. Bhargava, and P. Gunzel. 1993. Serum lipoprotein patterns in rats, dogs and monkeys including method comparison and influence of menstrual monkeys. *European Journal of Clinical Chemistry and Clinical Biochemistry* 31:633–637.

Leininger-Muller, B., and G. Siest. 1996. The rat, a useful model for pharmacological studies on apoliporotein E. *Life Sciences* 58:455–467.

Levine, B. S. 1995. Animal clinical pathology. In *CRC handbook of toxicology,* ed. M. J. Derelanko and M. A. Hollinger, pp. 517–537. Boca Raton, FL: CRC Press.

Levy, R. 1981. Cholesterol, lipoproteins, apoproteins, and heart disease. *Clinical Chemistry* 27:653–662.

Lind, B. M., R. Littbarski, G. Hohlbach, and K. O. Moller. 1990. Long-term investigations of serum cholesterol, serum triglyceride and HDL cholesterol in heritable hyperlipidemic rabbits. *Zeitschrift für Versuchstierkunde* 33:245–249.

Lombardi, B. 1966. Fatty liver. Considerations on the pathogenesis of fatty liver. *Laboratory Investigations* 15:1–20.

Mahley, R. W., and K. S. Holcombe. 1977. Alterations of the plasma lipoproteins and apoproteins following cholesterol feeding in rats. *Journal of Lipid Research* 18:314–324.

Maldonado, E. N., J. R. Romero, B. Ochoa, and M. I. Aveldano. 2001. Lipid and fatty acid composition of canine lipoproteins. *Comparative Biochemistry and Physiology B* 128:719–729.

Mazer, N. A., and M. C. Carey. 1984. Mathematical model of biliary lipid secretion: A quantitative analysis of physiological and biochemical data from man and other species. *Journal of Lipid Research* 25:932–953.

McIntosh, G. H., F. H. Bulman, R. J. Illman, and D. L. Topping. 1984. The influence of age, dietary cholesterol and vitamin C deficiency on plasma cholesterol concentration in the marmoset. *Nutrition Reports International* 29:673–682.

Meier, U., and A. M. Gressner. 2004. Endocrine regulation of energy metabolism: Review of pathobiochemical and clinical aspects of leptin, ghrelin, adiponectin, and resistin. *Clinical Chemistry* 50:1511–1525.

Moestrup, S. K., and L. B. Nielsen. 2005. The role of the kidney in lipid metabolism. *Current Opinions in Lipidology* 16:301–306.

Moffatt, R. J., and B. Stamford. 2005. *Lipid metabolism and health.* Boca Raton, FL: CRC Press.

Molgulkoc, R., A. K. Baltaca, E. Oztekin, A. Ozturk, and A. P. Sivrikaya. 2005. Short-term thyroxine administration leads to lipid peroxidation in renal and testicular tissues of rats with hypothyroidism. *Acta Biologica Hungarica* 56:225–232.

Mortensen, A., and H. Frandsen H. 1997. Blood lipids in young and adult Watanabe heritable hyperlipidemic (WHHL) and adult normolipidemic rabbits. *Scandinavian Journal of Laboratory Animal Science* 24:47–53.

Mortishire-Smith, R. J., G. L. Skiles, J. W. Lawrence, S. Spence, A. W. Nicholls, B. A. Johnson, and J. K. Nicholson. 2004. Use of metabonomics to identify impaired fatty acid metabolism as the mechanism of drug-induced toxicity. *Chemical Research in Toxicology* 17:165–173.

Moslen, M. T., and C. V. Smith. 1992. *Free radical mechanisms of tissue injury.* Boca Raton, FL: CRC Press.

Nauck, M., G. R. Warnick, and N. Rifai. 2002. Methods for measurement of LDL-cholesterol: A critical assessment of direct measurement by homogeneous assays versus calculation. *Clinical Chemistry* 48:2236–2254.

Noel, A-P., R. Dupras, and A-M. Fillion. 1983. The activity of cholesteryl ester hydrolysis in the enzymatic determination of cholesterol: Comparison of five enzymes obtained commercially. *Clinical Chemistry* 129:464–471.

Nonoyama, T., and R. Fukuda. 2008. Drug-induced phospholipidosis—Pathological aspects and its prediction. *Journal of Toxicology and Pathology* 21:9–24.

Okazaki, M., K. Sasamoto, T. Muramatsu, and S. Hosaki. 1997. Evaluation of precipitation and direct methods for HDL-cholesterol assay by HPLC. *Clinical Chemistry* 43:1885–1890.

Oppermann, P., G. Hubner, and D. Ehlers. 1983. Zur trennung der lipoproteine des rattenserums mit hilfe der dikelektrophorese. *Zeitschrift für Medizinische Laboratoriums Diagnostik* 24:200–203.

Overturf, M. L., and D. S. Loose-Mitchell. 1992. In vivo model systems: The choice of experimental animal model for the analysis of lipoproteins and atherosclerosis. *Current Opinions in Lipidology* 3:179–185.

Reasor, M. J., and S. Kacew. 2001. Drug-induced phospholipidosis: Are there functional consequences? *Experimental Biology and Medicine* 226:825–830.

Reed, R. G. 1997. In search of the ideal measure of high-density lipoprotein. *Clinical Chemistry* 43:1809–1810.

Reddy, J. K., and R. Chu. 1994. Peroxisome proliferator-induced pleiotropic responses: Pursuit of a phenomenon. *Annals of the New York Academy of Sciences* 804:176–201.

Reddy, J. K., and T. Hashimoto. 2001. Peroxisomal beta-oxidation and peroxisome proliferator-activated receptor alpha: An adaptive metabolic system. *Annual Review of Nutrition* 21:193–230.

Reddy, J. K., and N. D. Lalwani. 1987. Carcinogenesis by hepatic peroxisome proliferators: Evaluation of the risk of hypolipidemic drugs and industrial plasticizers to humans. *CRC Critical Reviews in Toxicology* 12:1–58.

Richmond, W. 1992. Analytical reviews in clinical biochemistry: The quantitative analysis sof cholesterol. *Annals of Clinical Biochemistry* 29:577–597.

Rifai, N., G. R. Warnick, and M. K. Dominiczak, eds. 2000. *Handbook of lipoprotein testing,* 2nd ed. Washington, D.C.: AACC Press.

Rifai, N., G. R. Warnick, J. R. McNamara, J. D. Belcher, G. F. Grinstead, and I. D. Frantz. 1992. Measurement of low-density-lipoprotein cholesterol in serum: A status report. *Clinical Chemistry* 38:150–160.

Roberts, L. J., J. P. Fessel, and S. S. Davies. 2005. The biochemistry of the isoprostane, neuroprostane, and isofuran pathways of lipid peroxidation. *Brain Pathology* 15: 143–148.

Ross, R. 1986. The pathogenesis of atherosclerosis. *New England Journal of Medicine* 314:488–500.

Sampson, M., M. Ruddel, and R. J. Elin. 1994. Effects of specimen turbidity and glycerol concentration on nine enzymatic methods for triglyceride determination. *Clinical Chemistry* 40:221–226.

Shiff, T. S., P. S. Roheim, and H. A. Eder. 1971. Effects of high sucrose diets and 4-aminopyrazolopyrimidine on serum lipids and lipoproteins in the rat. *Journal of Lipid Research* 12:596–603.

Sjoblom, L., and A. Eklund. 1989. Determination of HDL-cholesterol by precipitation with dextran sulfate and magnesium chloride: Establishing optimal conditions for rat plasma. *Lipids* 24:532–534.

Tabacchi, M. H., and A. Kirsey. 1973. Influence of dietary lipids on plasma and hepatic lipids and on blood clotting properties in rats fed oral contraceptives. *Journal of Nutrition* 103:1270–1278.

Tall, A. R. 1993. Plasma cholesteryl ester transfer protein. *Journal of Lipid Research* 34:1255–1274.

Temmerman, A. M., R. J. Vonk, K. Niezen-Koning, R. Berger, and J. Fernandes. 1989. Effects of dietary cholesterol in the Mongolian gerbil and the rat; a comparative study. *Laboratory Animals* 23:30–35.

Tengstrand Baronas, E., J-W. Lee, C. Alden, and F. Y. Hsieh. 2006. Biomarkers to monitor drug-induced phospholipidosis. *Toxicology and Applied Pharmacology* 216:72–76.

Terpstra, A. H., and A. C. Beynen. 1984. Density profile and cholesterol concentration of serum lipoproteins in experimental animals and human subjects on hypercholesterolemic diets. *Comparative Biochemistry and Physiology B* 77:523–528.

Tong, V., X. W. Tong, T. K. Chang, and F. S. Abbott. 2005. Valproic acid. I. Time course of lipid peroxidation markers, liver toxicity and valproic acid metabolites in rats. *Toxicological Science* 86:427–435.

Trautwein, E. X., K. Forgbert, D. Reickhoff, and H. F. Erbesdobler. 1999. Impact of β-cyclodextrin and resistant starch on bile acid metabolism and fecal steroid excretion in regard to their hypolipidemic action in hamsters. *Biochimica et Biophysica Acta* 1437:1–12.

Tschantz, J-C., and G. I. Sunahara. 1993. Microaffinity chromatographic separation and characterization of lipoprotein fractions in rat and Mongolian gerbil serum. *Clinical Chemistry* 39:1861–1867.

Tuten, T., K. A. Robinson, and D. S. Sgoutas. 1993. Discordant results for triglycerides in pig sera. *Clinical Chemistry* 39:125–128.

Uchida, K., Y. Nomura, M. Kadowaki, H. Takase, K. Takano, and N. Takeuchi. 1978. Age related changes in cholesterol and bile acid metabolism in rats. *Journal of Lipid Research* 19:544–551.

van Lenten, B. J., and P. S. Roheim. 1982. Changes in the concentrations and distributions of apolipoproteins of the aging rat. *Journal of Lipid Research* 23:1187–1195.

van Zutphen, L. P. M., and M. G. C. W. den Bieman. 1981. Cholesterol response in inbred strains of rats, *Rattus norvegicus*. *Journal of Nutrition* 111:1833–1838.

Warnick, G. R., and J. J. Albers. 1978. A comprehensive evaluation of the heparin-manganese precipitation procedure for estimating high density lipoprotein cholesterol. *Journal of Lipid Research* 19:65–76.

Warnick, G. R., M. Nauck, and N. Rifai. 2001. Evolution of methods for measurement of HDL-cholesterol: From ultracentrifugation to homogenous assays. *Clinical Chemistry* 47:1579–1596.

Wasan, K. M., V. B. Grossie, and G. Lopez-Berestein. 1994. Effects of intralipid infusion on rat serum proteins. *Laboratory Animals* 28:138–142.

Watanabe, Y. 1980. Serial inbreeding of rabbits with hereditary hyperlipidemia (WHHL-rabbit). *Atherosclerosis* 36:261–268.

Watson, T. D. G., and J. Barrie. 1993. Lipoprotein metabolism and hyperlipidemia in the dog and cat: A review. *Journal of Small Animal Practice* 34:479–487.

Weingand, K. W., and B. P. Daggy. 1991. Effects of dietary cholesterol and fasting on hamster plasma lipoprotein lipids. *European Journal of Clinical Chemistry and Clinical Biochemistry* 29:425–428.

Weingand, K. W., and C. L. Hudson. 1989. Accurate measurement of total plasma triglyceride concentrations in laboratory animals. *Laboratory Animal Science* 39:453–454.

Wenk, M. R. 2005. The emerging field of lipidomics. *Nature Reviews Drug Discovery* 4:594–610.

Wiebe, D. A., and J. T. Bernert. 1984. Influence of incomplete cholesteryl ester hydrolysis on enzymic measurements of cholesterol. *Clinical Chemistry* 30:352–356.

Wolford, S. T., R. A. Schroer, F. X. Gohs, P. P. Gallo, M. Brodeck, H. B. Falk, and R. Ruhren. 1986. Reference range data base for serum chemistry and hematology values in laboratory animals. *Journal of Toxicology and Environmental Health* 8:161–188.

Wu, G., G. Olivecrona, and T. Olivecrona. 2003. The distribution of lipoprotein lipase in rat adipose tissue. *Journal of Biological Chemistry* 278:11925–11930.

Xia, Z., E-L. Appelkvist, J. W. Depierre, and L. Nassberger. 1997. Tricyclic antidepressant-induced lipidosis in human monocytes in vitro as well as monocyte derived cell line, as monitored by spectrofluorimetry and flow cytometry after staining with Nile red. *Biochemical Pharmacology* 53:1521–1532.

Zambon, A., S. Bertocco, N. Vitturi, V. Polentarutti, D. Viancello, and G. Crepaldi. 2003. Relevance of hepatic lipase to the metabolism of triacylglycerol-rich lipoproteins. *Biochemical Society Transactions* 31:1070–1074.

Zambon, A., S. I. Hashimoto, and J. D. Brunzell. 1993. Analysis of techniques to obtain plasma for measurement of levels of free fatty acids. *Journal of Lipid Research* 34:1021–1028.

Zimetbaum, P., W. H. Frishman, and S. Kahn. 1991. Effects of Gemfibrozil and other fibric
    acid derivatives on blood lipids and lipoproteins. *Journal of Clinical Pharmacology*
    31:25–37.
Zimmerman, A. W., and J. H. Veerkamp. 2002. New insights into the structure and function of
    fatty acid-binding proteins. *Cellular and Molecular Life Science* 59:1096–1116.

10 Assessment of Endocrine Toxicity

Section 10.1: General Endocrinology

10.1.1 INTRODUCTION

The endocrine system plays an important role in regulating major physiological functions, including growth and development, reproduction, some metabolic processes, and reactions to external stimuli (e.g., behavior such as fight and flight responses). The system is a complex network of glands, hormones, and receptors and it is interlinked with the nervous system, which provides rapid electrical signals to organs and tissues; the endocrine system is slower and based on chemical messengers (i.e., hormones). The endocrine glands secrete hormones into the blood or other extracellular fluids; these are then distributed to target organ receptors. While the endocrine glands secrete their hormones into the bloodstream, exocrine hormones are secreted through ducts and transported to the target organ or into the gastrointestinal tract. Hormones produced by effector cells, which then act on receptors in adjacent cells, are described as having paracrine effects; for hormones produced and acting on the same cell, the effects are described as autocrine.

The hormones circulate around the body and modulate cellular and organ function by binding to receptor proteins within the target cells or on the cell surfaces; the binding process then triggers complex signal transduction pathways or the altered regulation of genes with a resultant action on the cellular metabolism. Peptide hormone receptors often are transmembrane proteins that function via intracellular messengers such as cyclic AMP, inositol 1.4.5. triphosphate (IP3), and calcium. Sometimes these receptors are described as G-protein receptors or sensory receptors (Zhou et al. 1994; Ekena et al. 1996; Woodman 1997; Harris, Katzenellenbogen, and Katzenellenbogen 2002; Gurnell and Chatterjee 2004; Millar et al. 2004; Sandler et al. 2004; Cheng 2005; Gudermann, Nurwakagari, and Ben-Menahem 2005; Shank and Pascal 2005). The cellular responses depend on the receptor and cell type and the effects of other hormones to which that cell may also be exposed; some hormones may stimulate the activity of one cell type but suppress that of a different cell type. Certain cells specifically producing hormones in the adenohypophysis are termed corticotrophs (ACTH), gonadotrophs (FSH and LH), thyrotrophs (TSH), somatotrophs (GH) and lactotrophs (prolactin).

Hormones may be polypeptides of variable lengths (e.g., short peptides such as vasopressin) or of longer lengths forming proteins (e.g., growth hormone, insulin). Other hormones are steroids (e.g., estrogens and androgens), eicosanoids derived from amino acids (e.g., the iodothyronines), or biogenic amines (e.g., epinephrine, norepinephrine).

The half lives of hormones differ with some having very short half lives of less than a few minutes e.g. ACTH, epinephrine and nor-epinephrine, with other hormones e.g., erythropoietin having half lives of about 2-3 h in the mouse and 8-10h in the dog. (see Woodman,1997 and Reimers,1999 for detailed descriptions of animal hormone structures and properties). The binding of circulating T3 and T4 to plasma proteins differs, and for the hormones that are bound to plasma proteins, any factors affecting protein synthesis and the ratio of free:total hormone levels must be considered when interpreting data.

Hormones are found in several tissues and organs including:

adipose tissue: leptin, adiponectin, resistin;
adrenal medulla: epinephrine, norepinephrine;
adrenal cortex: aldosterone, corticosterone, cortisol;
bone: osteocalcin;
duodenum: gastric inhibitory peptide, cholescytokinin, secretin, motilin;
ileum: enteroglucagon;
gonads: testes; testosterone, inhibin;
ovary: estradiol, progesterone, activin, relaxin;
heart: brain natriuretic peptide (BNP), atrial natriuretic peptide;
kidney: erythropoietin, renin, calcitriol, prostaglandins;
liver: insulin-like growth factor;
pancreas: glucagon, insulin, somatostatin (GH);
parathyroids: calcitonin;
pineal gland: melatonin;
placenta: estrogen, progesterone , placental lactogen;
posterior pituitary: oxytocin;
stomach: gastrin, ghrelin; and
thymus: thymosin, thymopoietin.

The hypothalamic releasing hormones act on the production and release of the trophic hormones by the pituitary, and these trophic hormones then act on the other endocrine glands such as the thyroids, adrenals, gonads and pancreas. Hormones of interest are listed in Tables 10.1.1. and 10.1.2. There are some minor spelling differences to be found in the terminology used (e.g., estrogen—oestrogen, gonadotropin —gonadotrophin).

One of the most obvious hormonal species differences is for glucocorticoids, where corticosterone is the major corticoid in rats and mice—unlike in dogs, where cortisol is the major glucocorticoid. The peak plasma concentrations also differ, with canine cortisol values occurring in the morning and rat corticosterone occurring during the night. The small molecular weight proteins T3, T4, and cortisol are structurally identical across the species, but other hormones (e.g., TSH glycoproteins)

TABLE 10.1.1
Trophic and Releasing Hormones and Their Abbreviations

Hypothalamus

Arginine vasopressin precursor

Corticotrophin (corticotrophic) releasing hormone (CRH)

Follicle-stimulating hormone releasing hormone (FRH)

Gonadotrophin releasing hormone (GnRH)

Luteinizing-hormone releasing hormone (LRH)

Somatotrophin releasing hormone, somatocrinin (SRH or GRH)

Somatotrophin release inhibitory factor (STH, SRIF, or GIH)

Thyrotrophin (thyrotrophic) releasing hormone (TRH)

Prolactin inhibitory hormone (PIH or factor PIH)

Prolactin releasing hormone (PRH)

Adenohypophysis (anterior pituitary)

Arginine vasopressin (AVP)

Adrenocorticotrophic hormone (ACTH or corticotrophin)

Folliotrophin or follicle stimulating hormone (FSH)

Luteotrophin or luteinizing hormone (LH)

Somatotrophin or growth hormone (GH)

Thyrotrophin or thyroid stimulating hormone (TSH)

Prolactin (PRL)

TABLE 10.1.2
Some Primary Hormones of Interest and Their Actions

Endocrine Gland	Hormones	Target Organ	Main Actions
Hypothalamus	Releasing or inhibiting hormones CRH, FRH, GnRH, LRH, SRH, STH, TRH, PIH, PRH	Anterior pituitary	Control of the production and release of other hormones
Adenohypophysis	AVP	Kidney	Retention of water Vasoconstrictor
	ACTH	Adrenal cortex	Synthesis of corticosteroids
	FSH	Gonads	Control of ovarian and estrus cycle Promotes testicular Sertoli cells to produce androgen binding protein
	LH	Gonads	Control of ovarian and estrus cycle Control of testicular Leydig cells to produce testosterone

204 | Animal Clinical Chemistry

TABLE 10.1.2 (CONTINUED)
Some Primary Hormones of Interest and Their Actions

Gland	Hormones	Target	Main Actions
	GH	Many tissues	Stimulates growth and cell reproduction. Controls release of hepatic insulin-like growth factor
	TSH	Thyroids	Controls production of iodothyronines
	PRL	Mammary glands	Promotes milk production
Adenohypophysis			
Thyroid	Tri-iodothyronine T3 Thyroxine, T4	Many tissues	Control of metabolic rate Influences development and reproduction
Adrenal cortex	Glucocorticoids (e.g., corticosterone and cortisol) Mineralcorticoids (e.g., aldosterone)	Many tissues	Affects inflammation and protein synthesis Electrolyte balance
Adrenal medulla	Epinephrine (adrenaline)	Many tissues	Glycogenolysis Lipid mobilization Smooth muscle contraction Cardiac function, vasodilation
	Norepinephrine (noradrenaline)		Vasoconstriction, arteriole contraction
Pancreas	Insulin	Liver, adipose tissue, muscle, and many other tissues	Increases glucose utilization Prevents excessive glycogenolysis in liver and muscle
	Glucagon	Liver, adipose tissue, muscle, and many other tissues	Acts on carbohydrate, fat, and protein metabolism to prevent hypoglycemia
Gonads	Sex steroids (e.g., testosterone, progesterone, estradiol)	Gonads and accessory sex organs	Reproductive function and sexual development

vary in structure across the species. Rats, mice, and hamsters have two different insulins—I and II—and these react poorly with some human insulin antibodies compared to dog and rabbit insulins. Guinea pig insulin shows poor cross-reactivity in immunoassays for human and rodent insulins.

There are a number of feedback mechanisms in the endocrine system whereby low circulating hormone concentrations will trigger additional hormone production and secretion, if the circulating hormone concentration is too high then the rates of production and secretion are reduced under normal physiological conditions. Figure 10.1.1. illustrates the general feedback pathways among the hypothalamus,

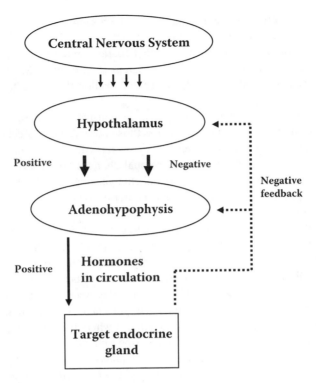

FIGURE 10.1.1   Linkages between the adenohypophysis and endocrine glands.

adenohypohysis and endocrine glands. This interplay between regulating and coun-
ter-regulating feedback loops makes it difficult to monitor molecular endocrine
changes when they occur.

10.1.2   TOXIC EFFECTS

Effects of xenobiotics on endocrine organs may become apparent as toxicity or
functional impairment. Adverse effects on the endocrine organs are often due to
exaggerated responses that can be predicted from knowledge of the pharmacological
action of the compound that has been administered at therapeutic dosages or above.
Compounds such as oral contraceptives, which are similar to endogenous hormones,
may mimic a hormone's physiological effects, or structurally similar compounds
may block the receptor sites.

Endocrine toxins can be broadly categorized as those that exert a direct effect
on the hormone-receptor mechanism or those that act via an indirect action. These
include (Thomas 1994, 1995, 1998; Harvey 1996; Atterwill and Cockburn 1997;
Capen 1997; Thomas and Colby 1997; Harvey, Rush, and Cockburn 1999; Rosol et
al. 2001; Houck and Kavlock 2008). These include:

inhibition of the enzymes involved in the biosynthesis of the hormone;
interference in the uptake of the hormone by the target organ;

interference with the release mechanism for the hormone;
alteration of capacity of carrier proteins;
alteration of hormone catabolism (e.g., via hepatic or renal pathways); and
interaction with a secondary messenger system (e.g., cyclic AMP); several of
    these are exemplified in thyroid toxicity (see Section 10.2).

Some endocrine organs appear to be more responsive or vulnerable to xenobiotics; this may result in rapid responses such as those observed for catecholamines and glucocorticoids. The majority of adverse toxic effects caused by xenobiotics require longer periods of exposure before the hormonal changes are observed (e.g., effects on the pituitary gland or following hormonal changes related to hepatic microsomal enzyme induction). Endocrine changes may be hypo- or hyperfunctional due to suppression or following stimulation.

The susceptibility of the endocrine tissues to compound-induced lesions has been shown to be ranked in the following decreasing order of frequency: adrenal, testes, thyroid, ovary, pancreas, pituitary, and parathyroid (Ribelin 1984; Woodman 1988; Thomas and Colby 1997); about 90% of all toxic effects on the endocrine system involve the adrenals, gonads, and thyroid glands. Enhanced hormone secretion appears to promote tumor formation in some cases, and it is important to separate these effects from other possible toxic effects in long-term rat studies where there is a higher spontaneous incidence of usually benign multiple endocrine tumors compared to other species. Some xenobiotics may affect several endocrine glands—for example, by altering both gonadal and thyroid hormones via the pituitary gland or changes of iodothyronines in response to glucocorticoids and the effects of iodothyronines on insulin secretion.

Toxic effects on the endocrine glands may be classified as primary, secondary, or indirect, where primary toxicity occurs when xenobiotics act directly on the endocrine gland. In secondary endocrine toxicity, toxic effects on other organs alter the hormonal imbalance and cause changes within the endocrine gland (e.g., hepatic enzyme induction alters the circulating levels of iodothyronines, causing the thyroid glands to respond with changes in this tissue and hormone synthesis). With stress responses caused by general toxic effects, endocrine changes may occur (e.g., with the adrenals), and this may be described as indirect toxicity. Some effects on the endocrine organs may be associated with other biochemical changes, such as perturbations of electrolyte balance or carbohydrate metabolism, and assessment of nutritional status is important when interpreting results of hormones such as insulin, parathyroid hormone, and calcitonin. Nutritional status can have marked effects via plasma proteins on hormones, which are bound to various protein fractions in the circulation. Xenobiotics also can displace some of the relatively weakly albumin-bound hormones.

Age is an important factor in the assessment of toxic effects on endocrine organs. The developing endocrine system in immature animals appears to be generally more susceptible to toxic compounds than in mature animals—particularly the pituitary–gonadal axis. For some studies, it may be preferable to use male rather than female animals, thus avoiding the several metabolic effects of the estrus cycle.

An endocrine disrupter is an exogenous xenobiotic or mixture absorbed into the body that disturbs the endocrine system by altering normal hormone levels, halting or stimulating the production of hormones, or changing the way hormones travel through the body, thus affecting hormonal control mechanisms (Kohrle 2008). The term *endocrine disrupting chemicals* (EDCs) is used to describe test chemicals, although the terms *endocrine-active compounds* (EACs) and *endocrine mimic* also are used to describe these compounds in which adverse effects and risks are uncertain. The hormonal actions of these chemicals are many times weaker than the hormones present naturally in the body. These xenobiotics work through several different mechanisms, which include:

an agonistic effect where the xenobiotic mimics the biological activity of a hormone by binding to a cellular receptor, which initiates the normal cellular response to the naturally occurring hormone at the wrong time or to an excessive extent;

an antagonistic response where the xenobiotic may bind to the receptor and prevents binding of the natural hormone and normal activation of the receptor;

binding to transport proteins in the blood, thus altering the circulating levels of natural hormones; and

altering metabolic processes and affecting the synthesis or catabolism of the natural hormones.

Compounds that are endocrine disrupters include natural animal hormones released into the environment, plant toxins or phytoestrogens, synthetic hormones present in sewage water and used for medical treatment (e.g., diethylstilbestrol), and several chemicals, including some pesticides and polychlorinated biphenols (PCBs). Endocrine disrupters enter the environment often as a by-product of many chemical and manufacturing processes and through waste disposal routes. Some evidence now suggests that effects of thyroid hormones and the immune system occur in addition to the disruptions of hormones that play a major part in the control of reproduction and development.

10.1.3 LABORATORY INVESTIGATIONS

Various methods can be used to detect toxic effects on endocrine function:

1. measurement of endocrine organ mass (absolute and relative to body weight)
2. histological examination of endocrine organ
3. measurement of circulating hormones
4. immunocytochemical examination of endocrine organ
5. surgical removal (e.g., ectomy of reproductive organs)
6. specific function tests
7. in vitro assays
8. indirect biochemical tests

When endocrine organ toxicity occurs, much of the initial diagnosis relies on the recognition of change in organ structure, relative organ mass, and appearance by the histopathologist. Additionally, clinical observations such as fluid intake or lethargy can be useful, and effects on growth or reproductive function can be important clues in endocrine toxicology. Of the previously listed investigations, those numbered 3–7 are generally selected when further characterization of the mechanistic effect is required following initial studies or when the structure of the compound strongly suggests a possible toxic effect. Some hormone measurements may be included as biomarkers in toxicology studies of therapeutic agents that are directed at making alterations of endocrine metabolism.

The use of in vivo bioassays (e.g., hyperglycemia) as a measure of insulin in an intact animal or organ is largely historic because the hormones can be measured directly, but in vitro bioassays or bioassays using endocrine responsive tissue cell cultures can be useful in screening compounds. These assays can measure changes of adenylate cyclase, intracellular calcium, and phosphoinositol metabolites.

Ideally, hormone assays should be evaluated in animal models where effects with test compounds or surgical removal have been described sufficiently well by other investigators. Alternatively, evidence from histopathology examinations can be correlated with hormone measurements in studies where there are marked effects on the target organ and relevant hormone.

10.1.3.1 HORMONE ASSAYS

A number of methodologies are available for the analysis of hormones; most of these use immunoassays in one format or another, although the biogenic amines (epinephrine and norepinephrine) and steroid hormones may be measured by other techniques, such as high-performance liquid chromatography or spectrophotometric/fluorimetric assays after chemical extraction (e.g., corticosterone—Sargent 1985, or gas liquid chromatography/mass spectrometry—Shu, Chou, and Lin 2003). The range of hormone immunoassays has improved over the last decade, and although the development of radioimmunoassay was an important landmark in measuring animal hormones (Reimers and Lamb 1991), other immunoassay formats have been developing.

The current technologies include radioimmunoassay (RIA), with two antibodies (double antibody methods); radioimmunoassay, with separation steps using activated charcoal or polyethylene glycol; immunoradiometric (IRMA), where the radiolabel is attached to the antibody; enzyme linked immunosorbent assays (ELISA; Webster et al. 1990); luminescence with bead assays; chemiluminescence (Reimers, Salerno, and Lamb 1996; Singh et al. 1997; Lee et al. 1998); and electrochemiluminescence (Golla and Seethala 2004) with microarrays. ELISA assays were originally unsuitable for even simple hormone assays, but now some assays have been developed with various detection systems (e.g., horseradish peroxidase, acetyl cholinesterase, or biotin detection systems). Perhaps the most rapid developments have occurred with insulin assays for rat and mouse, where the development has been largely driven by research into potential therapies for diabetes. Not every manufacturer of animal hormone assays is able to provide every hormone assay, and manufacturers may offer different technologies for various hormones to provide suitable assays. In validating hormone assays, precision, accuracy, sensitivity, and specificity need to be examined (see Chapter 13 and CLSI guidelines 1994, 2004a, 2004b, 2005, 2008a, 2008b).

Antibodies developed for hormone assays can be monoclonal antibodies or polyclonal antibodies; there is a greater degree of nonspecificity for these polyclonal antibodies, which can recognize several parts of the hormone molecules. In some assays, two monoclonal antibodies are directed against separate antigenic determinants on the hormone molecule (e.g., rat insulin). Ideally, a homologous immunoassay should be used when the antiserum and standards are available for the particular species being studied because the antibody to a specific hormone of one species may often fail to recognize or bind to the corresponding hormone in another species. As a general rule, antisera for low molecular mass hormones, such as the steroids, thyroxine, tri-iodothyronine, catecholamines, or small peptides, will recognize the hormone in several species. More than 30 species share the same sequence for the first 24 of the 40 amino acid residues of ACTH, so most antisera for ACTH will give satisfactory results in these immunoassays, although this hormone can be very unstable (Hegstad, Johnston, and Pasternak 1990). These structural similarities allow several antisera to human hormones to be used with other species, particularly nonhuman primates.

As the molecular masses and amino acid sequences of the protein hormones increase, the cross-reactivity of antisera in the different species becomes more problematic, and homologous antisera are required (Miller and Valdes 1992; Valdes and Miller 1992). Several homologous reagents are commercially available (e.g., prolactin, thyrotrophin, luteotrophin, and follitrophin for rats, and canine thyrotrophin). Some very specialized centers are able to produce suitable antisera given purified hormones, but this is a time-consuming process and the majority of toxicology laboratories use antisera from external suppliers who often can provide information on cross-reactivity.

The lack of suitable specific standards when using heterologous assays may mean acceptance of a compromise situation where hormonal changes can be demonstrated but values are expressed in terms of hormone standards obtained from another species. Some additional validation can be obtained by preparation of serial dilutions of unknown samples when they are added to the antiserum and hormone standards used for the calibration curve; the results of dilution should run parallel to the standard curve (i.e., dilutional parallelism). When "human" hormone kits are used for measuring animal hormones, the dynamic range for human assays may be inappropriate due to the different plasma hormone concentrations in the other species. If the test plasma hormone concentrations are at the lower end of the calibration curve, measurements will be less precise than measurements made in the middle of the measuring range. In such cases, the range of calibrators may require adjustment. For example, plasma thyroxine (T4) levels are lower in dog, rat, and cat compared with human plasma T4 levels, and the presence of total T4 in one third of "normal" canine samples was not detectable using a radioimmunoassay kit for human T4 (Eckersall and Williams 1983). Thus, assays may require modification to allow for species variations in hormone levels where an assay can be applied for more than one species.

Immunoassays are subject to some effects and interferences unique to immunoassay and some common to all chemical assays (Wu 2000). Establishment of an assay should include some assessment of antibody interference, signal interference, and matrix and hook effects. Interference may be caused by cross-reactivity or by an endogenous metabolite (e.g., in steroid hormone immunoassays) or a xenobiotic (or metabolite) with a similar structure; this problem occurs more frequently in competitive binding assays. Antibodies present in samples may bind to reagent antibodies—for example, when humans produce antibodies to therapeutic mouse monoclonal antibodies, which then interfere with assays based on mouse monoclonal antibodies. These possible interferences should be considered when studying any therapeutic protein (Levinson 1997). The hook effect describes a state where an antigen excess saturates all the binding sites of the antibody without forming complexes, thus leading to falsely negative/low values.

Matrix effects may be due to xenobiotics and/or metabolites that alter the magnitude of the reaction detection system (e.g., peroxidase/chromogen reactions, fluorescence, or luminescence) by increasing or by decreasing the reaction signal. The different biological matrices that exist between species can cause problems in heterologous assays; interactions occurring between the antibody and the plasma protein variations between the transport binding proteins of different species may also affect the assay (e.g., thyroid hormones; see Section 10.2). Additional recovery experiments can be performed with known levels of hormones added to the sample matrix. When feline insulin levels were measured with five commercial human insulin assay kits, the results were satisfactory with some kits; however, some data indicated a lack of "dilutional parallelism" and matrix effects were found with two of the kits (Lutz and Rand 1993).

Some hormones are stable when stored, while others (e.g., ACTH) are remarkably unstable; such hormones require careful collection procedures (Reimers et al. 1983; Hegstad et al. 1990; Hegstad-Davies 2006). Cyclical freezing and thawing of samples should be avoided because this denatures proteins. Collection procedures may have a marked effect on hormone level, most commonly due to stress (rats—Wuttke and Meites 1970; Ajika, Krulick, and McCann 1972; Dohler et al. 1977; Gartner et al. 1980; rabbits—Toth and January 1990; dogs—Garnier et al. 1990; monkeys—Torii et al. 1993). Some of these effects are discussed in Chapter 12.

10.1.3.2 CHRONOBIOCHEMISTRY

Some hormones show cyclical or seasonal rhythms, so the timing of blood sampling is a critical factor (Kreiger 1979). Apart from the obvious periodic changes in the levels of sex hormones, particularly in females, variations of other hormones occur in several species. Circadian variations for TSH, T3, and T4 in rats (Jordan et al. 1980) and for testosterone and cortisol in dogs (Plant 1981; Gordon and Lavie 1985; Palazzolo and Quadri 1987; Orth, Peterson, and Drucker 1988; Fukuda et al. 1988; Fukuda 1990) have been described. LH, FSH, prolactin, and testosterone have been shown to follow annual rhythms in male monkeys (Beck and Wuttke 1979; Torii and Nigi 1994) and rats (Wong et al. 1983). Episodic or pulsatile secretions of plasma prolactin and LH have been observed in rats (Kempainnen and Sartin 1984; Levine and Duffy 1988; Mistry and Voogt 1989). When cyclical changes do occur (e.g., in the estrus cycle), not all animals will be at the same stage of the cycle, so it may be necessary to take several samples during the cycle. For hormones with circadian rhythms, samples should be taken from a group of animals during a short period within the day; this may be at peak times or not for some species.

REFERENCES

Atterwill, C. K., and A. Cockburn. 1997. Introduction to endocrine toxicology. In *Endocrine toxicology*, ed. C. K. Atterwill and J. D. Flack, pp. 1–11. Cambridge: Cambridge University Press.

Capen, C. C. 1997. Mechanistic data and risk assessment of selected toxic end points of the thyroid gland. *Toxicologic Pathology* 25:39–48.

Cheng, S. Y. 2005. Thyroid hormone receptor mutations and disease: Beyond thyroid hormone resistance. *Trends in Endocrinology and Metabolism* 16:176–182.

Ekena, K., K. E. Weis, J. A. Katzenellenbogen, and B. S. Katzenellenbogen. 1996. Identification of amino acids in the hormone binding domain of human estrogen receptor important in estrogen binding. *Journal of Biological Chemistry* 27:20053–20059.

Gudermann, T., P. Nurwakagari, and D. Ben-Menahem. 2005. Hormone binding to the follicle-stimulating-hormone receptor—Crystal clear! *Experimental Clinical Endocrinology and Diabetes* 113:245–247.

Gurnell, M., and V. K. Chatterjee. 2004. Nuclear receptors in disease: Thyroid receptor beta, peroxisome-proliferators-activated receptor gamma and orphan receptors. *Essays in Biochemistry* 40:169–190.

Harris, H. A., J. A. Katzenellenbogen, and B. S. Katzenellenbogen. 2002. Characterization of the biological roles of the estrogen receptors, ER-alpha and ER-beta, in estrogen target tissues in vivo through the use of an ER-alpha-selective ligand. *Endocrinology* 143:4172–4177.

Harvey, P. W., ed. 1996. *The adrenal in toxicology*. London: Taylor & Francis.

Harvey, P. W., K. C. Rush, and A. Cockburn, eds. 1999. *Endocrine and hormonal toxicology*. Chichester, England: John Wiley & Sons Ltd.

Houck, K. A., and R. J. Kavlock. 2008. Understanding mechanisms of toxicity: Insights from drug discovery research. *Toxicology and Applied Pharmacology* 227:163–178.

Kohrle, J. 2008. Environment and endocrinology: The case of thyroidology. *Annales d'Endocrinologie* 69:116–122.

Millar, R. P., Z. I. Lu, A. J. Pawson, C. A. Flanagan, K. Morgan, and S. R. Maudsley. 2004. Gonadotrophin-releasing hormone receptors. *Endocrine Reviews* 25:235–275.

Reimers, T. J. 1999. Hormones. In *The clinical chemistry of laboratory animals*, ed. W. F. Loeband and F. W. Quimby, pp. 455–501. Boca Raton, FL: Taylor & Francis.

Ribelin, W. E. 1984. Effects of drugs and chemicals upon the structure of the adrenal gland. *Fundamental and Applied Toxicology* 4:105–119.

Rosol, T. J., J. T. Yarrington, J. Latendresse, and C. C. Capen. 2001. Adrenal gland: Structure, function and mechanisms of toxicity. *Toxicologic Pathology* 29:41–48.

Sandler, B. et al. 2004. Thyroxine-thyroid hormone receptor interactions. *Journal of Biological Chemistry* 279:55801–55808.

Shank, L. C., and B. M. Paschal. 2005. Nuclear transport of steroid hormone receptors. *Critical Reviews in Eukaryotic Gene Expression* 15:49–73.

Thomas, J. A. 1994. Actions of drugs/chemicals on nonreproductive endocrine organs. *Toxic Substances Journal* 8:957–962.

———. 1995. Gonadal-specific metal toxicology. *Metal Toxicology* 16:413–445.

———. 1998. Drugs and chemicals that affect the endocrine system. *International Journal of Toxicology* 17:12–38.

Thomas, J. A., and H. D. Colby, eds. 1997. *Endocrine toxicology*, 2nd ed. Boca Raton, FL: CRC Press.

Woodman, D. D. 1988. The use of clinical biochemistry for assessment of endocrine system toxicology. In *The use of clinical biochemistry in toxicologically relevant animal models and standardization and quality control animal biochemistry*, ed. P. Keller and E. Bogin, pp. 63–77. Basle, Switzerland: Hexagon–Roche.

————. 1997. *Laboratory animal endocrinology: Hormonal action, control mechanisms and interactions with drugs.* Chichester, England: John Wiley & Sons Ltd.

Zhou, Z-X., C-I. Wong, M. Sar, and E. M. Wilson. 1994. The androgen receptor: An overview. *Recent Progress in Hormone Research* 49:249–274.

Laboratory Investigations

Clinical and Laboratory Standards Institute Guidelines http://www.clsi.org/.

CLSI. 1994. LA1- A2. *Assessing the quality of radioimmunoassay systems, 2nd ed.* Approved guideline.

CLSI. 2004a. EP17-A. *Protocols for determination of limits of detections and limits of quantitation.* Approved guideline.

CLSI. 2004b. ILA23-A. *Radioimmunoassay and enzyme, fluorescence and luminescence immunoassays.* Approved guideline.

CLSI. 2005. EP14-A2. *Evaluation of matrix effects, 2nd ed.* Approved guideline.

CLSI. 2008a. ILA 21-A2. *Clinical evaluation of immunoassays, 2nd ed.* Approved guideline.

CLSI. 2008b. ILA 30-A. *Immunoassay interference by endogenous antibodies.* Approved guideline.

Ajika, D., L. Krulick, and S. M. McCann. 1972. The effect of pentobarbital (Nembutal) on prolactin release in the rat. *Proceedings of the Society for Experimental Biology and Medicine* 141:203–205.

Dohler, K-D., A. von zur Muhlen, K. Gartner, and U. Dohler. 1977. Effect of various blood sampling techniques on serum levels of pituitary and thyroid hormones in the rat. *Journal of Endocrinology* 74:341–342.

Eckersall, P. D., and M. E. Williams. 1983. Thyroid function tests in dogs using radioimmunoassay kits. *Journal of Small Animal Practice* 24:525–532.

Garnier, F., E. Benoit, M. Virat, R. Ochoa, and P. Delatour. 1990. Adrenalcortical response in clinically normal dogs before and after adaptation to a housing environment. *Laboratory Animals* 24:40–43.

Gartner, K., D. Büttner, K. Döhler, R. Friedel, J. Lindena, and I. Trautschold. 1980. Stress response of rats to handling and experimental procedures. *Laboratory Animals* 14:267–274.

Golla, R., and R. Seethala. 2004. A sensitive and robust high-throughput electrochemiluminescence assay for rat insulin. *Journal of Biomolecular Screening* 9:62–70.

Hegstad, R. L., S. D. Johnston, and D. M. Pasternak. 1990. Effects of sample handling on adrenocorticotrophin concentration measured in canine plasma using a commercially available radioimmunoassay kit. *American Journal of Veterinary Research* 51:1941–1947.

Hegstad-Davies, R. L. 2006. A review of sample handling considerations for reproductive and thyroid hormone measurement in serum and plasma. *Theriogenology* 66:592–598.

Lee, D. E., V. J. Salerno, S. V. Lamb, and T. J. Reimers. 1998. Clinical evaluation of immunlite chemiluminescent immunoassays in total thyroxine (TT4) thyrotropin (TSH) and free-thyroxine (FT4) in dog serum. *Clinical Chemistry* 44 (Suppl.): A108.

Levinson, S. S. 1997. Test interferences from endogenous antibodies. *Journal of Clinical Ligand Assay* 20:180–189.

Lutz, T. A., and J. S. Rand. 1993. Comparison of five commercial radioimmunoassay kits for the measurement of feline insulin. *Research in Veterinary Science* 55:64–69.

Miller, J. J., and R. Valdes. 1992. Methods for calculating cross-reactivity in immunoassay. *Journal of Clinical Immunoassay* 15:97–107.

Reimers, T. J., and S. V. Lamb. 1991. Radioimmunoassay of hormones in laboratory animals for diagnostics and research. *Laboratory Animals* 20:32–38.

Reimers, T. J., J. P. McCann, R. G. Cowan, and P. W. Concannon. 1983. Effect of storage, hemolysis, and freezing and thawing on concentrations of thyroxine, cortisol and insulin in blood samples. *Proceedings of the Society for Experimental Biology and Medicine* 170:509–516.

Reimers, T. J., V. J. Salerno, and S. V. Lamb. 1996. Validation and application of solid-phase chemiluminescent immunoassays for the diagnosis of endocrine diseases in animals. *Comparative Hematology International* 6:170–175.

Sargent, R. N. 1985. Determination of corticosterone in rat plasma by HPLC. *Journal of Analytical Toxicology* 9:20–21.

Shu, P-Y., S-H. Chou, and C-H. Lin. 2003. Determination of corticosterone in rat and mouse plasma by gas chromatography-selected ion monitoring mass spectrometry. *Journal of Chromatography B* 783:93–101.

Singh, A. K., Y. Jiang, J. T. White, and D. Spassova. 1997. Validation of nonradioactive chemiluminescent immunoassay methods for the analysis of thyroxine and cortisol in blood samples obtained from dogs, cats and horses. *Journal of Veterinary Diagnostic Investigation* 9:261–268.

Torii, R., N. Kitagawa, H. Nigi, and N. Ohsawa. 1993. Effects of repeated restraint stress at 30-minute intervals during 24-hour serum testosterone, LH and glucocorticoid levels in male Japanese monkeys (*Macaca fuscata*). *Experimental Animals* 42:67–73.

Toth, L. A., and B. January. 1990. Physiological stabilization of rabbits after shipping. *Laboratory Animal Science* 40:384–387.

Valdes, R., and J. J. Miller. 1992. Increasing the specificity of immunoassays. *Journal of Clinical Immunoassay* 15:87–96.

Webster, H. V., A. J. Bone, K. A. Webster, and T. J. Wilkin. 1990. Comparison of an enzyme linked immunosorbent assay (ELISA) with a radioimmunoassay for the measurement of rat insulin. *Journal of Immunological Methods* 134:95–100.

Wu, J. T. 2000. *Quantitative immunoassay: A practical guide for assay establishment.* Washington, D.C.: AACC Press.

Wuttke, W., and J. Meites. 1970. Effects of ether and pentobarbital on serum prolactin and LH levels in proestrous rats. *Proceedings of the Society for Experimental Biology and Medicine* 135:648–652.

Chronobiochemistry

Beck, W., and W. Wuttke. 1979. Annual rhythms of luteinizing hormone, follicle stimulating hormone, prolactin and testosterone in the serum of male rhesus monkeys. *Journal of Endocrinology* 83:131–139.

Fukuda, S., H. Nagashima, K. Morioka, and J. Aoki. 1988. Fluctuations in peripheral serum testosterone levels within a day, with age and by sexual stimulation in male beagle dogs bred indoors. *Jikken Dobutsu* 37:381–386.

Fukuda, S. 1990. Circadian rhythm of serum testosterone levels in male beagle dogs—Effects of lighting time zone. *Experimental Animals* 39:65–68.

Gordon, C. R., and P. Lavie. 1985. Day–night variations in urine excretions and hormones in dogs: Role of autonomic innervation. *Physiology and Behavior* 35:175–181.

Jordan, D., B. Rousset, F. Ferrin, M. Fournier, and J. Orgiazzi. 1980. Evidence of circadian variations in serum thyrotrophin, 3,5,3'-triiodothyronine, and thyroxine in the rat. *Endocrinology* 107:1245–1248.

Kempainnen, R. J., and J. J. Sartin. 1984. Evidence for episodic but not circadian activity in plasma concentrations of adrenocorticotrophin, cortisol and thyroxine in dogs. *Endocrinology* 103:219–226.

Kreiger, D. T. 1979. *Endocrine rhythms.* New York: Raven Press.

Levine, J. E., and M. T. Duffy. 1988. Simultaneous measurement of luteinizing hormone (LH)-releasing hormone and follicle-stimulating hormone release in intact and short-term castrate rats. *Endocrinology* 122:2211–2221.

Mistry, A., and J. L. Voogt. 1989. Role of serotonin in nocturnal and diurnal surges of prolactin in the pregnant rat. *Endocrinology* 125:2875–2880.

Orth, D. N., M. E. Peterson, and W. D. Drucker. 1988. Plasma immunoreactive propiomelanocortin peptides and cortisol in normal dogs and dogs with Cushing's syndrome: Diurnal rhythm and responses to various stimuli. *Endocrinology* 122:1250–1262.

Palazzolo, D. L., and S. K. Quadri. 1987. The effects of aging on the circadian rhythm of serum cortisol in the dog. *Environmental Gerontology* 22:379–387.

Plant, T. M. 1981. Time courses of concentrations of circulating gonadotrophin, prolactin, testosterone and cortisol in adult male rhesus monkey (*Macacca mulatta*) throughout the 24-h light-dark cycle. *Biology of Reproduction* 25:244–252.

Torii, R., and H. Nigi. 1994. Hypothalamo–pituitary–testicular function in male Japanese monkeys (*Macaca fuscata*) in nonmating season. *Jikken Dobutsu* 43:381–387.

Wong, C-C., K-D. Dohler, H. Geerlings, and A. von zur Muhlen. 1983. Influence of age, strain and season on circadian periodicity, gonadal and adrenal hormones in the serum of male laboratory rats. *Hormone Research* 17:202–215.

Section 10.2: Assessment of Thyroid Toxicity

10.2.1 STRUCTURE, BIOCHEMISTRY, AND PHYSIOLOGY

Located in the neck region, the thyroid is one of the largest endocrine organs. It contains the follicular cells, which synthesize and secrete the thyroid hormones, and the larger parafollicular cells (or C cells) dispersed among the follicles, which secrete the hormone calcitonin. The functional unit of the thyroid gland is the follicle, which is normally spherical with an outer layer of follicular cells surrounding a colloid containing primarily thyroglobulin. The blood flow to the thyroid via the carotid and thyroid arteries is greater than for many other major organs, and the thyroid tissue is highly vascularized; the blood flow to the thyroid is estimated to be approximately twice that supplied to kidneys.

The main function of the thyroid gland is to synthesize, store, and release thyroid hormones, which require the trapping of iodide by the thyroid gland for hormone synthesis. Dietary iodine is absorbed as iodides or iodates from the gastrointestinal tract, and the iodide in the blood is taken into the follicles by an iodide pump at the basement membrane of the follicular cell. This iodide active transport or pump mechanism works against a concentration gradient, where the iodide content is much higher in the thyroid gland, and under the influence of thyroid stimulating hormone. Approximately 20% of the total iodide in the body is stored in the thyroid gland, and it is highly conserved by the body. The main route for excretion of iodide is via the kidneys.

Thyroglobulin is a glycoprotein with a molecular mass of about 660 kDa that is synthesized within the follicular cell. After the trapping of iodide, thyroperoxidase within the follicle cell oxidizes the iodide, which becomes attached to the phenyl groups at the 3- and/or 5-positions of the tyrosyl residues of thyroglobulin to form monoiodotyrosine (MIT) or di-iodotyrosine (DIT). These iodination reactions occur mainly at the apical follicular cell membrane and colloid interface, with further iodinations forming thyroxine (3,5,3',5',tetraiodothyronine: T_4) or tri-iodothyronine (3,5',3-triiodothyronine: T_3). Iodinated thyroglobulin incorporating T_3 and T_4 is stored within the follicular colloid. Under the influence of thyrotrophin (thyroid stimulating hormone: TSH), proteases (cathespins) from the thyroidal lysosomes act on colloid droplets containing the thyroglobulin with iodothyronines to release T_3, T_4, MIT, and DIT. The MIT and DIT are largely degraded by microsomal tyrosine deiodinases, and the iodide is conserved. T_4 may also be deiodinated to small quantities of an inactive form—reverse T_3 (rT_3)—within the thyroid, although rT_3 is formed mainly in peripheral tissues (see Figure 10.2.1).

T_3, T_4, and rT_3 are released from the basement membrane of the follicle and enter the blood, where they are bound to carrier proteins synthesized by the liver. These proteins are alpha-globulins called thyroxine binding globulins (TBGs), transthyretin

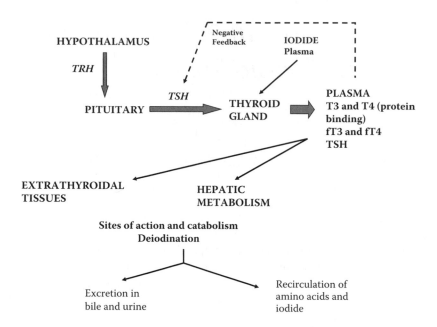

FIGURE 10.2.1 Outline of thyroid hormone metabolism.

(or thyroxine binding prealbumin: TBPA), and albumin; two of these thyroxine binding proteins are described by their electrophoretic mobilities. The binding of the hormones with proteins increases the molecular size, which helps to retain the hormones within the circulation and thus acts as a reservoir of active hormones available for delivery to target cells. Although albumin acts in most species as a low affinity binding protein, there are a number of variations between the species (Tanabe, Ishii, and Tamaki 1969; Refetoff, Robin, and Fang 1970; Larsson, Pettersson, and Carlstrom 1985; Savu et al. 1989; Emerson et al. 1990; Vranckx et al. 1990, 1994). Thyroxine binding globulin is largely absent from or at very low concentration in the plasma of adult rat, mouse, guinea pig, and rabbit, so the hormones are mainly transported by albumin. In dog plasma there are at least three globulins (TBGs) and TBPA, which are present together with albumin, but the levels of TBG are lower than in man (Ferguson 1995). Less than 1% of the total active iodothyronines in blood are present in the free (or unbound) forms; the bound fractions act as a storage buffer and help to maintain the concentration of the free forms.

Thyroid hormones enter the extrathyroidal tissues by the action of specific transporters: the organic anion transport protein (OATP) and the monocarboxylic transporter (MCT8) (Ekins et al. 1994; Friesema et al. 1999, 2005). Within some cells, deiodinating enzymes can remove an iodine atom from the T_4 or T_3 molecules and thereby modify the sensitivity of a cell to the actions of the thyroid hormones. The cellular actions of the thyroid hormones are mediated by nuclear receptor proteins, which bind to DNA and regulate transcription with at least two types of genes that encode these receptors (Barettino, Ruiz, and Stunnenberg 1994); these also provide a negative feedback action on the hypothalamic–pituitary axis. T_4 is sometimes considered to be a prohormone for T_3 because the majority of effects due to thyroid hormones are mediated through T_3, with a high proportion of circulating T_3 formed by deiodination of T_4 in the liver and kidneys.

In extrathyroidal tissues, the thyroid hormones are catabolized in a series of deiodination, oxidative, or conjugation reactions. Deiodination of circulating T_4 occurs mainly in the liver and kidney by type I deiodinases with either 5′-deiodination yielding T_3 or 5-deiodination yielding inactive rT_3. The production of reverse T_3 is thought to be another extrathyroidal control mechanism regulating the delivery of free T_3 to the tissues. Type II deiodinases carry out 5′-deiodination in the cerebral cortex and brown adipose tissues.

Some thyroid hormones are conjugated in the liver and excreted in the bile as sulfates or glucuronides, while small amounts of free hormones and the iodoacetic acid form break down products (Hood and Klaassen 2000a, 2000b; Klaassen and Hood 2001). The half-lives of T_4 and T_3 are much shorter in laboratory animals (16 and 6 h in the dog and rat, respectively) than for humans, where the half-life of circulating T_4 is approximately 5–7 days and is about 1–2 days for T_3.

Thyroid hormone production is governed by the actions of the hypothalamic–pituitary–thyroid axis (HPT axis). Thyrotropin releasing hormone (TRH) synthesized by the hypothalamus is transported to the anterior pituitary, where TRF stimulates thyrotrophic cells to produce thyrotrophin (TSH). TSH is a glycoprotein with a short half-life of less than 20 min; it is one of three pituitary glycoprotein hormones with alpha- and beta-subunits. These three pituitary glycoproteins (luteotrophin, folliotrophin, and TSH) share the same alpha-subunit.

The TSH then binds to a number of specific receptors on the thyroid follicular cell through several binding domains. The binding of TSH activates adenylate cyclase and leads to the accumulation of cAMP with the release of thyroid hormones. TSH can increase the production of iodothyronines through iodide uptake and effects on the synthesis, storage, and release actions involving thyroglobulin; these actions increase hormone production. To maintain circulating hormone levels and production within narrow limits, there are negative feedback mechanisms on both the hypothalamus and pituitary, with free T_4 acting to suppress both TSH and TRF production. If the plasma T_3 and T_4 levels decrease, the hypothalamus responds by increasing TRH and TSH, which in turn increases the hormone production. Conversely, when plasma T_3 and T_4 increase, the production of TSH decreases and the rates of hormone production fall.

The thyroid regulates many aspects of metabolism, including tissue metabolic rate and oxygen consumption, protein synthesis, mitochondrial oxidative phosphorylation, and carbohydrate metabolism (including gluconeogenesis, lipid metabolism, and bone metabolism) by altering calcium levels and bone resorption mechanisms. Thyroid hormones are essential for normal development and for maintenance of normal physiological functions; there is a complex regulation system for thyroid hormones.

10.2.2 TOXICOLOGICAL EFFECTS

Although changes of thyroid hormone levels are generally considered to be adverse, some debate continues about the degree of thyroid disruption induced by particular toxicants as to whether the changes are adaptive or adverse. This is particularly important with respect to the development of thyroid tumors. Understanding the mechanisms of thyroid toxicity of different toxicants can help to predict the risks associated with an adverse effect (Atterwill, Jones, and Brown 1992; Capen 1997, 1998, 1999; Connors 1997).

Hyperthyroidism describes overactive thyroid tissue with increased circulation of plasma T_3 and T_4, and where TSH will be low in primary hyperthyroidism: in hypothyroidism there is insufficient production of thyroid hormones and this is accompanied by increased TSH as the APT strives to increase hormone production.

Thyrotoxic xenobiotics may act by more than one mechanism: some of the mechanisms and some example compounds are:

- inhibition of the iodide pump by anions of a similar size to iodide; example compounds are bromide, perchlorate, pertechnetate, chlorate, selenocyanate, and thiocyanate;
- inhibition of thyroperoxidase/iodide oxidation (Taurog, Dorris, and Doerge 1996; Darras et al. 1998); example compounds are amphenazone, carbamazole, cobalt, p-aminosalicylic acid, some imidazoles, phenylbutazone, phenylindanedione, propylthiouracil, resorcinol, thiocyanate, and thiourea;
- interference with iodination and the formation of mono- and di-iodothyronines; example compounds are aromatic amines, polyhydric phenols, and thioamides;
- inhibition of TSH secretion; example compounds are dopamine, some corticosteroids, and hydrocortisone;
- altered plasma protein binding of thyroid hormones (Brouwer et al. 1990; Brouwer and van den Berg 1996; Chauhan, Kodavanti, and McKinney 2000); example compounds are fatty acids, estrogens, phenytoin, and salicylates; perturbations of plasma proteins (e.g., hepatotoxicity) will affect plasma protein binding;
- alteration of T_4 to T_3 conversion in extrathyroidal tissues; example compounds are amiodarone, erythrosine, and propranolol;
- reduction of T_3 uptake by the extrathyroidal tissues; example compounds are some anabolic steroids; and
- altered hepatic metabolism associated with enzyme induction, mainly through uridine diphosphate glucuronosyl transferase increasing clearances of T_3 and T_4 (Barter and Klaassen 1992, 1994; Hood and Klaassen 2000a, 2000b; Hood et al. 2003); example compounds are phenobarbitone, phenytoin, naphthoflavone, some halogenated dioxins, and polychlorinated and polybrominated biphenyl compounds.

Mechanisms whereby the pituitary is the primary cause of thyrotoxicosis are less common than the aforementioned and other mechanisms of thyroid toxicity.

The natural response to lowered levels of plasma thyroid hormones is for TSH production to increase with rapid growth of the thyroid gland and increased thyroglobulin synthesis. In the rat, the thyroid gland becomes desensitized to the effects of more TSH, and the weight of the thyroids stops increasing to the same extent. During this plateau period, some thyroid cells mutate and this leads to the development of thyroid tumors if dosing of the test compound continues. If the administration of the test compound ceases during this period, progression to tumor formation may be reversed. Several antithyroid xenobiotics have been shown to be carcinogenic to the thyroid gland in these two-stage rodent carcinogenesis models (Hill et al. 1989; Kanno et al. 1990; Atterwill et al. 1992; Onodera et al. 1994; Davies 1996; Takagi et al. 2002). The in vivo rodent model remains an important tool in evaluating exogenous compounds that may be endocrine disrupters (DeVito et al. 1999; OECD 2006a).

10.2.3 LABORATORY INVESTIGATIONS

In several OECD test guidelines (2006a, 2006b), the relevant toxicological study endpoints include thyroid weight and histology together with T_4, T_3, and TSH. The guidelines emphasize that the endpoints should be planned to obtain measures at the times of optimal effects. Although thyroid toxicants are often defined as compounds that alter circulating levels of thyroid hormone, identification of thyroid-toxic chemicals is largely dependent on histopathology rather than hormone levels. However, preclinical hormone measurements can be bridged to clinical studies if the samples are collected appropriately.

A number of commercially available assays are now available for some common laboratory animals (e.g., mouse, rat, and dog). These assays are based on chemiluminescence, enzyme linked immunosorbent (ELISA) colorimetric assays, and radioimmunoassay. For the iodothyronines (e.g., total T_3 and T_4), a wide choice of assays designed for human samples is available; these can be used across species because the molecule structures are common (Anderson, Nixon, and Akasha 1988; Daminet et al. 1999; Mooney, Shiel, and Dixon 2008). Some assays require adjustments to ensure that the majority of samples are measured within a suitable range because the plasma values vary across the species (Table 10.2.1). When these assays are used, there may be problems associated with calibration materials because external quality assessment schemes continue to show minor and sometimes major differences between assays produced for hormone analyses. With all of these immunoassays, the reagents must be shown to be suitable for the species being studied. Reports of

---

TABLE 10.2.1
Expectable Thyroid Hormone and TSH Ranges in Three Species

Species	T_3 (ng/dL)	fT_3 (pg/dL)	T_4 (µg/dL)	fT_4 (ng/dL)	TSH (ng/mL)
Mouse	80–120		3–8		1–3
Rat	30–120	180–270	4–7	0.25–5	1–10
Dog	40–160		1.5–4	0.6–3.0	0.3–0.6

Notes: See Appendix C for explanation of the term *expectable ranges.*
    Conversion factors for triiodothyronine (T_3) (molecular mass 651): ng/dL × 0.01536 = nmol/L; thyroxine (T_4) (molecular mass 777): ng/dL × 12.87 = nmol/L. Some conversion factors between ng/mL and µLU/mL for thyroid stimulating hormone (TSH) are provided by some assay kit suppliers, but should be used with caution.

interferences due to the presence of heterophilic antibodies (antibodies to other species) are rare but should be considered when therapeutic monoclonal antibodies are studied.

The choice of available assays is narrower for free T_3 and free T_4 assays, and the measurements are more difficult because of the relatively low concentrations of these hormones; therefore, these assays have been less commonly applied. Different methods for determining the free hormone levels include or omit extraction procedures. Direct methods, where free hormone is measured in the presence of bound hormone and proteins with free binding sites, can be problematic because the equilibrium between the free and bound fractions may be altered under the conditions of the assay. In addition, the different protein binding properties of different species may affect these analyses. Assays such as T_3 uptake that estimated the available binding sites and protein bound iodide are largely obsolete.

Assays for TSH present a different challenge because its structure varies between species and the discrimination between lower concentrations within the reference range and the suppressed levels found in hyperthyroidism was poor with some earlier reagents. However, recently introduced reagents are better (Spencer and Wang 1995; Pohlenz et al. 1999).

Thyroid hormones show marked diurnal variations in rats, dogs, and monkeys, so the times for sample collections are critical if moderate changes are to be detected (Leppaluoto, Ranta, and Tuomisto 1974; Jordan et al. 1980; Gianella-Neto, Quabbe, and Witt 1981; Ottenweiler and Hedge 1982; Ferguson 1988; Bruner, Scott-Moncrieff, and Williams 1998). Several publications give data for intra- and interanimal variations for rats and dogs (Reimers et al. 1990; Jensen and Høier 1996; Iversen et al. 1999). Stress may also affect hormone levels. For thyroid hormone assessment, Davies (1993) suggested that samples should be collected at necropsy within a 1-h period and that at least 20 rats per group were needed; however, this number can be reduced by careful study design and sampling procedures. The analysis of samples from large numbers of rodents without reference to appropriate sample timing may yield misleading and variable results. In dogs given phenobarbitone for 27 weeks, thyroid hormone changes were evident for at least 1–4 weeks after treatment (Gieger et al. 2000). When thyroid hormone results are interpreted, reference should be made to the plasma protein concentrations because of their thyroid hormone binding properties and the effects on potential protein binding sites (Panciera and Johnston 2002).

10.2.3.1   OTHER THYROID MEASUREMENTS

Although various tests, including plasma radiolabeled T_3 uptake (Halmolsky et al. 1959) and T_4 clearance (Davies 1993), responses to exogenous TSH (Meij, Mol, and Rijnberk 1996), and perchlorate uptake tests (Atterwill et al. 1987), have been described, tests are not commonly employed in toxicology studies. In vitro measurements are useful in mechanistic studies and for screening compounds for potential effects on thyroid tissue (Brown et al. 1986; Atterwill et al. 1987; Atterwill and Aylward 1995; Hood and Klaassen 2000a). Other effects associated with thyroid toxicants include plasma lipids with hypothyroidism associated with hypercholesterolemia, while hyperthyroidism is associated with hypocholesterolemia and hypercalcemia (Benvenga and Robbins 1993; Dixon, Reid, and Mooney 1999).

10.2.4   CALCITONIN

Calcitonin (thyrocalcitonin) is produced in the parafollicular (or C) cells of the thyroid gland from a prohormone: procalcitonin (Copp 1994; Woodman 1997). Procalcitonin and calcitonin are stored within the C cells before the release of calcitonin from secretory granules or degradation of excess calcitonin within the C cells. Calcitonin is a straight chain polypeptide composed of 32 amino acid residues with a single disulphide bridge and a molecular mass of approximately 3 kDa. Although the amino terminal group of calcitonins is similar across species, the remaining parts of the molecules differ considerably between species. However, rat and human calcitonins share 94% homology. Calcitonin has a short half-life in both the rat and the dog (Habener el al. 1971; Hazewinkel et al. 1999).

Calcitonin is secreted continuously under conditions of normocalcemia, and the synthesis of calcitonin is increased when the calcium concentrations in plasma and intracellular fluids increase. Hypermagnesemia has a similar effect on calcitonin production. In hypocalcemia, the production of calcitonin falls. The gastrointestinal hormones—gastrin, glucagon, cholecystokinin, and secretin—and high dietary calcium also stimulate calcitonin production. Long-term hypercalcemia may cause hyperplasia of the C cells.

Calcitonin acts on receptors in bone osteoclasts with a resulting reduction of bone resorption, and it also acts on the renal tubular reabsorption of phosphate. The phosphaturic effects are accompanied by diuresis and increased excretion of other electrolytes. Calcitonin and parathyroid hormone act as a dual negative feedback mechanism in controlling calcium in intra- and extracellular fluids. The range of calcitonin assays suitable for laboratory animals is limited, but the hormone can be measured by two-site radioimmunometric assays (Moukhtar et al. 2005).

REFERENCES*

General

Bently, P. J. 1998. *Comparative vertebrate endocrinology,* 3rd ed. Cambridge: Cambridge University Press.

Braverman, L. E., and R. D. Utiger, eds. 2004. *Werner and Ingbar's the thyroid: A fundamental and clinical text,* 9th ed. Philadelphia: Lippincott–Williams & Wilkins.

Connors, J. M. 1997. Physiology of the thyroid gland and agents affecting its secretion. In *Endocrine toxicology.* Target Organ series, ed. J. A. Thomas, pp. 43–68. Boca Raton, FL: CRC Press.

Gittoes, N. J., and J. A. Franklin. 1995. Drug-induced thyroid disorders. *Drug Safety* 13:46–55.

Iatropoulos, M. J. 1994. Endocrine considerations in toxicologic pathology. *Experimental and Toxicological Pathology* 45:391–410.

---

* Some references not cited in the text are included for background reading.

Reece, W. O. 2005. *Functional anatomy and physiology of domestic animals,* 3rd ed., pp. 457–473. Philadelphia: Lippincott, Williams & Wilkins.

Sterling, K., and J. H. Lazarus. 1977. The thyroid and its control. *Annual Review of Physiology* 39:349–371.

Thomas, J. A., ed. 1997. *Endocrine toxicology.* Target Organ series. Boca Raton, FL: CRC Press.

Woodman, D. D. 1997. Thyroid and parathyroid hormones. In *Laboratory animal endocrinology,* pp. 214–218. Chichester, England: John Wiley & Sons Ltd.

Other References

Andersen, S., N. H. Bruun, K. M. Pedersen, and P. Laurberg. 2003. Biologic variation is important for interpretation of thyroid function tests. *Thyroid* 13:1069–1078.

Anderson, R. R., D. A. Nixon, and M. A. Akasha. 1988. Total and free thyroxine and tri-iodothyroine in blood serum of mammals. *Comparative Biochemistry and Physiology* 89A:401–404.

Atterwill, C. K., and S. P. Aylward. 1995. Endocrine toxicology of the thyroid for industrial compounds. In *Toxicology of industrial compounds,* ed. H. Thomas, R. Hess, and F. Waechter, pp. 257–380. London: Taylor & Francis.

Atterwill, C. K., P. Collins, C. G. Brown, and R. F. Harland. 1987. The perchlorate discharge test for examining thyroid function in rats. *Journal of Pharmacological Methods* 18:199–203.

Atterwill, C. K., C. Jones, and C. G. Brown. 1992. Thyroid gland II. Mechanisms of species dependent thyroid toxicity, hyperplasia and neoplasia induced by xenobiotics. In *Endocrine toxicology,* ed. C. K. Atterwill and J. D. Flack, pp. 137–182. Cambridge: Cambridge University Press.

Barettino, D., M. D. M. Ruiz, and H. G. Stunnenberg. 1994. Characterization of the ligand-dependent transactivation domain of thyroid hormone receptor. *EMBO Journal* 13:3039–3049.

Barter, R. A., and C. D. Klaassen. 1992. UDP-glucuronosyltransferase inducers reduce thyroid hormone levels in rats by an extrathyroidal mechanism. *Toxicology and Applied Pharmacology* 113:36–42.

———. 1994. Reduction of thyroid hormone levels and alteration of thyroid function by four representative UDP-glucuronosyltransferase inducers in rats. *Toxicology and Applied Pharmacology* 128:9–17.

Benvenga, S., and J. Robbins. 1993. Lipoprotein–thyroid hormone interactions. *Trends in Endocrinology and Metabolism* 4:194–198.

Brouwer, A., E. Klassonwehler, M. Bokdam, D. C. Morse, and W. A. Traag. 1990. Competitive inhibition of thyroxine binding to transthyretin by monohydroxy metabolites of 3,4,3′,4′-tetrachlorobiphenyl. *Chemosphere* 20:1257–1262.

Brouwer, A., and K. J. van den Berg. 1996. Binding of a metabolite of 3,4,3′,4′-tetrachlorobiphenyl to transthyretin reduces serum vitamin A transport by inhibiting the formation of the protein complex carrying both retinol and thyroxin. *Toxicology and Applied Pharmacology* 85:301–312.

Brown, C. G., K. L. Fowler, P. J. Nicholls, and C. Atterwill. 1986. Assessment of thyrotoxicity using in vitro cell culture systems. *Food Chemistry and Toxicology* 24:557–562.

Bruner, J. M., J. C. Scott-Moncrieff, and D. A. Williams. 1998. Effect of time of sample collection on thyroid stimulating hormone concentrations in euthyroid and hypothyroid dogs. *Journal of the American Veterinary Association* 212:1572–1575.

Capen, C. C. 1997. Mechanistic data and risk assessment of selected toxic end points of the thyroid gland. *Toxicologic Pathology* 25:39–48.

———. 1998. Correlation of mechanistic data and histopathology in the evaluation of selected toxic endpoints of the endocrine system. *Toxicology Letters* 102–103:405–409.

————. 1999. Thyroid and parathyroid toxicology. In *Endocrine and hormonal toxicology,* ed. P. W. Harvey, K. Rush, and A. Cockburn. Chichester, England: John Wiley & Sons Ltd.

Chauhan, K. R., P. R. Kodavanti, and J. D. McKinney. 2000. Assessing the role of ortho-substitution on polychlorinated biphenyl binding to transthyretin, a thyroxine transport protein. *Toxicology and Applied Pharmacology* 162:10–21.

Clément, S., S. Refetoff, B. Robaye, J. E. Dumont, and S. Schurmans. 2001. Low TSH requirement and goiter in transgenic mice overexpressing IGF-I andIGF-Ir receptor in the thyroid gland. *Endocrinology* 142: 5131–5139.

Daminet, S., M. Paradis, K. R. Refsal, and C. Price. 1999. Short-term influence of prednisone and phenobarbital on thyroid function in euthyroid dogs. *Canadian Veterinary Journal* 40: 411–415.

Darras, V. M., K. A. Mol, S. Van der Geyten, and E. R. Kuhn. 1998. Control of peripheral thyroid hormone levels by activating and inactivating deiodinases. *Trends in Comparative Endocrinology and Neurobiology* 839:80–86.

Davies, D. T. 1993. Assessment of rodent thyroid endocrinology: Advantages and pitfalls. *Comparative Hematology International* 3:142–152.

————. 1996. Thyroid endocrinology. In *Animal clinical chemistry: A primer for toxicologists,* ed. G. O. Evans. London: Taylor & Francis.

DeVito, M. et al. 1999. Screening methods for thyroid hormone disruptors. *Environmental Health Perspectives* 107:407–415.

Dixon, R. M., S. W. Reid, and C. T. Mooney. 1999. Epidemiological, clinical, hematological and biochemical characteristics of canine hypothyroidism. *Veterinary Record* 145:481–487.

Ekins, R. P., A. K. Sinha, M. R. Pickard, I. M. Evans, and F. al Yatama. 1994. Transport of thyroid hormones to target tissues. *Acta Medica Austriaca* 21:26–34.

Emerson, C. H., J. H. Cohen, R. A. Young, S. Alex, and S. L. Fang. 1990. Gender-related differences of serum thyroxine-binding proteins in the rat. *Acta Endocrinology Copenhagen* 123:72–78.

Ferguson, D. C. 1988. The effects of nonthyroidal factors on thyroid function test in dogs. *Compendium of Continuing Education for the Practicing Veterinarian* 10:1365–1377.

————. 1995. Free thyroid hormone measurement in the diagnosis of thyroid disease. In *Current veterinary therapy. XII,* ed. J. D. Banagura and R. W. Kirk. Philadelphia: W. B. Saunders Co.

Friesema, E. C. et al. 1999. Identification of thyroid hormone transporters. *Biochemical and Biophysical Research Communications* 254:497–501.

Friesema, E. C., J. Jansen, C. Milici, and T. J. Visser. 2005. Thyroid hormone transporters. *Vitamins and Hormones* 70:137–167.

Gianella-Neto, D., H-J. Quabbe, and I. Witt. 1981. Pattern of thyrotrophin and thyroxine plasma concentrations during the 24-h sleep–wake cycle in the male rhesus monkey. *Endocrinology* 109:2144–2151.

Gieger, T. L., G. Hosgood, J. Taboada, K. J. Wolfsheimer, and P. B. Mueller. 2000. Thyroid function and serum hepatic enzyme activity in dogs after phenobarbitone administration. *Journal of Veterinary Internal Medicine* 14:277–281.

Hamolsky, M. W., A. Golodetz, and A. S. Freedberg. 1959. The plasma protein-thyroid hormone complex in man. III. Further studies on the use of the *in vitro* red blood cell uptake of I_{131} triiodothyronine as a diagnostic test of thyroid function. *Journal of Clinical Endrocrinology and Metabolism* 19:101–116.

Hill, R. N., L. S. Erdreich, O. E. Paynter, P. A. Roberts, S. L. Rosenthal, and C. F. Wilkinson. 1989. Thyroid follicular carcinogenesis: Review. *Fundamental and Applied Toxicology* 12:629–637.

Hood, A., M. L. Allen, Y. Liu, J. Liu, and C. D. Klaassen. 2003. Induction of T(4) UDP-GT activity, serum thyroid stimulating hormone, and thyroid follicular cell proliferation in mice treated with microsomal enzyme inducers. *Toxicology and Applied Pharmacology* 188:6–13.

Hood, A., R. Hashmi, and C. D. Klaassen. 1999. Effects of microsomal enzyme inducers on thyroid follicular cell proliferation, hyperplasia, and hypertrophy. *Toxicology and Applied Pharmacology* 160:163–170.

Hood, A., and C. D. Klaassen. 2000a. Differential effects of microsomal enzyme inducers on in vitro thyroxine (T(4)) and triiodothyronine (T(3)) glucuronidation. *Toxicological Science* 55:78–84.

————. 2000b. Effects of microsomal enzyme inducers on outer-ring deiodinase activity toward thyroid hormones in various rat tissues. *Toxicology and Applied Pharmacology* 163:240–248.

Iversen, L., A. L. Jensen, R. Høier, and H. Aaes. 1999. Biological variation of canine serum thyrotrophin (TSH) concentration. *Veterinary Clinical Pathology* 28:16–19.

Jensen, A. L., and R. Høier. 1996. Evaluation of thyroid function in dogs by hormone analysis: Effects on data of biological variation. *Veterinary Clinical Pathology* 25:130–134.

Jordan, D., B. Rousset, F. Perrin, M. Fournier, and J. Orgiazzi. 1980. Evidence for circadian variations in serum thyrotrophin 3,5,3′-triiodothyronine and thyroxine in the rat. *Endocrinology* 107:1245–1248.

Kanno, J., C. Matsuoka, K. Furyta, H. Onodera, H. Miyajima, A. Maekama, and Y. Hayashi. 1990. Tumor promoting effect of goitrogens on the rat thyroid. *Toxicologic Pathology* 18:239–246.

Klaassen, C. D., and A. M. Hood. 2001. Effects of microsomal enzyme inducers on thyroid follicular cell proliferation and thyroid hormone metabolism. *Toxicologic Pathology* 29:34–40.

Larsson, M., T. Pettersson, and A. Carlstrom. 1985. Thyroid hormone binding in serum of 15 vertebrate species: Isolation of thyroxine-binding globulin and prealbumin analogs. *General Comparative Endocrinology* 58:360–375.

Leppaluoto, J., T. Ranta, and J. Tuomisto. 1974. Diurnal variation of serum immunoassayable thyrotrophin (TSH) in the rat. *Acta Physiologica Scandinavica* 90:699–702.

Meij, B. P., J. A. Mol, and A. Rijnberk. 1996. Thyroid stimulating hormone responses after single administration of thyrotrophin-releasing hormone and combined administration of four hypothalamic releasing hormones in beagle dogs. *Domestic Animal Endocrinology* 13:465–468.

Mooney, C. T., R. E. Shiel, and R. M. Dixon. 2008. Thyroid hormone abnormalities and outcome in dogs with non-thyroidal illness. *Journal of Small Animal Practice* 49:11–16.

OECD. 2006a. Detailed review paper on thyroid hormone disruption assays, no. 57. Series on testing and assessment. Paris: OECD.

————. 2006b. Report on the validation of updated guideline 407: Repeat dose 28-oral toxicity study in laboratory rats, no. 59. Series on testing and assessment. Paris: OECD.

Onodera, H., K. Mitsumori, M. Takahashi, T. Shimo, K. Yasuhara, K. Kitaura, M. Takahashi, and Y. Hayahsi. 1994. Thyroid proliferative lesions induced by antithyroid drugs in rats are not always accompanied by sustained increase in serum TSH. *Journal of Toxicological Sciences* 19:227–234.

Ottenweiler, J. E., and G. A. Hedge. 1982. Diurnal variations of plasma thyrotrophin, thyroxine and triiodothyronine in female rats are phase shifted after inversion of the photoperiod. *Endocrinology* 111:509–514.

Panciera, D. L., and S. A. Johnston. 2002. Results of thyroid tests and concentrations of plasma proteins in dogs administered etodalac. *American Journal of Veterinary Research* 62:1492–1495.

Pohlenz, J., A. Maqueem, K. Cua, R. E. Weiss, J. van Sande, and S. Refetoff. 1999. Improved radioimmunoassay for measurement of mouse thyroptrophin in serum: Strain differences in thyrotrophin concentration and thyrotroph sensitivity to thyroid hormone. *Thyroid* 9:1265–1271.

Refetoff, S., N. I. Robin, and U. S. Fang. 1970. Parameters of thyroid function in serum of 16 selected vertebrate species a study of PBI, serum T4, free T3 and the pattern of T4 and T3 binding in serum protein. *Endocrinology* 86:793–805.

Reimers, T. J., D. F. Lawler, P. M. Sutaria, M. T. Correa, and H. N. Erb. 1990. Effects of age, sex and body size on serum concentrations of thyroid and adrenocortical hormones in dogs. *American Journal of Veterinary Research* 3:454–457.

Savu, L., R. Vranckx, M. Maya, D. Gripois, M. F. Blouquit, and E. A. Nunez. 1989. Thyroxine-binding globulin and thyroxine-binding prealbumin in hypothyroid and hyperthyroid developing rats. *Biochimica et Biophysica Acta* 992:379–384.

Spencer, C. A., and C. C. Wang. 1995. Thyroglobulin measurement. Techniques, clinical benefits, and pitfalls. *Endocrinology and Metabolism Clinics of North America* 24:841–863.

Takagi, H., K. Mitsumori, H. Onodera, M. Nasu, T. Tamura, K. Yasuhara, K. Takegawa, and M. Hirose. 2002. Improvement of a two-stage carcinogenesis model to detect modifying effects of endocrine disrupting chemicals on thyroid carcinogenesis in rats. *Cancer Letters* 178:1–9.

Tanabe, Y., T. Ishii, and Y. Tamaki. 1969. Comparison of thyroxine-binding plasma proteins of various vertebrates and their evolutionary aspects. *General Comparative Endocrinology* 13:14–21.

Taurog, A., M. L. Dorris, and D. R. Doerge. 1996. Minocycline and the thyroid: Antithyroid effects of the drug, and the role of thyroid peroxidase in minocycline-induced black pigmentation of the gland. *Thyroid* 6:211–219.

Vranckx, R., M. Rouaze-Romet, L. Savu, P. Mechighel, M. Maya, and E. A. Nunez. 1994. Regulation of rat thyroxine-binding globulin and transthyretin: Studies in thyroidectomized and hypophysectomized rats given tri-iodothyronine or/and growth hormone. *Journal of Endocrinology* 142:77–84.

Vranckx, R., L. Savu, M. Maya, and E. A. Nunez. 1990. Characterization of a major development regulated serum thyroxine-binding globulin in the euthyroid mouse. *Biochemical Journal* 271:373–379.

Calcitonin

Copp, D. H. 1994. Calcitonin: Discovery, development and clinical applications. *Clinical and Investigative Medicine* 17:268–277.

Crass, M. F., and L. V. Avioli. 1994. *Calcium regulating hormones and cardiovascular function.* Boca Raton, FL: CRC Press.

Habener, J. F., F. R. Singer, L. J. Deftos, R. M. Neer, and J. T. Potts. 1971. Explanation for unusual potency of salmon calcitonin. *Nature: New Biology* 232:91–92.

Hazewinkel, H. A., I. Schoenmakers, D. Pelling, M. Snijdelaaar, J. Wolfswinkel, and J. A. Mol. 1999. Biological potency and radioimmunoassay of canine calcitonin— Calibration by international collaborative study. *Domestic Animal Endocrinology* 17:333–344.

Moukhtar, M. S., D. Tharoud, A. Julliene, D. Raulais, C. Calmettes, and G. Milhaud. 2005. Immunological similarity of human and rat calcitonin confirmed by immunofluorescent methods. *Cellular and Molecular Life Science* 30:1420–1471.

Newsome, F.E., R. K. O'Dor, C. O. Parkes, and D. H. Copp. 1973. A study of the stability of calcitonin biological activity. *Endocrinology* 92:1102–1106.

Woodman, D. D. 1997. Thyroid and parathyroid hormones. In *Laboratory animal endocrinology*, pp. 214–218. Chichester, England: John Wiley & Sons Ltd.

Section 10.3: Other Endocrine Glands

10.3.1 INTRODUCTION

This section discusses some of the tests for assessing the functionality and toxic injury to several of the endocrine glands other than the thyroid glands. It is important to recognize and distinguish hormonal changes due to direct or indirect toxicities from dysfunctional endocrine changes due to exaggerated pharmacology or changes that occur spontaneously.

10.3.2 ADRENAL GLANDS

These glands are situated adjacent to the kidneys and have several distinct anatomical zones that are functionally different. The outer adrenal cortex has three distinct zones: the outer zona glomerulosa, the intermediate zona fasciculate, and the inner zona reticularis, which adjoins the central adrenal medulla.

10.3.2.1 ADRENAL CORTEX

Within the adrenal cortex, the zona glomerulosa is the site of mineralocorticoid production, which includes aldosterone, so this zone is therefore associated with electrolyte homeostasis (see Chapter 6). The inner two cortical zones secrete glucocorticoids, adrenal androgens, estrogens, and progesterone, but the rates of synthesis for both estrogens and androgens are lower than in the gonads. Some of the zonal differences are related to steroidogenic enzyme systems involving the members of the cytochrome (CYP) P450 family. In the adrenal mitochondrial and microsomal fractions, a number of the CYP 11, 17, 19, and 21 subsets of the cytochrome family affect various adrenal steroid hydroxylase enzymes. However, these biochemical functions are not totally separate because cells may slightly alter their location and function within the adrenal cortex. The adrenal glands secrete androstenedione, dihydroepiandrosterone (DHEA), and its sulfate (DHEAS), which are converted in peripheral tissues to the potent androgens testosterone and 5α-testosterone; the adrenal androgens are also precursors for estrogen synthesis in some other tissues.

The biosynthesis and secretion of these adrenal cortical hormones are influenced by the hypothalamus–pituitary axis and the adrenocorticotrophic hormone (ACTH) and its associated feedback mechanisms (Figure 10.3.1). The secretions of ACTH are pulsatile, and they are influenced more by the central nervous system and the pituitary gland than the glucocorticoid feedback mechanisms.

The glucocorticoids influence the metabolism of carbohydrates, lipids, and proteins in the liver, muscle, and adipose tissues; these steroids promote gluconeogenesis,

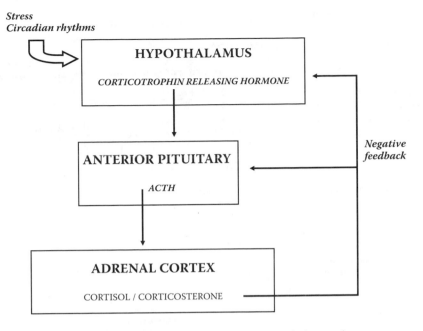

Stress
Circadian rhythms

HYPOTHALAMUS

CORTICOTROPHIN RELEASING HORMONE

ANTERIOR PITUITARY

ACTH

Negative feedback

ADRENAL CORTEX

CORTISOL / CORTICOSTERONE

FIGURE 10.3.1   Simplified pathways for the hypothalamus–pituitary axis.

glycogen storage, and fatty acid metabolism. The glucocorticoids also have anti-inflammatory actions inhibiting the accumulation of leukocytes and the adhesion of neutrophils at sites of inflammation, and these properties underlie the application of glucocorticoids as anti-inflammatory treatments.

The two primary glucocorticoids of interest are the structurally similar corticosterone and cortisol, and there are some species differences in the proportions of these two glucocorticoids (Figure 10.3.2). In the rat and mouse, corticosterone is the principal glucocorticoid; cortisol is the principal glucocorticoid in dog, nonhuman primates, guinea pigs, and humans. Corticosterone is higher in female rats compared to males, and the values change during the estrus cycle; they are highest in the late proestrus stage. Corticosterone levels are lower in rats aged about 2 years (Carnes et al. 1994). More marked responses to ACTH are observed in female rats compared to male rats (Rivier 1994). In hamsters, both cortisol and corticosterone are secreted, but with higher levels of corticosterone, and the proportions of these two glucocorticoids change during the day (Albers et al. 1985; Ottenweller et al. 1985); the daily values show similar patterns to other nocturnal rodents. The adrenal gland to body weight ratio is relatively large, and the primary glucocorticoid is cortisol in the guinea pig, making this species a useful model for assessing adrenal toxicity (Colby 1987, 1988), although there is a high rate of interconversion between cortisol and cortisone (Manin, Tournaire, and DeLost 1982).

The circulating levels of adrenal cortical hormones in rats depend on several factors, including age, season, and strain (Wong et al. 1983; Carnes et al. 1994), gender

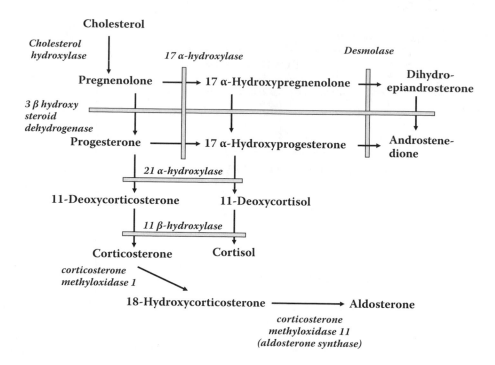

FIGURE 10.3.2 Steroid biosynthesis in the adrenal cortex. The relevant enzymes are in italics and boxes indicate where the enzymes catalyze more than one reaction.

and light (Critchlow et al. 1963; Buckingham, Dohler, and Wilson 1978), handling and environment (Barrett and Stockham 1963; Dunn and Scheving 1971; Dohler et al. 1978; Jurcovicova et al. 1984), and circadian rhythm (Ottenweller et al. 1979; D'Agostino, Vaeth, and Henning 1982; Jones et al. 1987). In the mouse, there is a diurnal variation with maximal values occurring at the start of the dark cycle for males and later in the dark cycle for females (Scheving et al. 1983). In dogs, a circadian rhythm is not always apparent (Johnston and Mather 1978), but episodic secretion of cortisol and ACTH has been reported (Kemppainen and Sartin 1984; Orth, Peterson, and Drucker 1988).

These steroid hormones are sparingly soluble in aqueous media and are transported in plasma mainly bound to proteins, but it is the free (or unbound) hormone levels that are important for the biological activity in the target tissues. Corticosteroids are bound to plasma proteins including transcortin (corticosteroid binding globulin: CBG) and albumin, and these proteins have differing affinities and binding capacities for the corticoids. Transcortin is synthesized in the liver and it is an alpha-1-globulin with a molecular mass of about 53 kDa. It appears to be present in most species (Seal and Doe 1965; Hsu and Kuhn 1988), and the binding capacities of CBG vary across the species (Gayrard, Alvinerie, and Toutain 1996.) In the mouse, corticosterone circulates as free and bound forms with about 99% bound to CBG or albumin; in the dog, the free fraction has been estimated to be about 10% of the total plasma cortisol (Meyer and Rothuizen 1993).

10.3.2.2 ADRENAL MEDULLA

The adrenal medulla forms part of the sympathetic nervous system and is the primary site for the production of the catecholamines—epinephrine (adrenaline) and norepinephrine (noradrenaline), which are primary hormones (also called biogenic amines). The cells of the medulla are arranged in lobules and the medulla contains chromaffin cells, which are modified postganglionic cells of the sympathetic nervous system. The medulla produces catecholamines from tyrosine and their structures contain catechol and amine groups (Figure 10.3.3).

The hormone epinephrine is synthesized in the medulla and released into the bloodstream, whereas norepinephrine is synthesized and stored in sympathetic nerve endings and acts as a neurotransmitter. Glucocorticoids from the adrenal cortex stimulate the conversion of norepinephrine to epinephrine, and these two catecholamines are released from the adrenal glands in response to stress. The actions of catecholamines are mediated through adrenergic receptors, which may alter the function of blood vessels, heart, intestine, ureter, eye pupils, and several other tissues. Alpha-adrenergic receptors are associated with excitatory responses and beta-adrenergic receptors are associated with inhibitory responses, although there are some exceptions; there are subsets of both alpha- and beta-receptors (Carmichael and Stoddard 1992).

The catecholamines affect most of the body's tissues by altering blood flow and energizing tissues, particularly in fight/flight responses. Within the blood,

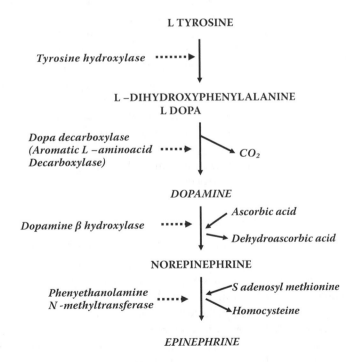

FIGURE 10.3.3 Catecholamine synthesis.

approximately 50% of the catecholamines are loosely bound to plasma albumin. Dopamine is another neurotransmitter/biogenic amine synthesized from tyrosine in the adrenal medulla and in nervous tissue; this amine is catabolized by mono-amine oxidase and catechol-O-methyl transferase to homovanillic acid, which is excreted in the urine. Epinephrine and norepinephrine are catabolized primarily in the liver, but breakdown also occurs in several other tissues. These catecholamines are excreted mainly as unconjugated 3-methoxy-4-hydroxymandelic acid (VMA) and 3-methoxy-4-hydroxyphenylglycol (MOPG).

10.3.2.3 TOXIC EFFECTS ON THE ADRENALS

The adrenal glands are supplied by a good vascular system, and the high tissue lipid content assists the entry and transport of xenobiotics (including fat-soluble xenobi-otics) into the adrenal tissues. In addition, enzymes—particularly the cytochrome P450s—may metabolize xenobiotics to more potent toxic metabolites or reduce the potential toxicity caused by the xenobiotic by inactivation. The toxic effects may be localized to specific regions, cause more generalized necrosis, or be a general-ized effect that follows necrosis initially within a zone of the cortex. Several differ-ing mechanisms affecting steroid metabolism can cause adrenal cortex toxicities (Ribelin 1984; Szabo and Lippe 1989; Harvey 1996; Colby et al. 1997; Rosol et al. 2001).

Example compounds affecting the adrenal cortex include acrylonitrile, amino-gluthemide, amytriptyline, aniline, carbon tetrachloride (Colby et al. 1994), chloro-form, cimetidine, etomidate, domperidone, fluphenazine, glycyrrhizin, ketoconazole (Loose et al. 1983), methanol, parathion, pentabarbitone, phencyclidine, pyra-zole, spironolactone, tamoxifen, and urethane (Colby and Longhurst 1992; Szabo and Sandoz 1997). Amytriptyline and cimetidine reduce corticosterone secretion, whereas pentobarbitone and phencyclidine increase its secretion. Etomidate inhib-its 11β- and 17α-hydroxylating reactions. Spironolactone affects cytochrome P450 enzymes (Kossor et al. 1991), and domperidone blocks cortisol secretion. Some ACAT inhibitors cause adrenal cytotoxicity (Wolfgang et al. 1995).

Example compounds affecting the adrenal medulla include acrylonitrile, cysteam-ine, dichloromethane, malathion, estrogens, and thiouracil.

10.3.2.4 LABORATORY INVESTIGATIONS FOR ADRENAL CORTEX

Severe toxic effects on the adrenals cause metabolic changes, which may be detected by measurements of plasma glucose, electrolytes, cholesterol, and proteins without resorting to the measurement of plasma hormones or urinary hormones or using adrenal function tests. Some additional information that may indicate adrenal tox-icities can be gained from fluid balance and hematology, where the blood leuko-cyte values may suggest responses to inflammation or stress. In the dog, plasma alkaline phosphatase may be induced by excessive steroid production (see Chapter 2). As a consequence of hepatic toxicity or excessive renal loss of protein, some hormonal alterations can be caused by changes to plasma binding proteins. The control mechanisms for the glucocorticoids and mineralocorticoids are essentially independent of each other, but both may be affected in severe adrenal toxicity.

Plasma cortisol and corticosterone may be measured by various methods, including chemiluminescence, radioimmunoassays, enzyme linked immunosorbent assays, and fluorimetry (for examples, see Ginel et al. 1998 and Russell et al. 2007). Measurements of basal plasma cortisol or corticosterone and following administration of ACTH (or synthetic analogues) can be used as a functional test for the adrenals; the use of adrenal functional measurements has been advocated for rats and dogs (Feldman 1983; Garnier et al. 1990; Wolfgang et al. 1995; Kemppainen, Behrend, and Busch 2005; Harvey, Everett, and Springall 2007). The ACTH procedures require careful sample timing, and this can be achieved more readily in canine studies, where the animal numbers are generally smaller than those in rodent studies.

To avoid hormonal changes due to blood collection procedures, alternative non-invasive measurements using urine and feces have been suggested, particularly by investigators of stress caused in mice and rats by animal husbandry and other experimental procedures. These methods can produce highly variable results because of sampling procedures, even though these do not involve blood collection (Macleod and Shapiro 1988; Touma et al. 2003) Furthermore, urine corticosterone measurements have been suggested as a measure of stress-mediated immunological changes in rats, particularly for compounds that target the central nervous system and produce nonspecific stress responses, which may be accompanied by altered immunological parameters (Pruett et al. 2008).

Urinary corticoid measurements (in 17–24 h, but not short-term samples) can be used to assess adrenocortical function as alternatives to blood sampling techniques (Hilfenhaus 1977). The use of urinary measurements over a timed period may provide a better indication of corticosteroid metabolism in contrast to the fluctuations observed in plasma measurements. Although some reports in the literature use randomly collected urine for veterinary clinical diagnosis, these measurements are not suitable for toxicological studies. Older methods for urinary 17-hydroxycorticosteroids have been replaced by cortisol or corticosterone measurements.

For ACTH measurements, although there are small differences in amino acid sequences, most antibodies appear to react across several species, and several immunoassays have been used and reported in the literature. Plasma ACTH assays are problematic because the samples need to be carefully collected, separated promptly, and stored at low temperatures using ice. The proteinase inhibitor aprotinin has been used to reduce sample degradation (Kemppainen, Clark, and Peterson 1994; Scott-Moncrieff et al. 2003).

There are functional tests in which ACTH or glucocorticoid measurements can be made following the administration of metyrapone, which inhibits adrenal 11β-hydroxylase activity and causes a transient reduction in cortisol synthesis and increased secretion of 11-deoxycortisol (Orth et al. 1988), or dexamethasone suppression tests. However, these are not commonly employed in toxicological studies.

It is perhaps a little surprising that improved analytical methods (e.g., high-performance liquid chromatography, proton resonance mass spectrometry) have not led to a reexamination of catecholamines as markers of stress and adrenal medullary function.

10.3.3   GONADS

Reproductive toxicology may be defined as any adverse effect on any aspect of male or female sexual structure or function, including conception and lactation, which may interfere with the production and development of normal offspring to maturity (Witorsch 1995). It is important to recognize the importance of reproductive and teratology studies in the detection of toxicants to the reproductive system (ICH 2005) and perhaps how little used are the biochemical measurements of the hormones that drive the reproductive systems in these regulatory studies.

10.3.3.1   OVARIES

The hormonal control of the female reproductive system involves several hormones of the hypothalamic–pituitary–ovarian axis. The hypothalamic secretion of a decapeptide—gonadotrophin releasing hormone (GnRH; also sometimes termed luteinizing hormone releasing factor: LHRH)—acts in a pulsatile manner to stimulate the release of follitrophin (or follicle stimulating hormone: FSH) and luteotrophin (luteinizing hormone or lutropin: LH) from the anterior pituitary gland. These two gonadotrophins (FSH and LH) are dimeric glycoproteins of similar molecular mass. The alpha-monomer is identical for FSH, LH, and thyroid stimulating hormone (TSH), although the beta-monomers differ, and both LH and FSH have short half-lives of less than 30 min (Figure 10.3.4).

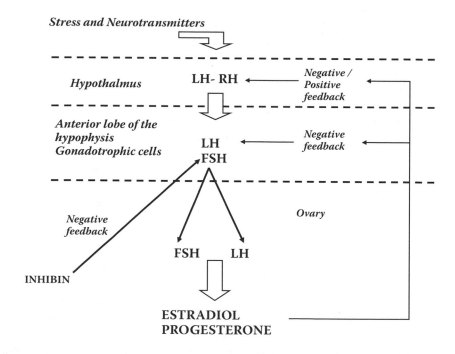

FIGURE 10.3.4   Schematic diagram for hormonal regulation in females.

Within the ovary are three functional units: the follicle, the oocyte, and the corpus luteum. LH targets the thecal cells, corpus luteum, promotion of ovulation, and differentiation of luteal cells (luteinization). FSH affects the maturation of the follicles and stimulates steroid hormone production by the granulosa cells. Ovarian production of estrogens occurs in the follicles, corpus luteum, and the placenta. This is driven by the production of androgens in the ovarian thecal cells by LH, followed by conversions of testosterone to estradiol and androstenedione to estrone by aromatase enzymes. The estrogens have similar structures and are also produced in the adrenal glands and adipose tissue, but mainly in the ovaries. The estrogens interact with estrogen receptors in various tissues. There are several positive and negative feedback mechanisms in the female hormonal regulation pathways (Woodman 1997).

Other hormones involved in the female reproductive system include androgens, gestagens, and prolactin. The androgens modulate production and secretion of the hypophyseal gonadotrophins. Gestagens include the steroid progesterone, which is synthesized in the corpus luteum and placenta, and progesterone acts in the uterus to control the secretory transformation of the endometrium. Prolactin is a single chain polypeptide, and its hypophyseal synthesis and release are controlled by neuronal dopamine, prolactin inhibiting factor (PIF), and prolactin releasing factor (PRF).

In laboratory animals, the estrous and menstrual cycles vary in their duration and frequency; these cycles are much shorter in mice, rats, and hamsters (approximately 4 days) compared to humans (Donham and Stetson 1991; Chattopadhyay et al. 1999). There are several rhythmic patterns of the plasma reproductive hormones, together with natural episodic/pusatile changes (e.g., LH is secreted in a pulsatile manner and these pulses can cause plasma levels to vary by more than several-fold from baseline values) (Moor and Younglai 1975). Reproductive senescence occurs in older animals (e.g., in rodents where female rats develop irregularities in their estrous cycle at about 10 months of age).

10.3.3.2 Testes

The mammalian testis can be functionally separated into the seminiferous tubules and interstitial region with its Leydig cells (or interstitial cells). The major function of the Leydig cells is the maintenance of spermatogenesis, which is partially mediated by the production of testosterone and dihydrotestosterone. Androgens (which have structural similarities with estrogens) govern maturation and the maintenance of the male sexual characteristics, and testosterone is the principal androgen; some androgens are produced by the adrenal glands (Mooradian, Morley, and Korenman 1987). Androgens also have an effect on hepatic microsomal cytochrome P450 enzymes.

In the seminiferous tubules, there are two major cell types: the spermatogonial and the Sertoli cells. The functions of the Sertoli cells include the synthesis of androgen binding proteins, controlling nutrition for the developing sperm cells, and maintenance of the blood–testis barrier. The endocrine control of testicular function is mainly exercised by LH (also called interstitial cell stimulating hormone: ICSH) and FSH; the Leydig and Sertoli cells are the primary targets for LH and FSH, respectively, but the homeostatic control of this hypothalamo–pituitary–testicular (HPT) axis is complex, with several overlapping functions and feedback mechanisms at different sites (Woodman 1997) (Figure 10.3.5). A number of other local regulating factors include inhibin and pro-opiomelanocortin metabolites, and neuropeptides and prolactin also appear to act together with LH and FSH in regulating testosterone metabolism (Lindzey et al. 1994). However, the hormonal control of the reproductive system is less complex compared to females.

In plasma, testosterone and its active metabolite 5α-dihydrotestosterone circulate as free steroids and as fractions that are protein bound, mainly to albumin. Both testosterone and estradiol are bound to sex hormone binding globulin (SHBG; which also has been called testosterone-estradiol binding globulin: TEBG). This protein is a hepatic glycoprotein that shows greater affinity for androgens. SHBG appears to be absent from plasma in rats and mice and shows different binding preferences in non-human primates (primarily 17β-hydroxyandrogens and estradiol) and in dogs and rabbits (primarily androgens) (Corvol and Bardin 1973; Danzo and Joseph 1994). The Sertoli cells produce an androgenic binding glycoprotein (ABP) that is very similar to SHBG (Gunsalus, Musto, and Bardin 1978; Bardin et al. 1981; Gunsalus et al. 1981; Spitz et al. 1985). The hepatic production of the major urinary protein in male rats—alpha$_{2u}$-globulin—is influenced by androgens (Swenberg 1993), and there are interactions between testosterone and the renal production of erythropoietin (Foresta et al. 1995; Malgor et al. 1998).

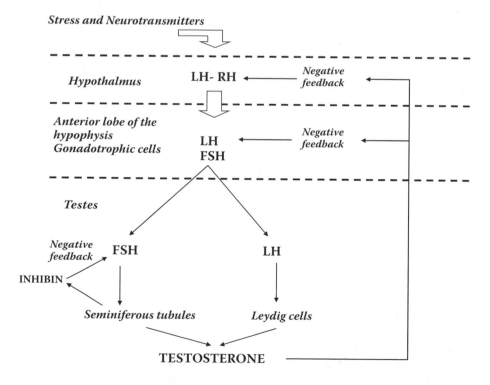

FIGURE 10.3.5   Schematic diagram for hormonal regulation in males.

Rats exhibit circadian rhythms for plasma testosterone (Kalra and Kalra 1977; Mock, Norton, and Frankel 1978). Episodic fluctuations of this hormone have been reported in rabbits (Moor and Younglai 1975), dogs (de Palaitis, Moore, and Falvo 1978; Fukuda et al. 1988), and rhesus monkeys (Michael, Setchell, and Plant 1974; Plant 1981).

10.3.3.3 Toxic Effects

Xenobiotics may act directly because they possess a structural similarity to endogenous compounds (e.g., acting as antagonists or agonists of gonadotrophic hormones) or because of a general toxic effect (e.g., tissue necrosis observed with alkylating agents). Some toxins act indirectly by affecting the enzymes involved in steroid synthesis and in hepatic metabolism. Although the levels of cytochrome P450s and mixed function oxidases are lower in the testes and ovaries compared to the liver, these enzymes can be important in local biotransformations of xenobiotics to more toxic metabolites (Lovekamp-Swan and Davis 2003; Fan et al. 2004). Compounds may also cause toxicity via the neuroendocrine centers by influencing the production of gonadotrophic hormones (James, Crook, and Heywood 1979; Mattison and Thomford 1989) and via effects of the thyroid glands. Sometimes the causation of the toxicity may not be the most obvious candidate mechanism; for example, the toxicity observed in dogs given estrogens is due to bone marrow suppression rather than the estrogenic action on the gonads (Johnson 1989).

In ovarian toxicity, the granulosa cells, thecal cells, and oocytes may all be targeted by toxins, and there may be inhibitory effects on ovulation, ovum transport, fertilization, or implantation (Haney 1985; Jarrell et al. 1988; Mattison et al. 1990; Woodman 1997; Mitchell et al. 2004; Hoyer 2005). Perturbations due to xenobiotics can occur in various stages of hormonal regulation, including synthesis, release and storage, transport and clearance, receptor recognition and binding, and postreceptor activation.

Example compounds include heptachlor and ketoconazole (affect hormone synthesis); lead and cadmium (interfere with steroidogenic enzymes); tributylin, erythrosine, and rose Bengal (affect ovarian microsomal aromatase); endosulphan, lindane, and malathion (affect hormone release and storage); DDT analogs (affect hormone transport and clearance); 2,2,-bis-4-hydroxyphenyl propane and some PPARs (affect ovarian P450s) (Lovekamp-Swan and Davis 2003); phenobarbitone and clofibrate (increase hepatic metabolism of estradiol and progesterone); atachlor, aldrin, dieldrin nafoxidine, tamoxifen, and paradichorobenzene (affect hormone receptors); and meclofenamate (reduces progesterone release).

Although a large number of diverse compounds have been reported to affect the male reproductive system, only a few of the underlying mechanisms for these compounds have been elucidated. Again, disruption of the male reproductive system can occur in various stages: synthesis, release and storage, transport and clearance, receptor recognition and binding, and postreceptor activation of hormones and spermatogenesis.

Some example compounds include aminogluthethimide cyanoketone and ketoconazole (affect hormone synthesis); lithium (interferes with steroidogenic enzymes); endosulphan, lindane, and malathion (affect hormone release and storage); DDT analogs (affect hormone transport and clearance); phenobarbitone and clofibrate (increase hepatic metabolism of androgens); cyproterone, dicaboximide metabolites, and the p,p′DDE metabolite of DDT (affect hormone receptors); and some phthalates, desethylamiodarone, hexane-2,5 dione, and 2-methoxyacetaldehyde (affect spermatogenesis cells). Most heavy metals acting on the testes primarily affect the germ cells, although they also may have some effects on the Sertoli cells. Cadmium primarily affects the endothelial cells of the vasculature (Biswas et al. 2001). A few compounds (e.g., some phthalates, 2,5-hexanedione, and dinitrobenzene) affect Sertoli cells (Boekelheide et al. 2003), and severe reductions of nutritional supply to the Sertoli cells also can affect their function.

10.3.4 LABORATORY INVESTIGATIONS

A number of suitable immunoassays and radioimmunoassays are available for measuring the major hormones testosterone, estrogen, LH, and FSH. Some of these assays may need adjustments to ensure that the majority of values fall within the optimal part of the measuring range because the ranges differ between laboratory animal species. Given the similarities in the structures of FSH and LH, some assays can be used for both rats and mice if the antisera are suitable (Jarrell et al. 1988). A number of methods have been described that use gas liquid or liquid chromatography combined with mass spectrometry, which can be used to measure several of the steroid hormones. The development of various contraceptives has often been helped by these hormone measurements as biomarkers of efficacy rather than markers of toxicity in animal models.

Although the masses and histopathology of the testes, epididymes, and sperm morphology are the primary indicators of possible toxic effects on the male reproductive system (Lanning et al. 2002; Creasy 2003), the measurement of circulating hormones and some other biomarkers and enzymes can assist in the diagnosis of testicular toxicity. Some hormones, such as inhibin, change in severe testicular toxicity, but inhibin is less useful as a marker of mild toxicity. The use of hormone measurements potentially should increase as suitable antibodies and methodologies become available, but they will still be limited by the considerable physiological inter- and intra-animal variations (episodic/pulsatile and chronobiochemical effects).

The application of several of the current hormone measurements does little to extend the histopathological findings for many endocrinological toxins. However, given the continued interest in "endocrine disrupters" (see Section 10.1), measurements of circulating levels of one or more hormones together with other specific indicators of endocrine organ function can be useful tools in defining the level at which functional impairment occurs and the progression of the lesions, as well as distinguishing among alterations of function, experiment stress, and effects due to toxic injury. The potential effects of sex hormone perturbations on immune function should also be considered and vice versa when the immune system is compromised (Luster, Pfeifer, and Tucker 1985).

The timing of sample collections is particularly critical for hormone measurements when effects on the female reproductive system are studied in smaller laboratory animals, given the shorter estrous cycles and pusatile/episodic changes of plasma hormones. Dealing with a group of female animals within study groups when they may be at different parts of the estrus requires a different approach to treatment groups when the experimental data are analyzed. An additional problem can be the temporal changes in the estrus cycle in these animals, which may be caused by the test compound. It is always important to consider the relative maturity of the animals in a study of effects on the reproductive systems of both sexes (Rehm 2000; Goedken, Kerlin, and Morton 2008).

Alternative approaches to hormone measurements have included the measurement of enzymes such as LDH-C4 and creatine. Several enzymes are specific to the testis, including lactate dehydrogenase isozyme LDH-C4 or LDH-X; this enzyme is synthesized at a particular stage of germ cell development, and it has been investigated and suggested as a target for contraceptive vaccines (Meistrich et al. 1977; Wheat et al. 1977; Wheat and Goldberg 1983). Increases of plasma LDH-C4 have been reported in several studies of acute testicular toxicity in the rat, where it is not normally detected in circulating blood (Haqqi and Adhami 1982; Itoh and Ozasa 1985; Reader, Shingles, and Stonard 1991). Creatinuria has been suggested as a marker of testicular damage because increases of urine creatine have been reported for several testicular toxicants (Gray et al. 1990; Moore et al. 1992; Timbrell 2000), but creatinuria is not specific for testicular injury because it has been observed in animal models of lead and cadmium poisoning where there has been no evidence of testicular injury. Proteomics may lead to the identification of other biomarkers of testicular toxicities (e.g., glutathione transferases, glyceraldehyde-3-phosphate dehydrogenase, phosphatidyl ethanolamine binding protein, and heat shock protein) (Yamamoto et al. 2005).

REFERENCES

The Adrenals

Albers, H. E., L. Yogev, R. B. Todd, and B. D. Goldman. 1985. Adrenal corticoids in hamsters: Role in circadian timing. *American Journal of Physiology* 248:R434–38.

Barrett, A. M., and M. A. Stockham. 1963. The effect of housing conditions and simple experimental procedures upon the corticosterone level in the plasma of rats. *Journal of Endocrinology* 26:97–105.

Buckingham, J. C., K. D. Dohler, and C. A. Wilson. 1978. Activity of the pituitary–adrenocortical system and thyroid gland during the estrous cycle of the rat. *Journal of Endocrinology* 78:359–366.

Carmichael, S. W., and S. L. Stoddard. 1992. *The adrenal medulla, 1989–1991.* Boca Raton, FL: CRC Press.

Carnes, M., B. M. Goodman, S. J. Lent, H. Vo, and R. Jaeckels. 1994. Coincident plasma ACTH and corticosterone time series: Comparisons between young and old rats. *Experimental Gerontology* 29:625–643.

Colby, H. D. 1987. The adrenal cortex. In *Clinical endocrine physiology,* ed. G. A. Hedge, H. D. Colby, and R. L. Goodman, pp. 127–159. Philadelphia: W. B. Saunders.

———. 1988. Adrenal gland toxicity: Chemically induced dysfunction. *Journal of the American College of Toxicology* 7:45–69.

Colby, H. D., and P. A. Longhurst. 1992. Toxicology of the adrenal gland. In *Endocrine toxicology,* ed. C. K. Atterwill and J. D. Flack, pp. 243–258. Cambridge: Cambridge University Press.

Colby, H. D., H. Purcell, S. Kominami, S. Takemori, and D. C. Kossor. 1994. Adrenal activation of carbon tetrachloride: Role of microsomal P450 isozymes. *Toxicology* 94:31–40.

Colby, H. D. et al. 1997. Toxicology of the adrenal cortex: Role of metabolic activation. In *Endocrine toxicology,* 2nd ed., ed. J. A. Thomas and H. D. Colby. New York: Taylor & Francis.

Critchlow, V., R. A. Liebelt, M. Bar-Sela, W. Mountcastle, and H. S. Lipscomb. 1963. Sex difference in the resting pituitary–adrenal function in the rat. *American Journal of Physiology* 205:807–815.

D'Agostino, J. B., G. F. Vaeth, and S. J. Henning. 1982. Diurnal rhythm of total and free concentrations of serum corticosterone in the rat. *Acta Endocrinologica (Copenhagen)* 100:85–90.

Dohler, K. D., C. C. Wong, D. Gaudssuhn, A. von zur Muhlen, K. Gartner, and U. Dohler. 1978. Site of blood sampling in rats as a possible source of error in hormone determinations. *Journal of Endocrinology* 79:141–142.

Dunn, J., and L. Scheving. 1971. Plasma corticosterone levels in rats killed sequentially at the "trough" or "peak" of the adrenocortical cycle. *Journal of Endocrinology* 49:347–348.

Feldman, E. C. 1983. Comparison of ACTH response and dexamethasone suppression as screening test in canine hyperadrenocorticism. *Journal of the American Veterinary Medical Association* 182:506–510.

Garnier, F., E. Benoit, M. Virat, R. Ochoa, and P. Delatour. 1990. Adrenal cortical response in clinically normal dogs before and after adaptation to a housing environment. *Laboratory Animals* 24:40–43.

Gayrard, V., M. Alvinerie, and P. L. Toutain. 1996. Interspecies variations of corticosteroid-binding globulin parameters. *Domestic Animal Endocrinology* 13:35–45.

Ginel, P. J., A. Perez-Rico, P. Moreno, and R. Lucena. 1998. Validation of a commercially available enzyme-linked immunosorbent assay (ELISA) for the determination of cortisol in canine plasma samples. *Veterinary Research Communications* 22:179–185.

Harvey, P. W., ed. 1996. *The adrenal in toxicology.* London: Taylor & Francis.

Harvey, P. W., D. J. Everett, and C. J. Springall. 2007. Adrenal toxicology: A strategy for assessment of functional toxicity to the adrenal cortex and steroidogenesis. *Journal of Applied Toxicology* 27:103–115.

Hilfenhaus, M. 1977. Urinary excretion of corticosterone as a parameter of adrenal cortical function in rats. *Naunyn-Schmiedebergs Archives of Pharmacology* 297 (Suppl. 11): R41.

Hsu, B. R., and R. W. Kuhn. 1988. The role of the adrenal in generating the diurnal variation in circulating levels of corticosteroid-binding globulin in the rat. *Endocrinology* 122:421–426.

Johnston, S. D., and E. C. Mather. 1978. Canine plasma cortisol (hydroxycortisone) measured by radioimmunoassay; clinical absence of diurnal variation and results of ACTH stimulation and dexamethasone suppression tests. *American Journal of Veterinary Research* 39:1766–1770.

Jones, M. K., W. P. Weisenburger, I. G. Sipes, and D. H. Russell. 1987. Circadian alterations in prolactin, corticosterone, and thyroid hormone levels and down-regulation of prolactin receptor activity by 2,3,7,8-tetrachlorodibenzo-p-dioxin. *Toxicology and Applied Pharmacology* 87:337–350.

Jurcovicova, J., M. Vigas, P. Klir, and D. Jezova. 1984. Response of prolactin, growth hormone and corticosterone to morphine administration or stress exposure in Wistar–AVN and Long–Evans rats. *Endocrinologica Experimentia* 18:209–214.

Kemppainen, R. J., T. P. Clark, and M. E. Peterson. 1994. Preservative effect of aprotinin on canine plasma immunoreactive adrenocorticotrophic concentration. *Domestic Animal Endocrinology* 11:355–362.

Kemppainen, R. J., E. N. Behrend, and K. A. Busch. 2005. Use of compounded adrenocorticotrophic hormone (ACTH) for adrenal function testing in dogs. *Journal of the American Animal Hospital Association* 41:368–372.

Kemppainen, R. J., and J. L. Sartin.1984. Evidence for episodic but not circadian rhythm in plasma concentrations of adrenocorticotrophin, cortisol and thyroxine in dogs. *Journal of Endocrinology* 103:219–226.

Kossor, D. C., S. Kominami, S. Takemori, and H. D. Colby. 1991. Role of steroid 17-alpha-hydroxylase in spironolactone mediated destruction of adrenal cytochrome p450. *Molecular Pharmacology* 40:321–325.

Loose, D. S., P. B. Kan, M. A. Jirst, T. A. Marcus, and D. Feldman. 1983. Ketoconazole blocks adrenal steroidogenesis by inhibiting cytochrome P450-dependent enzymes. *Journal of Clinical Investigation* 71:1495–1499.

Macleod, J. N., and B. H. Shapiro. 1988. Repetitive blood sampling in unrestrained and unstressed mice using a chronic indwelling right atrial catheterization apparatus. *Laboratory Animal Science* 38:603–608.

Manin, M., C. Tournaire, and P. DeLost. 1982. Measurement of the rate of secretion, peripheral metabolism and interconversion of cortisol and cortisone in adult conscious male guinea pigs. *Steroids* 39:81–88.

Meyer, H. P., and J. Rothuizen. 1993. Determination of the percentage of free cortisol in plasma in the dog by ultrafiltration. *Domestic Animal Endocrinology* 10:45–53.

Orth, D. N., M. E. Peterson, and W. D. Drucker. 1988. Plasma immunoreactive proopiomelanocortin peptides and cortisol in normal dogs and dogs with Cushing's syndrome: Diurnal rhythm and responses to various stimuli. *Endocrinology* 122:1250–1262.

Ottenweller, J. E., A. H. Meier, A. C. Russo, and M. E. Frenzke. 1979. Circadian rhythms of plasma corticosterone binding activity in the rat and mouse. *Acta Endocrinoligica (Copenhagen)* 91:150–157.

Ottenweller, J. E., W. N. Tapp, J. M. Burke, and B. H. Natelson. 1985. Plasma cortisol and corticosterone concentrations in the golden hamster (*Mesocricetus auratus*). *Life Sciences* 37:1551–1558.

Pruett, S., J. M. Lapointe, W. Reagan, M. Lawton, and T. T. Kawabata. 2008. Urinary corticosterone as an indicator of stress-mediated immunological changes in rats. *Journal of Immunotoxicology* 5:17–22.

Ribelin, W. E. 1984. Effects of drugs and chemicals upon the structure of the adrenal gland. *Fundamental and Applied Toxicology* 4:105–119.

Rivier, C. 1994. Stimulatory effect of interleukin-1 beta on the hypothalamic–pituitary–adrenal axis of the rat: Influence of age, gender and circulating sex steroids. *Journal of Endocrinology* 140:365–372.

Rosol, T. J., J. T. Yarrington, J. Latendresse, and C. C. Capen. 2001. Adrenal gland: Structure, function and mechanisms of toxicity. *Toxicologic Pathology* 29:41–48.

Russell, N. J., S. Foster, P. Clark, I. D. Robertson, D. Lewis, and P. J. Irwin. 2007. Comparison of radioimmunoassay and chemiluminescent assay methods to estimate canine blood cortisol concentrations. *Australian Veterinary Journal* 85:487–494.

Scheving, L. E., T. H. Tsai, E. W. Powell, J. N. Pasley, F. Halberg, and J. Dunn. 1983. Bilateral lesions of suprachiasmatic nuclei affect circadian rhythms in [3H]-thymidine incorporation into deoxyribonucleic acid in mouse intestinal tract, mitotic index of corneal eptithelium and serum corticosterone. *Anatomical Record* 205:239–249.

Scott-Moncrieff, J. C., M. A. Kosho, J. A. Brown, K. Hill, and K. R. Refsal. 2003. Validation of a chemiluminescent method enzyme immunometric assay for plasma adrenocorticotrophic hormone in the dog. *Veterinary Clinical Pathology* 32:180–187.

Seal, U. S., and R. P. Doe. 1965. Vertebrate distribution of corticosteroid-binding globulin and some endocrine effects on concentration. *Steroids* 5:827–841.

Szabo, S., and I. T. Lippe. 1989. Adrenal gland: Chemically induced structural and functional changes in the cortex. *Toxicologic Pathology* 17:317–329.

Szabo, S., and Z. Sandoz. 1997. Chemically induced lesions in the adrenal cortex. In *Endocrine toxicology,* 2nd ed., ed. J. A. Thomas and H. D. Colby, pp. 115–132. New York: Taylor & Francis.

Touma, C., N. Sachser, E. Most, and R. Paime. 2003. Effects of sex and time of day on metabolism and excretion of corticosterone in urine and feces of mice. *General Comparative Endocrinology* 130:267–278.

Wolfgang, G. H., D. G. Robertson, D. F. Welty, and A. L. Metz. 1995. Hepatic and adrenal toxicity of a novel lipid regulator in beagle dogs. *Fundamental and Applied Toxicology* 26:272–281.

Wong, C-C., K-D. Dohler, H. Geerlings, and A. von zur Muhlen. 1983. Influence of age, strain and season on circadian periodicity of pituitary, gonadal and adrenal hormones in the serum of male laboratory rats. *Hormone Research* 17:202–215.

The Gonads

Bardin, C. W., N. Musto, G. L. Gunsalus, N. Kotiten, S. L. Cheng, F. Larrea, and R. Becker. 1981. Extracellular androgen binding proteins. *Annual Review of Physiology* 43:189–198.

Biswas, N. M., R. Sen Gupta, A. Chattopadhyay, G. R. Choudhury, and M. Sarkar. 2001. Effect of atenolol on cadmium-induced testicular toxicity in male rats. *Reproductive Toxicology* 15:699–704.

Boekelheide, K. et al. 2003. 2,5-hexanedione-induced testicular injury. *Annual Review of Pharmacology and Toxicology* 43:125–127.

Chattopadhyay, S., S. Ghosh, S. Chaki, J. Debnath, and D. Ghosh. 1999. Effect of sodium arsenite on plasma levels of gonadotrophins and ovarian steroidogenesis in mature albino rats: Duration-dependent response. *Journal of Toxicological Sciences* 24:425–431.

Corvol, P., and C. W. Bardin. 1973. Species distribution of testosterone-binding globulin. *Biology of Reproduction* 8:277–282.

Creasy, D. M. 2003. Evaluation of testicular toxicity: A synopsis and discussion of the recommendations proposed by the Society of Toxicological Pathologists. *Birth Defects Research Part B. Developmental and Reproductive Toxicology* 68:408–415.

Danzo, B. J., and D. R. Joseph. 1994. Structure–function relationships of rat androgen binding protein/human sex-hormone binding globulins: The effect of mutagenesis on steroid-binding parameters. *Endocrinology* 135:157–167.

de Palaitis, L., J. Moore, and R. E. Falvo. 1978. Plasma concentrations of testosterone and LH in the male dog. *Journal of Reproduction and Fertility* 52:201–207.

Donham, R. S., and M. H. Stetson. 1991. The prepubertal golden hamster and the transition between daily and estrous cycle hormone rhythm. *Biology of Reproduction* 44:1108–1112.

Fan, L. Q., L. You, H. Brown-Borg, S. Brown, S. Edwards, and J. C. Corton. 2004. Regulation of phase I and phase II steroid metabolism enzymes by PPAR alpha activators. *Toxicology* 204:109–121.

Foresta, C., R. Mioni, P. Bordon, F. Gottardell, A. Nogara, and M. Rossato. 1995. Erythropoietin and testicular steroidogenesis: The role of second messengers. *European Journal of Endocrinology* 132:103–108.

Fukuda, S., H. Nagashima, K. Morioka, and J. Aoki. 1988. Fluctuations in peripheral serum testosterone levels within a day, with age and by sexual stimulation in male beagle dogs bred indoors. *Jikken Dobutsu* 37:381–386.

Goedken, M. J., R. L. Kerlin, and D. Morton. 2008. Spontaneous and age-related testicular findings in beagle dogs. *Toxicologic Pathology* 36:465–471.

Gray, J., J. K. Nicholson, D. M. Creasy, and J. A. Timbrell. 1990. Studies on the relationship between acute testicular damage and urinary and plasma certain concentration. *Archives of Toxicology* 64:443–450.

Gunsalus, G. L., F. Larrea, N. A. Musto, R. R. Becker, J. P. Mather, and C. W. Bardin. 1981. Immunoassay of androgen binding protein in blood: A new approach for study of the seminiferous tubule. *Science* 200:65–66.

Gunsalus, G. L., N. A. Musto, and C. W. Bardin. 1978. Androgen binding protein as a marker for Sertoli cell function. *Journal of Steroid Biochemistry* 15:99–106.

Haney, A. F. 1985. Effect of toxic agents on ovarian function. In *Endocrine toxicology*, pp. 181–210. Target Organ Toxicology series. New York: Raven Press.

Haqqi, T. M., and U. M. Adhami. 1982. Testicular damage and change in serum LDH isoenzyme patterns induced by multiple sublethal doses of apholate in albino rats. *Toxicology Letters* 12:199–205.

Hoyer, P. B. 2005. Damage to ovarian development and function. *Cell Tissue Research* 322:99–106.

ICH. 2005. S5(R2) Detection of toxicity to reproduction for medicinal products and toxicity to male fertility. International Conference on Harmonization of Technical Requirements for Registration of Pharmaceuticals for Human Use.

Itoh, R., and H. K. Ozasa. 1985. Changes in serum lactate dehydrogenase isozyme X activity observed after cadmium administration. *Toxicology Letters* 28:151–154.

James, R. W., D. Crook, and R. Heywood. 1979. Canine pituitary–testicular function in relation to toxicity testing. *Toxicology* 13:237–247.

Jarrell, J., D. R. Mattison, A. McMahon, and E. V. Younglai. 1988. An evaluation of the serum FSH as a biomarker for ovarian toxicity in the rat. *Reproductive Toxicology* 2:111–115.

Johnson, A. N. 1989. Comparative aspects of contraceptive steroids—Effects observed in beagle dogs. *Toxicologic Pathology* 17:389–395.

Kalra, P. S., and S. P. Kalra. 1977. Circadian periodicities of serum androgens, progesterone, gonadotrophins and luteinizing hormone-releasing hormone in male rats: The effects of hypothalamic differentiation, castration and adrenalectomy. *Endocrinology* 101:1821–1827.

Lanning, L. L., D. M. Creasy, R. E. Chapin, P. C. Mann, N. J. Barlow, K. S. Regan, and D. G. Goodman. 2002. Recommended approaches for evaluation of testicular and epididymal toxicity. *Toxicologic Pathology* 30:507.

Lindzey, J., M. Vijay Kumar, M. Grossman, C. Young, and D. J. Tindall. 1994. Molecular mechanism of androgen action. *Vitamins and Hormones* 49:383–432.

Lovekamp-Swan, T., and B. J. Davis. 2003. Mechanisms of phthalate ester toxicity in the female reproductive system. *Environmental Health Perspectives* 111:139–145.

Luster, M. I., R. W. Pfeifer, and A. N. Tucker. 1985. Influence of sex hormones on immunoregulation with specific references to natural and environmental estrogens. In *Endocrine toxicology*, ed. J. A. Thomas, pp. 67–85. Target Organ Toxicology series. New York: Raven Press.

Malgor, L. A., M. Valsecia, E. Vergés, and E. E. De Markowsky. 1998. Blockade of the in vitro effects of testosterone and erythropoietin on Cfu-E and Bfu-E proliferation by pretreatment of donor rats with cyproterone and flutamide. *Acta Physiologica Pharmacologica Therapeutic Latinoam* 48:99–105.

Mattison, D. R., D. R. Plowchalk, M. J. Meadows, A. Z. al-Juburi, J. Gandy, and A. Malek. 1990. Reproductive toxicity: Male and female reproductive systems as targets for chemical injury. *Medical Clinics of North America* 74:391–411.

Mattison, D. R., and P. J. Thomford. 1989. The mechanism of action of reproductive toxicants. *Toxicologic Pathology* 17:364–376.

Meistrich, M. L., P. K. Trostle, M. Frapart, and R. P. Erickson. 1977. Biosynthesis and localization of lactate dehydrogenase X in pachytene spermatocytes and spermatids of mouse testes. *Developmental Biology* 60:428–441.

Michael, R. P., K. D. Setchell, and T. M. Plant. 1974. Diurnal changes in plasma testosterone and studies on plasma corticosteroids in nonanaesthetized male rhesus monkeys.
Journal of Endocrinology 63:325–335.

Mitchell, A. E. et al. 2004. Evaluating chemical and other agent exposure for reproductive and developmental toxicity. *Journal of Toxicology and Environmental Health A*
67:1159–1314.

Mock, E. J., H. W. Norton, and A. I. Frankel. 1978. Daily rhythmicity of serum testosterone
levels in the male laboratory rat. *Endocrinology* 92:1111–1121.

Moor, B. C., and E. V. Younglai. 1975. Variations in peripheral level of serum LH and testosterone in adult male rabbits. *Journal of Reproduction and Fertility* 42:259–266.

Mooradian, A. D., J. E. Morley, and S. G. Korenman. 1987. Biological actions of androgens.
Endocrinology Review 8:1–28.

Moore, N. P., D. M. Creasy, T. J. Gray, and J. A. Timbrell. 1992. Urinary creatine profiles after
administration of cell-specific toxicants to the rat. *Archives of Toxicology* 66:435–442.

Plant, T. M. 1981. Tine courses of concentrations of circulating gonadotrophin, prolactin, testosterone and cortisol in adult male rhesus monkeys (*Macaca mulatta*) throughout the
24-h light–dark cycle. *Biology of Reproduction* 25:244–252.

Reader, S. C., C. Shingles, and M. D. Stonard. 1991. Acute testicular toxicity of 1:3 dini-
tro benzene and ethylene glycol monomethyl ether in the rat: Evaluation of biochemical effect markers and hormonal responses. *Fundamental and Applied Toxicology*
16:61–70.

Rehm, S. 2000. Spontaneous testicular lesions in purpose bred beagle dogs. *Toxicologic
Pathology* 28:782–787.

Spitz, I. M., G. L. Gunsalus, J. P. Mather, R. Thau, and C. W. Bardin. 1985. The effects of imi-
dazole carboxylic acid derivative, tolmidamine on testicular function. 1. Early changes
in androgen binding protein secretion in the rat. *Journal of Androgens* 6:161–178.

Swenberg, J. A. 1993. Alpha-2u-globulin nephropathy and renal tumors: Review of the cellular and molecular mechanisms involved and their implications for human risk assessment. *Environmental Health Perspectives* 99:313–349.

Timbrell, J. A. 2000. Urinary creatine as a biochemical marker of chemical induced testicular
damage. *Archiv za Higijenu Rada I Toksikologiju* 51:295–303.

Wheat, T. E., and E. Goldberg. 1983. Sperm specific lactate dehydrogenase C4: Antigenic
structure and immunosuppression of fertility. *Isozymes Current Topics in Biological and
Medical Research* 7:113–130.

Wheat, T. E., M. Hintz, E. Goldberg, and E. Margoliash. 1977. Analyses of stage specific
multiple forms of lactate dehydrogenase and of cytochrome c during spermatogenesis in
the mouse. *Differentiation* 9:37–41.

Witorsch, R. J. 1995. *Reproductive toxicology,* 2nd ed. Target Organ series. New York: Taylor
& Francis.

Woodman, D. D. 1997. *Laboratory animal endocrinology: Hormonal action, control mechanisms and interactions with drugs.* Chichester, England: John Wiley & Sons Ltd.

Yamamoto, T., T. Fukushima, R. Kikkawa, H. Yamada, and I. Horri. 2005. Protein expression
analysis of rat testes: Induced testicular toxicity with several reproductive toxicants.
Journal of Toxicological Sciences 30:111–126.

11 Assessment of Neurotoxicity

11.1 STRUCTURE AND PHYSIOLOGY

Within the brain there are several cell types, including neurons, glial cells, and endothelial cells. The neurons have a cell body with a nucleus, dendrites, axons, and terminals. The axons are insulated for the conduction of nerve impulses by layers that include myelin-containing cells, and along the surface of the nerve there are ion channels. The axon branches to provide numerous nerve terminals with synaptic vesicles containing neurotransmitters released by exocytosis. These transmitters include acetylcholine, some amino acids (e.g., glycine and glutamine), catecholamines, and serotonin. The glial cells are myelin-forming cells and the larger glial cells are termed astrocytes; these cells form a layer around the brain blood vessels and also play important roles in neuronal tricarboxylic cycle metabolism. The dendrites are numerous and receive messages via chemoreceptors.

The blood–brain barrier (BBB) is formed by endothelial cells around the blood capillaries associated with the astrocytes. These tightly packed endothelial cells are linked by tight junctions but are not fenestrated, unlike many other endothelial cells in the body. Xenobiotics and other endogenous compounds must cross the blood–brain barrier by passing through the endothelial cells, and this permeability is governed by the molecular size and the hydrophilic properties of a compound. Thus, selective protective mechanisms restrict the entry of many xenobiotics and also protect the brain from possible effects from circulating hormones and several neurotransmitters, thereby helping to maintain a relatively constant environment for the brain (Bakay, Sweeney, and Wood 1986; Davson and Segal 1996). There are some differences in the blood–brain barrier between species that affect the passage of endogenous substances and of xenobiotics (Reiber and Thiele 1983; Davson and Segal 1996). The choroidal cells of the choroid plexus provide a separate but similarly selective blood–cerebrospinal fluid barrier.

In the brain, the hypothalamus links the nervous system to the pituitary gland (hypophysis) and this acts on the endocrine system through a number of hypothalamic hormone releasing factors: neurohormones (see Chapter 10). The hypothalamus is responsible for the regulation of body temperature, hunger, and thirst and for chronobiological rhythms.

11.2 TOXIC EFFECTS

Neurotoxicity (or a neurotoxic effect) may be defined as an adverse change in the structure or function of the nervous system that results from exposure to a chemical, biological, or physical agent, where adverse implies an alteration from baseline that is toxicological and detrimental to the structure and function of the nervous system (OECD 2004; U.S. EPA 2007). Effects may be directly on the nervous system or by indirect actions on targets outside the nervous system that subsequently affect the nervous system. Indirect effects on the nervous system may result from insufficient blood, oxygen, or nutrient supply to the brain; thyroid dysfunction; or a result of hepatic or renal failure. Some neurotoxins injure the brain through the formation of free radicals, partly through actions on membrane lipids and the lack of enzymes to deal with the formation of free radicals. The effects of neurotoxicity may be reversible or irreversible depending on the mechanisms, duration, and levels of exposure.

Neurotoxicity can include effects on behavior and physiology, including motor function, sensory function, and cognitive function. These aspects are mainly studied in safety pharmacology, where the emphases are on functional and behavioral tests (e.g., functional observational battery; FOB) (OECD 2004), and neurotoxicity may or may not be associated with changes in neuropathology. Neurotoxins may target different parts of the neuron, and neuronopathies may involve injury to the neurones, followed by necrosis and loss; the effects may be broad or selective for a subpopulation of neurons.

In axonpathies, the primary sites of toxicity are the axons, which can lead to the degeneration of the axon together with the myelin surrounding the axon, but the cell body of the neurone can remain intact. Longer axons tend to be affected more often than shorter ones because of the increased sites available for adverse actions of neurotoxins. In myelinopathies, the reduction of myelin insulation alters the conduction of electrical impulses through the neurone. Toxicity associated with neurotransmission dysfunction can be caused by a number of mechanisms, including effects on uptake, storage, release, or degradation of the neurotransmitter; receptor binding; inactivation; receptor function; signal transduction; etc. (Abou-Donia 1992; Harry and Tilson 1999; Connell 2005). The receptors on the dendrites may be excited by neuron degeneration and exhibit excitotoxicity, and neurotoxins may act as receptor agonists or antagonists. Some enzyme measurements have proved to be useful in studies of xenobiotics, including several insecticides and pesticides and their effects on neurotransmission. Examples include the cholinesterases and neurotoxic esterase; unlike many of the other enzymes we measure in toxicology, it is the reduction of enzyme levels for cholinesterase, paraoxanase, and neurotoxic esterase that is important in defining toxic effects.

Neurotoxicology has always been a focus for environmental toxicology (e.g., monitoring for possible adverse effects with pesticides). However, interest within the pharmaceutical industry is increasing because the central nervous system (CNS) has several interesting therapeutic targets (e.g., Alzheimer's syndrome) and because of an awareness that preclinical studies often fail to predict adverse effects of drugs on the CNS when they are given to humans and animals.

11.2.1 CHOLINESTERASES

There are two main enzymes of interest. Acetylcholinesterase (AChE; EC 3.1.1.7) has an affinity for the substrate acetylcholine and it is found in the erythrocytes and nervous tissue. The enzyme is sometimes referred to as "true" cholinesterase, and it exists in differing polymorphic forms (Skau 1985). Butyrylcholinesterase (BuChE, acylcholine acylhydrolase, EC 3.1.1.8)—also known as pseudocholinesterase or non-specific cholinesterase—has affinities for the substrates butyrylcholine and/or propionylcholine, which are dependent on the animal species (Myers 1953; Ecobichon and Comeau 1973; Scarsella et al. 1979; Unakami et al. 1987; Evans 1990; Matthew and Chapin 1990; Woodard et al. 1994).

The enzyme choline acetyltransferase (EC 2.3.1.6) is the key enzyme in the synthesis of acetylcholine, whereas AChE is essential for the inactivation and regulation of acetylcholine at localized sites of neurotransmission. The mechanism of action of AChE involves an initial reaction where acetylcholine forms a complex with the enzyme, leading to acetylation and the release of choline. The reaction is reversible with the regeneration of de-acetylated enzyme.

The AChE enzymes are found in various locations within the CNS, including neuromuscular junctions, neuronal cell bodies, junctions between muscles and tendons, axons, muscles, and thymocytes. Inhibition of AChE can lead to prolonged cholinergic nerve impulses that can cause nerve and/or muscle injury. The accumulation of acetylcholine accumulation resulting from the enzyme inhibition can result in cognitive dysfunction or heightened sensitivity to cholinomimetic compounds. Choline itself can have significant agonist activity at certain acetylcholine receptor subtypes.

Butyrylcholinesterase occurs in the liver and at the motor endplates in muscle fibers and at synapses together with acetylcholinesterase (Silver 1974). It is estimated that approximately 15% of total cholinesterase activity in the nervous system is due to the nonspecific cholinesterase activity in some of the white matter (Ecobichon and Joy 1982), and the synthesis of this nonspecific cholinesterase occurs in the liver. Several organophosphorus compounds can react and phosphorylate acetylcholinesterase; carbamate ester compounds can carbamylate the enzyme, so both can inhibit the acetylcholinesterase.

Regulatory guidelines suggest it is essential to measure both cholinesterase activities in blood and brain and also to comment on the frequency of blood measurements in specific study designs (e.g., chronic toxicity studies) with brain tissue measurements made in all or some of the animals at necropsy, depending on the species (U.S. EPA 1984; OECD 2000, 2002) when performing toxicological studies of organophosphorus and carbamate esters. These measurements can be used to provide an index of xenobiotic absorption, the potential to cause an adverse effect on the nervous system, and possible reversibility of effects (Wills 1972; Padilla 1995). Cholinesterase levels are affected by age; effects of xenobiotics generally are more toxic in juvenile animals in comparison with adults (Lu, Jessup, and Lavallee 1965; Peet, Shiloff, and Clement 1987; Pope et al. 1991). Diet has also been shown to affect esterase activities (van Lith et al. 1992; van Lith and Beynen 1993).

For these studies, the dog and rat are species commonly studied, with the inclusion of concurrent control groups in the studies; with dogs, pretreatment baseline sampling on at least two occasions may be used to establish intra- and interindividual variations. A consensus view is that up to 20% difference from the mean baseline value within the "normal" variability for both brain and blood cholinesterases and above 20% inhibition is biologically significant (Gage 1967; Hackathorn et al. 1983; Lepage et al. 1985; Mason and Lewis 1989; JMPR 1998). However, this percentage value is dependent upon establishing the baseline for the chosen enzyme measurement, and there remains a regulatory debate about the significance of cholinesterase inhibition as an adverse finding in toxicity testing.

11.2.2   PARAOXANASE (PON1: EC 3.1.1.2)

This enzyme is important in its ability to metabolize organophosphates such as paraoxon and the association of the enzyme with high-density lipoprotein (HDL) and the protection of low-density lipoproteins from the effects of oxidative stress (Costa et al. 1990; Feingold et al. 1998; Costa and Furlong 2002; Costa et al. 2005; Costa, Vitalone, et al. 2005). The enzyme exists in several polymorphisms and it is synthesized mainly in the liver. The enzyme activity can be measured using paraoxon as substrate (Hasselwander et al. 1998). Although the measurement of the enzyme has been used mainly in monitoring the effects of pesticides, more recently the enzyme has received increased attention as a measure of hepatic injury (Gil et al. 1994; Hernandez et al. 1997; Ferre et al. 2002) and in the study of causation of atherosclerosis.

11.2.3   NEUROPATHY (OR NEUROTOXIC) TARGET ESTERASE

A small number of compounds cause a delayed neurotoxicity referred to as organophosphate-induced delayed polyneuropathy (OPIDP) (Lotti 1991; Johnson 1993; Vilanova, Barril, and Carrera 1993; Johnson and Glynn 1995; Harry and Tilson 1999; Jokanovic, Stukalov, and Kosanovic 2002). In this case, clinical signs of neurotoxicity (e.g., paralysis) do not develop until several days or weeks after dosing, although this OPIDP commences with the inhibition of the neuropathy target esterase (NTE) within a few hours after dosing. In cases of OPIDP, histopathological examination shows injury to peripheral nerves and spinal cord. This NTE may also be inhibited by carbamate esters, but this inhibition does not lead to OPIDP.

Of several avian species sensitive to OPIDP, the adult hen has been accepted as a suitable species for evaluating the potential hazards from organophosphorus esters (Johnson 1974; Johnson and Richardson 1983; Seifert and Wilson 1994; Glynn 1997). Other species, including rats, rabbits, guinea pigs, and hamsters, do not exhibit consistent delayed neurotoxic responses to the neuropathic organophosphorus compounds (e.g., tri-ortho cresyl phosphate).

11.2.4   GLIAL FIBRILLARY ACIDIC PROTEIN (GFAP)

Within the astrocytes is a major intermediate filament protein called glial fibrillary acidic protein (GFAP) that is important for structural stability of these cells (Smith, Perret, and Eng 1984; Eng 1985; O'Callaghan and Sriram 2005). In response to neuronal cell injury caused by xenobiotics, viruses, and bacteria, the astrocytes undergo both hypertrophy and proliferation—a process termed reactive gliosis, which affects astrocytes adjacent to and extending beyond the site of injury. This reactive gliosis is characterized by extensive synthesis of GFAP.

11.2.5 MYELIN BASIC PROTEIN (MBP)

Myelin is a major component of neural tissue lipids and contains unique proteins such as myelin basic protein. Changes in cellular lipid composition can reflect demyelination, where these changes may consist of a decrease in myelin or protein/lipid with an increase in water content accompanied by the appearance of cholesterol esters (Norton 1984). Myelin basic protein content or synthesis may be determined to quantify myelination in the brain or reactive synthesis secondary to a toxic insult (Conti et al. 1996; Hamano et al. 1996).

11.3 LABORATORY ASSESSMENT

The functional and structural diversity of the CNS leads to measurements that are equally diverse. Several measurements use plasma erythrocytes, urine, and cerebrospinal fluid. However, historically, these measurements have not been widely used in toxicology except for the cholinesterases.

11.3.1 CHOLINESTERASE ASSAYS

Current measurements of cholinesterase are based upon the hydrolysis of an ester by an enzyme (Wills 1972; Whittaker 1986). The measurements for AChE and BuChE enzymes are sensitive to pH, temperature, and substrate concentration, and these factors must be considered in order to optimize the assay for the relevant species. There are basically four different principles for these assays, which include: (1) methods based on the Ellman colorimetric assay and thiocholine substrates, (2) pH change, (3) radiometric methods, and (4) manometric methods. The most widely used techniques are the colorimetric assays based upon the use of acetyl- or propionyl-thiocholine(s) that are hydrolyzed to thiocholine and, when combined with 5,5-dithio-bis-2-nitrobenzoic acid (DTNB), produce a yellow color. The yellow-colored product has a large extinction coefficient and offers a highly sensitive method (Ellman et al. 1961).

The potentiometric technique involves the measurement of pH, which falls as acetic acid released by hydrolysis of the acetylated enzyme occurs; however, this method lacks sensitivity (Michel 1949). The radioisotopic method uses tritiated acetylcholine as substrate. The method is highly sensitive but requires a scintillation counter (Winteringham and Disney 1964; Johnson and Russel 1975). The manometric method is based upon the release of carbon dioxide evolved from the action of the bicarbonate in the system with the acid formed by hydrolysis of the ester (Augustinsson 1948).

Some significant pitfalls are associated with the measurement of cholinesterase, and these include the timings of sample collection and analysis. The time between blood and tissue sampling and assay should be minimized to prevent further inhibition

TABLE 11.1
Plasma Cholinesterase Activities[a] Measured Colorimetrically by Three Separate Substrate Methods in Four Species[b]

	Acetyl-Choline Substrate[c]	Butyryl-Choline Substrate[c]	Propionyl-Choline Substrate[c]
Rats, male and female	819 ± 544	340 ± 237	1047 ± 694
Male rats	456 ± 82	147 ± 29	484 ± 98
Female rats	1182 ± 367	533 ± 186	1611 ± 549
Rabbits, male and female	575 ± 78	1143 ± 1157	513 ± 174
Dogs, male and female	2559 ± 412	5071 ± 891	3175 ± 579
Humans, male	3511 ± 1195	7064 ± 2312	5436 ± 1850

Source: Evans, G. O. 1990. In *Fourth Congress of International Society for Animal Clinical Biochemistry,* p. 270. University of California, Davis.

Notes: Female rat values were higher than those for male rats, and the values for rats using the butyrylcholine substrate were lower than for the other two substrates. For rabbits, dogs, and humans, the values obtained using butyrylcholine were higher than those obtained with the other two substrates.

[a] IU/L.
[b] $n = 20$ per group.
[c] Mean value ± 1 SD.

of the enzyme by any free inhibitor or the reactivation of the inhibited enzyme when the incubation time for the assay must be minimized following dilution of the blood sample. If these conditions are not controlled, then the degree of inhibition of cholinesterase may be inaccurate (Wilhelm and Reiner 1973; Padilla and Hooper 1992; Padilla 1995; U.S. EPA 1996; Wilson et al. 1996).

Differences between the species toward the thiocholine substrates have been reported. Table 11.1 illustrates some observed differences with three species. For plasma pseudocholinesterase measurements, dog, rabbit, and man show higher substrate specificity for butyryl substrates, whereas rat, mouse, and hamster show higher specificity for propionyl substrates; all the species show less specificity toward benzoyl substrates. Female rats have higher values compared to males with all three substrates, and the cholinesterase levels in platelets are higher in rats compared to the very low levels in human platelets.

11.3.2   NEUROPATHY TARGET ESTERASE (OR NEUROTOXIC ESTERASE, NTE)

The assay of NTE uses hen brain tissue, which contains substantial esterase activity with phenyl valerate substrate. It should include the use of comparative compounds that are neurotoxic (e.g., mipafox) and non-neurotoxic (e.g., paraoxon) as inhibitors of the enzyme for comparative purposes (Johnson 1977; Johnson and Richardson 1983; Correll and Ehrich 1991; Richardson et al. 1993; Seifert and Wilson 1994).

11.3.3 GLIAL FIBRILLARY ACIDIC PROTEIN (GFAP)

This protein can also be measured by a detergent-based solid-phase radioimmunoassay (O'Callaghan and Miller 1985), immunobinding assay (Brock and O'Callaghan 1987), and ELISA methods (O'Callaghan 1991; Petzold et al. 2004). GFAP also may be measured by immunohistochemical procedures, which provide a semiquantitative estimation by light microscopy (Eng and De Armand 1983). Age-related increases of GFAP in rats and regional differences of GFAP in the brain have been reported (Dickens et al. 1993). Although quantification of cell specific markers can be helpful in identifying cell degeneration and immunohistochemistry can help localize the protein, these techniques may be poor predictors of the functional integrity of cells.

11.3.4 IN VITRO ASSAYS AND FUTURE ASSAYS

In the future, there may be greater utilization of cerebrospinal fluid and techniques such as proteomics and metabonomics (Ohta and Ohta 2002; van den Heuvel et al. 2003; Sukuzi et al. 2005). Collection of cerebrospinal fluid (CSF) is an invasive procedure generally reserved for terminal procedures. However, it is not commonly used in toxicology, and species differences in the blood–brain barriers are not well documented.

Several measurements require the collection of nervous tissue at necropsy and homogenization of the tissues prior to analysis; simple tissue procedures and associated measurements often do not indicate the localization of effects. Assays using tissue microdissection and in vitro cell cultures can help in the understanding of neurotoxic mechanisms, and these are being used more widely (Abdulla and Campbell 1992; Costa 1998; Harry et al. 1998). The development of assays such as neural gold protein, amyloid precursor protein, neuron specific enolase, heat shock proteins, and amyloid precursor proteins to study nervous diseases may find applications in some toxicology studies where the assays can be adapted for laboratory animals (de la Monte et al. 1997; Fitzpatrick et al. 2000; Rajdev and Sharp 2000).

REFERENCES

Neurotoxicity

Abou-Donia, M. B. 1992. *Neurotoxicology.* Boca Raton FL: CRC Press.
Bakay, R. A., K. M. Sweeney, and M. D. Wood. 1986. Pathophysiology of cerebrospinal fluid in head injury: Part 2. Biochemical markers for central nervous system trauma. *Neurosurgery* 18:376–382.
Connell, D. W. 2005. *Basic concepts of environmental chemistry,* 2nd ed. Boca Raton, FL: CRC Press Inc.
Davson, H., and M. Segal. 1996. *Physiology of the CSF and blood–brain barriers.* Boca Raton, FL: CRC Press Inc.
Harry, G. J., and H. A. Tilson. 1999. *Neurotoxicology,* 2nd ed. Target Organ Toxicology series. Boca Raton, FL: CRC Press Inc.
OECD. 2004. *Guidance document for neurotoxicity series on assessment and testing, no. 20.* Paris: OECD Environment Health and Safety Publications
Reiber, H., and P. Thiele. 1983. Species dependent variable in blood cerebrospinal fluid barrier function for proteins. *Journal of Clinical Chemistry and Clinical Biochemistry* 21:199–202.

U.S. EPA. 2007. 40 CFR Part 158. Data requirements for pesticides. Washington, D.C.: Environmental Protection Agency.

Cholinesterase

Augustinsson, K. B. 1948. Cholinesterases, a study in comparative enzymology. *Acta Physiologica Scandinavica* 15 (Suppl. 52): 1–192.

Ecobichon, D. J., and M. Comeau. 1973. Pseudocholinesterases of mammalian plasma: Physicochemical properties and organophosphate inhibition in eleven species. *Toxicology and Applied Pharmacology* 24:92–100.

Ecobichon, D. J., and R. M. Joy. 1982. *Pesticides and neurological disease.* Boca Raton, FL: CRC Press.

Ellman, G. L., K. D. Courtney, V. Andres, and R. M. Featherstone. 1961. A new and rapid colorimetric determination of acetylcholinesterase activity. *Biochemical Pharmacology* 7:88–95.

Evans, G. O. 1990. Species relationships for plasma acylcholine hydrolase using three different substrates. In *Fourth Congress of International Society for Animal Clinical Biochemistry*, p. 270. University of California, Davis.

Gage, J. C. 1967. The significance of blood cholinesterase activity measurements. *Residue Reviews* 18:159–173.

Hackathorn, D. R., W. J. Brinkman, T. R. Hathaway, T. D. Talbot, and L. R. Thompson. 1983. Validation of whole blood method for cholinesterase monitoring. *American Industrial Hygiene Association Journal* 44:547–551.

Johnson, C. D., and P. L. Russel. 1975. A rapid, simple radiometric assay for cholinesterase, suitable for multiple determinations. *Analytical Biochemistry* 64:229–238.

JMPR. 1998. Joint Meeting Pesticides Residues Report: IPCS–WHO.

Lepage, L., F. Schiele, R. Gueguen, and G. Siest. 1985. Total cholinesterase in plasma: Biological variations and reference ranges. *Clinical Chemistry* 31:546–550.

Lu, F. C., D. C. Jessup, and A. Lavallee. 1965. Toxicity of pesticides in young versus adult rats. *Food and Cosmetics Toxicology* 3:591–596.

Mason, H. J., and P. J. Lewis. 1989. Intra-individual variation in plasma and erythrocyte cholinesterase activities and the monitoring of uptake of organophosphate pesticides. *Journal of the Society of Occupational Medicine* 39:121–124.

Mathew, C. B., and C. L. Chapin. 1990. Spectrophotometric determination of circulating cholinesterases in rats. *Aviation Space and Environmental Medicine* 61:374–378.

Michel, H. O. 1949. An electrometric method for the determination of red blood cell and plasma cholinesterase activity. *Journal of Laboratory and Clinical Medicine* 34:1564–1568.

Myers, D. K. 1953. Studies on cholinesterase. 9. Species variation in the specificity pattern of the pseudo-cholinesterases. *Biochemistry Journal* 55:67–75.

OECD. 2000. *Guidance notes for analysis and evaluation of repeat-dose toxicity studies.* Series on testing and assessment no. 32 and series on pesticides no. 10. Paris: OECD.

———. 2002. *Guidance note on analysis and evaluation of chronic toxicity and carcinogenicity studies.* Series on testing and assessment no. 35 and series on pesticides no. 14. Paris: OECD.

Padilla, S. 1995. Regulatory and research issues related to cholinesterase inhibition. *Toxicology* 102:215–220.

Padilla, S., and M. J. Hooper. 1992. Cholinesterase measurements in tissues from carbamate-treated animals. Cautions and recommendations. *Proceedings of the U.S. EPA Workshop on Cholinesterase Methodologies,* pp. 63–81. Washington, D.C.: Office of Pesticide Residue Programs, U.S. Environmental Protection Agency.

Peet, S., J. D. Shiloff, and J. G. Clement. 1987. Relationship between age of mice, enzymes such as acetylcholinesterase, and aliesterase, and toxicity of soman (pinacolyl methylphosphonofluoridate). *Biochemical Pharmacology* 36:3777–3779.

Pope, C. N., T. K. Chakraborti, M. L. Chapman, J. D. Farrar, and D. Arthun. 1991. Comparison of in vivo cholinesterase inhibition in neonatal and adult rats by three organophosphorothioate insecticides. *Toxicology* 68:51–61.

Scarsella, G., G. Toschi, S. R. Bareggi, and E. Giacobini. 1979. Molecular forms of cholinesterase in cerebrospinal fluid, blood plasma and brain tissue of the beagle dog. *Journal of Neuroscience Research* 4:19–24.

Silver, A. 1974. The biology of cholinesterases 1974. In *Frontiers of biology,* vol. 36. Amsterdam: North Holland Publishing.

Skau, K. A. 1985. Acetylcholinesterase molecular forms in serum and erythrocytes of laboratory animals. *Comparative Biochemistry and Physiology* 80C:207–210.

Unakami, S., S. Suzuki, E. Nakanishi, K. Ichinohe, M. Hirata, and Y. Tanimoto. 1987. Comparative studies on multiple forms of serum cholinesterase in various species. *Experimental Animals* 36:199–204.

U.S. EPA. 1984. Pesticide assessment guidelines. Subdivision F, hazard evaluation: Human and domestic animals. 1991. Pesticide assessment guidelines. Subdivision F, addendum 10. Neurotoxicity series 81, 82, and 83.

———. 1996. OPP 00342. Standard operating procedures for measuring cholinesterases in rats and dogs exposed to nonreversible cholinesterase inhibitors. Washington, D.C.: Environmental Protection Agency.

van Lith, H. A., and A. C. Beynen. 1993. Dietary cholesterol lowers the activity of butyrylcholinesterase (EC 3.1.1.8.) but elevates that of esterase-1 (EC 3.3.1.1). *British Journal of Nutrition* 70:721–726.

van Lith, H. A., M. Haller, G. van Tintelen, L. F. van Zutphen, and A. C. Beynen. 1992. Plasma esterase-1(ES-1) activity in rats is influenced by the amount and type of dietary fat and butyrylcholinesterase activity by the type of dietary fat. *Journal of Nutrition* 122:2109–2120.

Whittaker, M. 1986. *Cholinesterase. Monographs in human genetics,* vol. II. Basle, Swizerland: Karger.

Wilhelm, K., and E. Reiner. 1973. Effect of sample storage on human blood cholinesterase activity after inhibition by carbamates. *Bulletin of the World Health Organization* 48:235–238.

Wills, J. H. 1972. The measurement and significance of changes in the cholinesterase activities of erythrocytes and plasma in man and animals. *CRC Critical Reviews in Toxicology* 1:153–202.

Wilson, B. W. et al. 1996. Factors in standardizing automated cholinesterase assays. *Journal of Toxicology and Environmental Health* 48:187–195.

Winteringham, F. P., and R. W. Disney. 1964. A simple method of estimating blood cholinesterase. *Laboratory Practice* 13:739–740.

Woodard, C. L., C. A. Calamaio, A. Kaminskis, D. R. Anderson, L. W. Harris, and D. G. Martin. 1994. Erythrocyte and plasma cholinesterase activity in male and female Rhesus monkeys before and after exposure to sarin. *Fundamental and Applied Toxicology* 23:342–347.

Paraoxanase

Costa, L. G., T. B. Cole, A. Vitalone, and C. E. Furlong. 2005. Measurement of paraoxanase (PON1) status as a potential biomarker of susceptibility to organophosphate toxicity. *Clinica Chimica Acta* 352:37–47.

Costa, L. G., and C. E. Furlong, eds. 2002. *Paraoxanase (PON1) in health and disease: Basic and clinical aspects.* Norwell, MA: Kluwer Academic Publishers.

Costa, L. G., B. E. McDonald, S. D. Murphy, G. S. Omenn, R. J. Richter, A. G. Motuslky, and C. E. Furlong. 1990. Serum paraoxanase and its influence on paraoxon and chlorpyrifos-oxon toxicity in rats. *Toxicology and Applied Pharmacology* 103:66–76.

Costa, L. G., A. Vitalone, T. B. Cole, and C. E. Furlong. 2005. Modulation of paraoxanase (PON1) activity. *Biochemical Pharmacology* 69:541–550.

Feingold, K. R., R. A. Memon, A. H. Moser, and C. Grunfeld. 1998. Paraoxanase activity in the serum and hepatic mRNA levels decrease during the acute phase response. *Atherosclerosis* 139:307–315.

Ferre, N., J. Camps, E. Prats, E. Vilella, A. Paul, L. Figuera, and J. Joven. 2002. Serum paraoxanase activity: A new additional test for the improved evaluation of chronic liver disease. *Clinical Chemistry* 48:261–268.

Gil, F., M. C. Gonzalvo, A. F. Hernández, E. Vilanueva, and A. Pla. 1994. Differences in the kinetic properties, effect of calcium and sensitivity to inhibitors of paraoxon hydrolase activity in rat plasma and microsomal fraction from rat liver. *Biochemical Pharmacology* 48:1559–1568.

Hasselwander, O., D. McMaster, D. G. Fogarty, A. P. Maxwell, D. P. Nicholls, and I. S. Young. 1998. Serum paraoxanase and platelet-activating factor acetylhydrolase in chronic renal failure. *Clinical Chemistry* 44:179–181.

Hernandez, A. F., M. C. Gonzalvo, F. Gil, E. Vilanueva, and A. Pla. 1997. Divergent effects of classical inducers on rat plasma and microsomal fraction paraoxanase and arylesterase. *Environmental Toxicology and Pharmacology* 3:83–86.

Neuropathy (Neurotoxic) Target Esterase

Correll, L., and M. Ehrich. 1991. A microassay method for neurotoxic esterase. *Fundamental and Applied Toxicology* 116:110–116.

Glynn, P. 1997. Neuropathy target esterase (NTE): Molecular characterization and cellular localization. *Archives of Toxicology* Suppl. 19:325–329.

Johnson, M. K. 1974. The primary biochemical lesion leading to the delayed neurotoxic effect of some organophosphorus esters. *Journal of Neurochemistry* 23:785–798.

———. 1977. Improved assay of neurotoxic esterase for screening organophosphates for delayed neurotoxicity potential. *Archives of Toxicology* 37:113–115.

———. 1993. Symposium introduction: Retrospect and prospects for neuropathy target esterase (NTE) and the delayed polyneuropathy (ODIDP) induced by some organophosphorus esters. *Chemical and Biological Interactions* 87:339–346.

Johnson, M. K., and P. Glynn. 1995. Neuropathy target esterase (NTE) and organophosphorus-induced polyneuropathy (ODIDP): Recent advances. *Toxicology Letters* 82–82:459–463.

Johnson, M. K., and R. J. Richardson. 1983. Biochemical endpoints: Neurotoxic esterase assay. *Neurotoxicology* 4:311–320.

Jokanovic, M., P. V. Stukalov, and M. Kosanovic. 2002. Organophosphate induced delayed polyneuropathy. *Current Drug Targets and CNS Neurological Disorders* 1:593–602.

Lotti, M. 1991. The pathogenesis of organophosphate polyneuropathy. *Critical Reviews in Toxicology* 21:465–487.

Richardson, R. J., T. B. Moore, U. S. Kayyali, and J. C. Randall. 1993. Chlorpyrifos: Assessment for potential for delayed neurotoxicity by repeated dosing in adult hens and monitoring of brain acetylcholinesterase, brain and lymphocyte neurotoxic esterase and plasma butylcholinesterase. *Fundamental and Applied Toxicology* 21:89–96.

Seifert, J., and B. W. Wilson. 1994. Solubilization of neuropathy target esterase and other phenyl valerate carboxylesterases from chicken embryonic brain by phospholipase A2. *Comparative Biochemistry and Physiology C* 108:337–441.

Vilanova, E., J. Barril, and V. Carrera. 1993. Biochemical properties and possible toxicological significance of various forms of NTE. *Chemical and Biological Interactions* 87:369–381.

Glial Fibrillary Acidic Protein

Brock, T. O., and J. P. O'Callaghan. 1987. Quantitative changes in the synaptic proteins, synapsin 1 and p38, and the astrocyte specific protein, GFAP, are associated with chemical-induced injury to the rat central nervous system. *Journal of Neuroscience* 7:931–942.

Dickens, A. D., L. J. Lea, J. A. Robinson, and I. Slack. 1993. Measurement of glial fibrillary acidic protein (GFAP) in the rat and validation of its use as a biochemical marker of neurotoxicity. *Comparative Hematology International* 3:57.

Eng, L. F. 1985. Glial fibrillary acidic protein: The major protein of glial intermediate filaments in differentiated astrocytes. *Journal of Neuroimmunology* 8:203–214.

Eng, L. F., and S. J. De Armand. 1983. Immunochemistry of the glial fibrillary acidic protein. In *Progress in neurobiology,* vol. 5, ed. H. M. Zimmerman, pp. 19–39. New York: Raven Press.

O'Callaghan, J. P. 1991. Quantification of glial fibrillary acidic protein: comparison of slot-immunobinding assays with a novel sandwich ELISA. *Neurotoxicology and Teratology* 13:275–281.

O'Callaghan, J. P., and D. B. Miller. 1985. Cerebellar hypoplasia in the Gunn rat is associated with quantitative changes in neurotypic and gliotypic proteins. *Journal of Pharmacology Experiments and Therapeutics* 234:522–533.

O'Callaghan, J. P., and K. Sriram. 2005. Glial fibrillary acidic protein and related glial proteins as biomarkers of neurotoxicity. *Expert Opinions in Drug Safety* 4:433–442.

Petzold, A., G. Keir, A. J. Green, G. Giovannoni, and E. J. Thompson. 2004. An ELISA for glial fibrillary acidic protein. *Journal of Immunology Methods* 287:169–177.

Smith, M. E., V. Perret, and L. F. Eng. 1984. Metabolic studies in vitro of the CNS cytoskeletal proteins: Synthesis and degradation. *Neurochemical Research* 9:1493–1507.

Myelin Basic Protein

In Vitro Assays and Future Assays

Abdulla, E. M., and I. C. Campbell. 1992. In vitro tests of neurotoxicity. *Journal of Pharmacological and Toxicological Methods* 29:69–75.

Conti, A. M., E. Scarpino, M. L. Malosio, A. M. Di Giulio, P. Baron, G. Scarlato, P. Mantegazzza, and A. Gorio. 1996. *In situ* hybridization study of myelin protein mRNA in rats with an experimental diabetic neuropathy. *Neuroscience Letters* 207:65–69.

Costa, L. G. 1998. Neurotoxicity testing: A discussion of in vitro alternatives. *Environmental Health Perspectives* 106 (Suppl. 2): 505–510.

de la Monte, S. M., K. Ghanbari, W. H. Frey, I. Behestti, P. Averback, S. L. Hauser, H. A. Ghanbari, and J. R. Wands. 1997. Characterization of the AD7C-NTP cDNA expression of a 41-kD protein in cerebrospinal fluid. *Journal of Clinical Investigation* 100:3093–3104.

Fitzpatrick, J., M. Munzar, M. Focht, R. Bibiano, and P. Averback. 2000. 7C Gold urinary assay of neural thread protein in Alzheimer's disease. *Alzheimer's Report* 3:155–159.

Hamana, K., N. Iwasaki, T. Takeya, and H. Takita. 1996. A quantitative analysis of rat central nervous system myelination using the immunochemical method for MBP. *Brain Research: Developmental Brain Research* 93:18–22.

Harry, G. J., M. Billingsley, A. Bruinink, I. L. Campbell, W. Classen, D. C. Dorman, C. Galli, D. Ray, R. A. Smith, and H. A. Tilson. 1998. In vitro techniques for the assessment of neurotoxicity. *Environmental Health Perspectives* 106 (Suppl. 1): 13–58.

Norton, W. T. 1984. Recent advances in myelin biochemistry. *Annals of the New York Academy of Sciences* 436:5–10.

Ohta, M., and K. Ohta. 2002. Detection of myelin basic protein in cerebrospinal fluid. *Expert Reviews in Molecular Diagnosis* 2:627–633.

Rajdev, S., and F. R. Sharp. 2000. Stress proteins as molecular markers of neurotoxicity. *Toxicologic Pathology* 28:105–112.

Sukuzi, Y., M. Tanaka, M. Sohmiya, S. Ichinose, A. Omori, and K. Okamoto. 2005. Identification of nitrated proteins in normal rat brain using a proteomic approach. *Neurological Research* 27:630–633.

van den Heuvel, L. P., M. H. Farhoud, R. A. Wevers, B. G. M. van Engelen, and J. A. M. Smeitink. 2003. Proteomics and neuromuscular disease: Theoretical concept and first results. *Annals of Clinical Biochemistry* 40:9–15.

12 Preanalytical Variables

12.1 INTRODUCTION

In designing studies and before the interpretation of data, it is important to consider some of the variables that can affect the data but are unrelated to the compound being tested because changes can occur in plasma and urine values due to normal biological variations. In addition to biological variations, other variations may be caused by analytical variation and the methodological variation that occurs when a study is performed.

Methodological variance is introduced by all of the experimental procedures used during a study. These variables should be considered when data are compared for the same test compound where the route of administration may differ or the study is repeated in another center using slightly different experimental procedures. In addition, there are some general considerations to be made in choosing the most suitable methodology for the selected species. Some variables within a study or between studies may be tightly controlled (e.g., species and strain), while others may be less well controlled. In this chapter and the following one, some of the preanalytical variables and some analytical variables are discussed. Preanalytical variations observed with human data (Young 2007) are much less than those for laboratory animals, mainly because of the biological component variations where environment, nutrition, and sample collection procedures have greater effects.

In this chapter some of the preanalytical factors are considered:

animals;
species, strain, age, gender, and pregnancy;
blood collection procedures;
volume, frequency, anticoagulant, collection site, and anesthesia;
environment, transportation, and stress;
nutrition and fluid balance; and
chronobiological rhythms.

12.2 SPECIES, STRAIN, AGE, GENDER, AND PREGNANCY

Several references for these variables—species, gender, and age—are also listed in Appendix A. Referenced compendiums of data often show diverse values for a single laboratory species obtained by different investigators and techniques, and this diversity is in part due to the use of different blood collection procedures and analytical techniques (Mitruka and Rawnsley 1977; Caisey and King 1980; Matsuzawa, Nomura, and Unno 1993; Loeb and Quimby 1999). There are some major differences between species for reference clinical chemistry values in healthy laboratory animals.

Some examples of differences between species include enzymes (e.g., lower-plasma alanine aminotransferase in the marmoset, higher-plasma alkaline phosphatase in the cynomolgus monkey), the proportion of intestinal alkaline phosphatase in rats in plasma, the lower-plasma bilirubin and gamma glutamyltransferase in rats, and the dominant high-density lipoprotein fraction in many of the smaller laboratory animals when compared to human plasma. Such differences are not confined to plasma (e.g., the urine protein alpha$_{2u}$-globulin found in male rat urine is not found in the urine from other species). These differences are not necessarily related to size or relative organ weight (Garattini 1981), although plasma creatinine is broadly related to muscle mass. Interspecies differences for clinical chemistry tests must be recognized in the same way that we recognize the different metabolic responses to xenobiotics in the various species.

12.2.1 STRAIN

Most laboratory animals are now purpose bred and genetically more uniform, but interstrain and breeder differences do occur (e.g., two hamster strains) (Maxwell et al. 1985). There are differences between published data for commonly used rat strains. Genetic differences may occur in healthy animals (e.g., glomerular filtration rates vary between inbred strains of rats; Hackbarth et al. 1981; Vadiei, Berens, and Luke 1990) and therefore may affect relative nephrotoxicities, while differences may become obvious only as the animals age. Palm (1998) reported that the incidence of chronic progressive nephrosis was much higher in one strain of Sprague–Dawley rats compared to rats of the same strain obtained from another supplier. Occasionally, some strains, such as diabetic Zucker rats or the hyperlipidemic Watanabe rabbit, may be chosen specifically to test for toxic effects of therapeutic agents, and the biochemical profiles of these animals will differ from the strains used for general toxicology studies.

Transgenic laboratory animals are mainly mice, which are useful to the pre-clinical scientists and pharmacologists, but for these investigations they remain a challenge, often with a reduced life span. There is a paucity of published data for these animals, and their plasma and urine biochemistry are not well characterized. Animals with inherited disorders occur in several species, but these animals are generally not used in toxicology studies. Some of the differences between strains found within published studies are no greater than data sets for the same strain obtained from different laboratories.

It is known that different rat strains differ in their metabolism—particularly in hepatic tissue reactions and therefore exposure to the test compound—so it should not be too surprising that clinical chemistry measurements may reflect these differences. When animal strains or suppliers are changed, new reference ranges should be established and compared with existing data.

12.2.2 Age

Figure 12.1 illustrates the relationships with age and when studies are usually performed during the life spans. Body and organ functions are maturing during the juvenile period/young adult period, when many rodent acute studies are performed. In later stages of rodent studies, organ function declines with impaired hormonal production and regulation. In neonates and geriatric animals, the ranges for many tests tend to show greater variation compared to late juveniles/mature adults.

Age-related changes have been described for rats (Nachbaur et al. 1977; Wolford et al. 1987; Petterino and Argentino-Storino 2006) and dogs (Andersen and Good 1970; Pickrell et al. 1974; Uchiyama, Tokoi, and Deki 1985). Plasma alkaline phosphatase is probably the best-known example of an age-dependent parameter: relatively high values during the early growth phase associated with osseous activity, followed by lower values in mature animals. Plasma creatinine values also tend to increase with age, reflecting changes in muscle mass and maturity and later alterations in the glomerular filtration rate. In rats, proteinuria (albuminuria) increases with age, with consequential changes of plasma proteins occurring at approximately 8–14 months of age (Neuhaus and Flory 1978). Age differences have been reported for urinary GGT in Wistar rats (Stoykova et al. 1983).

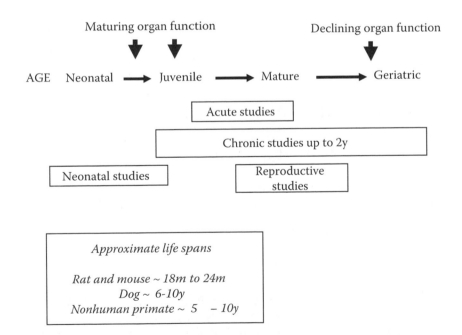

FIGURE 12.1 The relationship between animal age and study types.

12.2.3 GENDER

Occasionally, it may be useful to combine data for both genders when data are limited, but this must not disguise significant differences that may exist due to differing toxicities and metabolism between the two sexes. Apart from the obvious gender differences observed for the reproductive hormones, other plasma and urine parameters differ. Many of these differences in healthy animals are minor, and some of the published evidence is contradictory. An example of a marked difference is for plasma cholinesterase levels, which are much higher in female rats (see Table 11.1 in the preceding chapter). Urine outputs can vary between males and females (e.g., mice; Myers and Mackenzie 1985), and male rats excrete the major urinary protein, $alpha_{2u}$–globulin, which is at very low levels in female rat urine. Male mice also excrete a similar major urine protein to $alpha_{2u}$-globulin, and these are the dominant male urine proteins, unlike in larger species where albumin is the dominant protein. The excretion of the enzyme N-acetylglucosaminidase is higher in male rats and dogs (Nakamura et al. 1983; Funakawa et al. 1984).

12.2.4 PREGNANCY

Although current guidelines for reproductive toxicology studies do not require the inclusion of clinical chemistry, there is an increasing application of plasma chemistry measurements (for rats, see Papworth and Clubb 1995, LaBorde et al. 1999, and Liberati, Sansone, and Feuston 2004; for rabbits, see Bortolotti, Castelli, and Bontati 1989 and Palm 1997). Some of the published evidence is contradictory (e.g., for total cholesterol and triglycerides), but most investigators have found a decrease in plasma albumin, total protein, and glucose as the plasma volume expands during the pregnancy.

12.3 BLOOD COLLECTION PROCEDURES

When blood is collected, a number of factors need to be considered, particularly from the smaller animals. These factors include:

sample volume relative to total blood volume;
frequency of sampling;
site of sampling;
agents used for anesthesia or euthanasia;
time of sampling; and
use of anticoagulant.

Blood collection procedures can have a significant impact on study results, and a variety of collection sites is used, particularly for the smaller laboratory animals. Blood sampling procedures require skilled personnel, and it is not uncommon to see a higher incidence of poor-quality specimens when routine procedures have not been used or the operator is not sufficiently proficient. Some variations can be traced to individuals performing the collection procedures in slightly different ways and therefore producing different results (Fowler 1982). In some circumstances, it is extremely difficult to obtain samples (e.g., from animals where the blood circulation is severely affected or in extremis).

12.3.1 Volume, Frequency, and Site

Analytical developments during the last three decades have reduced the blood volumes required for the common plasma tests, but the blood sample volume collected must be sufficiently large to be a representative sample. Using very small volumes may be attractive but can yield atypical results, and this can be confirmed by the variable results obtained when taking a small number of serial samples, which are often partially affected by tissue fluid contamination. Although estimates vary for circulating blood volumes in the various species, these estimates are based on different techniques. A broad rule is that the blood volume is approximately 6–7% of the body volume (i.e., 60–70 mL/kg body weight for all species), and this can be used to calculate the approximate blood volume in the body. However, not all of this volume is available for collection because it is "trapped" in tissues, etc.

Guidance for the removal of blood, including routes and volumes, is provided by several publications (McGuill and Rowan 1989; BVA/FRAME/RSPCA/UFAW 1993; Diehl et al. 2001). Toxicokineticists should also be aware of the effects of blood removal on their measurements and their possible impact on combined toxicology studies (Hulse, Feldman, and Bruckner 1981; Tamura et al. 1990). For animals weighing more than 1 kg, repetitive blood sampling is rarely a problem, but for smaller animals the guidance of collecting less than 15% of total blood volume for a single sampling and less than 7.5% per week for repetitive sampling is a reasonable guideline. The volumes from conscious animals will be less than at necropsy; this is particularly important for smaller animals. The collection of 0.5 mL of blood from a 20-g mouse represents a 20% loss of blood volume for that animal. Repetitive sampling or excessive blood withdrawal may cause anemia and prejudice the outcome of a study (McGuill and Rowan 1989; Evans 1994). Toxicology laboratories have local procedures covering permitted blood volumes and frequency of collection, as well as local rules for animal welfare.

The choice of sampling site depends on the volumes of blood required for analysis and whether the sampling time is during or at the end of a study, when larger samples can usually be taken. The sites for blood collection used for different species vary, and sites are sometimes preferentially chosen on the basis of local experience with a technique, in the absence of data suggesting that one site is best.

The sites used for blood collection in different species include:

dog: jugular, femoral, saphenous, cephalic veins;
ferret: jugular or cephalic vein, abdominal vena cava;
gerbil: tail (coccygeal) vein, orbital-venous sinus, tail cut, or from the heart;
guinea pig: from the heart, or jugular or ear veins;
hamster: from the heart or jugular vein;
marmoset: femoral vein or coccygeal vein;
mouse: tail cut, tail vein, or from the heart;

rabbit: ear vein or artery, jugular vein, or from the heart;

rat: tail vein, retro-orbital venous plexus (sinus), sublingual vein, jugular vein, abdominal vena cava, abdominal aorta, and heart; and

monkey: femoral, cephalic, jugular, or saphenous veins, or from the heart.

When blood cannot be collected from the central veins of smaller laboratory animals, sites such as the retro-orbital plexus and tail are used. Some of these procedures can be carried out only at termination or may require anesthesia to allow interim sampling. In general, the collection of blood from dogs and most primates does not cause particular problems in terms of the sample volume required for core clinical chemistry tests, but the demand for and inclusion of additional biomarkers may require a compromise in study design.

Anesthetics should be chosen on the basis of causing minimal stress to the animal, minimal interference effects on the analyte, and minimal hazards to the operator through accidental injection, chemical toxicity of the anesthetic agents, or injuries caused by the animal's behavior during the procedure. Anesthetic agents used for rodents include halothane, ether, barbiturate, methoxyfluorane, and carbon dioxide. Frequently repeated anesthesia can affect the analyte values.

Multiple and excessive blood collections may in themselves cause hematological changes (e.g., anemia). Repeated or excessive blood sampling from the femoral veins in marmosets may lead to edema and hematoma at the site of collection. Even when available sample volumes are limited, pooling of samples prior to analysis should be avoided. Using more than one collection procedure within a study should be avoided if possible (e.g., in rodent studies, collecting interim samples by tail collection procedures but collecting the final sample by cardiac sampling at necropsy will result in differences when comparing the interim and final time day due in part to the two collection procedures). These procedural differences emphasize the need to interpret data cautiously when making comparisons between studies and to establish reference ranges using chosen procedures. Errors can be caused by poor sampling procedures, prolonged venous stasis, inadequate mixing with appropriate amounts of anticoagulant, and the presence of small blood clots.

Numerous methods and data have been published for the collection of blood from rats and mice (Riley 1960; Upton and Morgan 1975; Cardy and Warner 1979; Fowler, Brown, and Flower 1980; Archer and Riley 1981; Cochetto and Bjornsson 1983; Neptun, Smith, and Irons 1985; Suber and Kodell 1985; Conybeare et al. 1988; Dameron et al. 1992; Itumi et al. 1993; Matsuzawa et al. 1994; Bernardi et al. 1996; Walter 1999; Mahl et al. 2000; Nahas et al. 2000; Schnell et al. 2002). Values obtained from major blood vessels or cardiac puncture are less variable than those samples taken from the tail or retro-orbital plexus; this may be in part due to contamination with tissue fluid. Potassium, total protein, and several enzymes are higher in samples collected from the tail or the retro-orbital plexus. The use of carbon dioxide and, to a lesser extent, halothane increases plasma levels of glucose, potassium, and inorganic phosphate.

The use of restraining procedures may affect biochemical values in small and, to a lesser extent, large laboratory animals. Increased plasma alanine and aspartate aminotransferase activities associated with restraint during collection have been reported in mice and rats (Pearl, Balazs, and Buyske 1966; Swaim, Taylor, and Jersey 1985; Landi and Kissinger 1994; Sanchez et al. 2002). These effects on enzymes may be due to stress, tissue injury, glycogenolysis, or gluconeogenesis.

In dogs, the values obtained for common plasma tests were similar when collected from the cephalic and exterior jugular vein (Jensen, Wenck, and Koch 1994). On some occasions, the sampling needle may injure tissues and cause plasma enzyme elevations (e.g., with dogs) (Fayoll, Lefebvre, and Braun 1992). Ketamine as a sedative can alter plasma proteins and electrolytes when samples are taken from monkeys (Bennett et al. 1992), and this agent can cause local myotoxicity in marmosets (Davy et al. 1987) with increased plasma enzymes. As a general rule, any change of sedative or agent for euthanasia should be assessed for its potential to alter biochemical values and compared with previous data. Increased plasma enzymes are also seen with other xenobiotics given by intramuscular (i.m.) injections; these effects may be caused by the osmolality, pH, and volume of solution administered. The reaction may be also be caused by some excipients (Meltzer, Mrozak, and Boyer 1970; Gloor, Vorburger, and Schädelin 1977; Steiness et al. 1978; Surber and Dubach 1989).

Several of the blood collection procedures alter the plasma albumin and total protein concentrations, and these changes should be considered when interpreting toxicokinetic data, particularly when perturbations of plasma proteins occur (Hulse et al. 1981; Chou and Levy 1984; Tamura et al. 1990; Proost, Wierda, and Meijer 1996).

To avoid hemolysis during sample collection and transfer to the sample tube, the needle size should be chosen to suit the animal and collection site, and blood should be transferred to the sample tube without excessive force. Blood samples should be thoroughly mixed immediately with the anticoagulant after collection. However, samples that are mixed too vigorously can lead to red cell fragmentation and hemolysis.

12.3.2 ANTICOAGULANTS

The ongoing debate in human medicine (e.g., Zhang et al. 1998; Miles et al. 2004) about the use of serum or plasma for common clinical chemistry measurements is similar to the discussions in animal clinical chemistry, and the topic is repeatedly investigated. Broad guidance for the use of anticoagulants is available (ICCLS 2003). There are slight differences between plasma and serum, but these differences are generally small and much less than interindividual variations, except obviously for fibrinogen. Many laboratories use sample tubes designed for human pediatrics to collect samples from small laboratory animals (with volumes of less than 2 mL), and users should be aware that the label colors on commercially available tubes are not always the same.

Lithium heparinate (or heparin: with orange or green labels) is a suitable anticoagulant for most plasma measurements. Plasma or serum should be separated within 2 h of collection because erythrocytic glycolysis occurs and reduces the apparent levels of glucose. Potassium and several enzymes also leak from the erythrocytes if not promptly separated and increase the apparent concentrations. The anticoagulant sodium fluoride alone or in combination with potassium oxalate will halt this glycolysis. For several enzyme measurements, it is suggested that plasma rather than serum be used because of the release of erythrocytic enzymes during clotting processes (Korsrud and Trick 1973; Friedel and Mattenheimer 1970). Some enzymes are present at relatively high concentrations in erythrocytes compared to plasma and therefore may interfere with the measurements— for example, adenylate kinase in creatine kinase (CK) assays. If blood samples are not centrifuged with enough force to sediment platelets, then the platelets can release enzymes (e.g., creatine kinase) and lactate dehydrogenase, which affect the analysis results (Shibata and Kobayashi 1978; Evans 1985; Reimann, Knowlen, and Tvedten 1989; Aktas et al. 1994). With samples from mice, additional centrifugal force may be required to sediment the small erythrocytes. Blood samples for bilirubin assays should be protected from strong light because this will reduce levels.

Inappropriate use of anticoagulants and incorrect proportions of anticoagulant to blood volumes may also cause errors and yield serum rather than plasma when underfilled. Ethylenediamine tetracetic acid (K_2EDTA or K_3EDTA, or sequestrene— usually with a pink label) is the anticoagulant commonly used for full blood counts, but it is unsuitable for many of the common analytes; it has a marked effect on potassium because it is present in the anticoagulant and calcium due to the chelation of calcium by EDTA (Ceron et al. 2004). Sodium citrate used as an anticoagulant for blood coagulation measurements also chelates plasma calcium (sometimes the tube label is purple and sometimes the label is green). For some specialized assays, certain anticoagulants are preferred, and unpublished data suggest that, in some multiple analyses of samples by "multiplexing" assays, the use of a single anticoagulant may not be suitable for all assays.

The local laboratory should always be consulted as to the appropriate anticoagulant and sample collection tubes to be used. "Noncore" tests may require the use of other anticoagulants.

12.3.3 URINE COLLECTION

Various methods for urine collection from laboratory animals have been reviewed by Kurien, Everds, and Scofield (2004). Both the fluid balance of the animals and diuresis will affect the volumes of urine collected (Obatomi and Plummer 1993, 1997). The design of devices for separating urine and feces is a critical factor in reducing fecal contamination of urine because feces contains many substances, including enzymes, and may cause falsely raised values (Plummer and Wright 1970). Catheterization may be used as a collection procedure in dogs, but samples may become contaminated due to the collection procedure (see Chapter 4). Using well-designed metabolism cages, urine should be collected over fixed time periods; these periods are often more than 15–18 h overnight. The timing of the collection in relation to dosing and injury may produce differing results, and for nephrotoxicity studies, several collections should be made.

Urine specimens collected overnight at room temperature may lose carbon dioxide or become contaminated with ammonia-producing bacteria; this may be indicated by high-alkaline pH. If the urine is not fresh, pH values may also be unreliable. It is preferable not to use liquid preservatives (e.g., toluene), particularly with urine collections from small animals, because this introduces variable dilution effects. Collections using ice or cooling packs to chill the urine container may be required for some tests (e.g., enzymes). Urine contamination by cleaning fluids such as hypochlorite can lead to false positive results with test strips. Centrifuging urines other than for microscopy can reduce the levels of enzymes contained within cells and cell debris and minerals (e.g., inorganic phosphates).

12.3.4 SAMPLE STORAGE

When it is possible, assays should be performed on the same day as collection; inevitably, however, some samples have to be stored for analyses at a later date, and their stabilities vary. Storage should be at 4, –20, or –40°C, and the laboratory should evaluate the stabilities of analytes under their current operating conditions (Hirata, Nomura, and Tanimoto 1979; Falk 1981; Ito et al. 1998). Samples for ionized calcium and blood gases require additional collection and storage procedures to prevent change of pH and oxygen content (Pickrell, Light, et al. 1973; Pickrell, Mauderley, et al. 1973; Szenci, Brydl, and Bajcsy 1991).

Cyclical freezing and thawing of samples should be avoided because this denatures proteins. Urine enzymes and proteins are affected by storage at low temperatures; they are usually decreased by freezing and thawing processes. Urinary gamma glutamyl transferase is adversely affected by freezing, with a very marked loss of enzyme activity (Stokke 1974; Matteuchi et al. 1991; Berg et al. 1998).

12.3.5 HEMOLYSIS AND LIPEMIA

Observations of hemolysis and lipemia should always be recorded. Hemolysis is more frequently due to problems with sample collection rather than an effect of the test compound, and additional hematological data, if available, may be used to clarify this issue. Some examples of the effects of hemolysis are the increases of several plasma enzymes and potassium in most species (Chin, Tipton, and Kozbelt 1979; Czerwek and Bleuel 1981; Davy et al. 1984; Greenson, Farber, and Dubin 1989; O'Neill and Feldman 1989; Leard et al. 1990; Jacobs, Lumsden, and Grift 1992). In dogs, the effects of hemolysis on potassium are much less than in many other species because the erythrocytic potassium concentrations are similar to plasma levels (Coldman and Good 1967; Coulter and Small 1971). Hemolysis may also affect hormone levels (Reimers et al. 1991); for example, erythrocytic insulinases lower plasma insulin values (Sapin et al. 1998).

12.4 ENVIRONMENT, TRANSPORTATION, AND STRESS

The challenge of experimental refinement (one of the "3 Rs"; Rowan 1990) has led to investigations and observations on the effects of environment and transportation of animals, with suggested measures of these effects including stress. Several environmental factors, including caging density (i.e., numbers of animals per cage), lighting cycles, room temperature and humidity, cage bedding, environmental enrichment (e.g., toys, chew sticks, swings), cleaning procedures, etc., have been shown to affect animals and, in some cases, biochemical measurements (Fouts 1976; Gärtner et al. 1980; Riley 1981; Bickhardt et al. 1983; Dobrakovová and Jurčovičová 1984; Peng et al. 1989; Vadiei et al. 1990; Whary et al. 1993; Perez et al. 1997). Modern animal accommodation and animal care practices are designed to minimize but do not eliminate these effects. With today's breeding and animal care procedures, parasitic or viral infections are less likely to occur, but, when they are present, these infections may affect some measurements (e.g., plasma proteins).

Transportation within and between animal accommodation can affect some biochemical tests (Bean-Knudsen and Wagner 1987; Kuhn and Hardegg 1988; Drozdowicz et al. 1990; Garnier et al. 1990; Toth and January 1990; Kuhn et al. 1991; Tuli et al. 1995), and some rat and mouse studies have included plasma corticosterone and catecholamines as measures of stress (Garbus, Highman, and Atland 1967; Vogel 1987; Haemisch, Guerra, and Hurker 1999). Because blood sampling procedures can increase corticosterone, noninvasive fecal measurements have been advocated for measuring stress effects, but the results from fecal collections are variable (Eriksson 2004; Royo et al. 2004). Although some individual animals have a quiet disposition and show minimal stress responses, the behavior of some animals can be markedly affected by blood sampling procedures.

Except when blood samples may be essential—for example, in health screening for viral status on receipt of animals to new accommodation—it is preferable to allow a period of acclimatization prior to blood sampling to avoid some of the variations caused by housing changes, transportation, and dietary changes. During most studies, the animal room conditions will remain relatively constant, but stress effects in individual animals may occur and vary during toxicity studies, so their potential effects on biochemical data should be recognized.

12.5 NUTRITION AND FLUID BALANCE

Some laboratories require both rodents and dogs to be fasted prior to blood sample collections; although there is agreement concerning dogs, there is some debate about the fasting of rodents (Matsuzawa and Sakaume 1994; Waner and Nyska 1994). Possible short-term effects have been studied to determine the effects of overnight fasting (16–24 h) on rat plasma chemistry; these fasting effects include reduced plasma alkaline phosphatase; changes of urea, glucose, creatinine, and plasma proteins with hemoconcentration; and organ weight changes, although some of the reported effects vary (Jenkins and Robinson 1975; Apostoulou, Saidt, and Brown 1976; Kast and Nishikawa 1981; Pickering and Pickering 1984; Maejima and Nagase 1991). Depletion of hepatic glycogen by fasting in rats generally takes more than 24 h, and this period may extend to 48 h. In dogs, slight hemoconcentration may occur following an overnight fast. Postprandial increases for both plasma urea and creatinine have been reported in dogs, and these increases vary with diet (Street et al. 1968; Watson, Church, and Fairburn 1981; Evans 1987).

Longer-term studies in rats (Schwartz, Tornaben, and Boxhill 1973; Oishi, Ishi, and Hiraga 1979; Levin, Semler, and Ruben 1993; Slaughter et al. 1998), mice (Dancla and Nachbaur 1981), and cynomolgus monkeys (Yoshida et al. 1994) show effects due to dietary restrictions. Alterations of dietary protein can change the amounts of proteinuria in rats (Meyer, Kristiansen, and Wurtzen 1989; Macconi et al. 1997; Hammond and Janes 1998). Other reports show effects due to altering dietary fat content and minerals (Stonard, Samuels, and Lock 1984; Meijer, De Bruijne, and Beynen 1987; Bertani et al. 1989). Diets with mineral imbalance and altered protein content may cause nephrocalcinosis and affect proteinuria in some species, with associated changes in plasma and urine biochemistry (Stonard et al. 1984; Bertani et al. 1989; Meyer et al. 1989). Alterations of plasma thyroid hormones caused by diet are a less obvious example of diet-induced changes in the rat (Ingbar and Galton 1975; Cokelaere et al. 1996). Differing diets have been reported to affect longevity and tumor incidence rates in long-term carcinogenicity studies (Hart et al. 1995).

Unlike fats and carbohydrates, which are stored within the body, protein gains or losses can be more immediate indicators of nutritional changes affecting the animal. However, given that more than 50% of the body's albumin is located in extravascular spaces and the half-life of albumin, plasma albumin may take some time to fall, while some other smaller proteins synthesized in the liver may fall more quickly because they have shorter half-lives. Increased gluconeogenesis may occur following dietary alterations and lead to changes of the plasma aminotransferases.

Severe dehydration and reduction of plasma volume may become apparent through increased plasma protein and hematocrit values (Boyd 1981; Kutscher 1988). Alterations of fluid intake affect plasma electrolyte balance (Clausing and Gottschalk 1989; Boemke et al. 1990; Single et al. 1998). Simple observations of water intake together with urinary output are important when examining subjects for fluid balance perturbations.

Most of the references provided in this section are for studies in which deliberate manipulations of fluid and food intakes have occurred, which have then caused effects on plasma or urine chemistry values. As a result of severe toxicity, animals may alter their food and water intakes and these consumption data should be examined when interpreting laboratory data; this is particularly important when there is evidence of gastrointestinal, hepatic, or renal toxicity (Omaye 1986). Toxicity may exaggerate differences between dosed or treatment groups, and alterations of nutrition and fluid balance can also potentially alter the absorption or uptake of the test compound and changes in the rates of metabolism and/or detoxification, modify renal clearance, or change the competitive binding of proteins with the test compound and thus the overall toxicity findings.

Treatment prior to sequential blood sampling in toxicology studies should be similar in respect to food and water intake, and any effects on dietary and fluid intake should be considered when biochemical changes are interpreted. Any major changes of animal diets should be monitored for possible effect on plasma and urine chemistry.

12.6 CHRONOBIOCHEMICAL RHYTHMS

Periodic or cyclic variations and their effects on toxicology and pharmacology are being increasingly recognized, as many physiological measurements show some degree of change with time—within the day or month or over longer periods. Some of these changes may be small while others may be more obvious (Moore-Ede and

Sulzman 1983; Murphy and Campbell 1996; Arendt 1998). Periodic changes are observed for most plasma hormones and reproductive cycle hormones in particular. These hormonal changes may be short-term pulsatile changes or daily rhythms or follow longer-term cycles (see Chapter 10; Wong et al. 1983; Kempainnen and Sartin 1981; Fukuda et al. 1988; Orth, Peterson, and Drucker 1988; Nigi and Torii 1991; Torii and Nigi 1994).

Several different patterns affecting enzymuria in rats have been described; these patterns include daily and seasonal changes (Grotsch et al. 1985; Cal et al. 1987; Cambar, Dorian, and Cal 1987; Pariat et al. 1990; Do et al. 1992). These renal patterns become more complex with compounds such as aminoglycosides, which also show time-dependent toxicity changes (Batalla et al. 1994; Yamauchi et al. 1998; LeBrun et al. 1999).

To reduce variations associated with time, it is sensible to consider taking samples at the same time of day if numbers permit, particularly for hormone assays, or taking samples in a randomized order rather than from all control group animals followed by all animals within the treatment groups. The collection order should also be randomized if several individuals are responsible for collecting samples. Pooling of blood samples from several animals should be avoided because this procedure hides interanimal variation. The possible use of a wide range of procedures emphasizes the caution needed when comparing study data with reference ranges or published data, as well as the need for contemporary controls.

12.7   SUMMARY

Some of the preanalytical variables are controllable (e.g., species, strain, age range, and gender) when a study or series of studies is designed. Good practice in animal care minimizes stress and creates good sample collection procedures to reduce variations. When blood samples are to be taken from several treatment groups containing large numbers of animals, the order of sampling should be randomized. When the number of animals within a study is small, samples should be taken to measure intra-animal variations before and during the study. There is a need for careful examination of procedures and data when blood collection procedures are altered or baseline data appear to change markedly. The timing of blood or urine sampling in relation to the toxic insult is critically important. For example, following renal tubular damage or cardiac muscle injury, enzyme changes may occur rapidly in the early phase of a study, and measurements may have returned to normal or to pretreatment levels at the times scheduled for sample collection.

REFERENCES

Young, D. S. 2007. *Effects of preanalytical variables on clinical laboratory tests.* 3rd ed. Washington, DC: American Association of Clinical Chemistry Press.

Species, Strain, Age, Gender
Andersen, A. C., and L. S. Good, eds. 1970. *The beagle as an experimental dog.* Ames: The Iowa State University Press.

Bortolotti, A., D. Castelli, and M. Bontati. 1989. Hematology and serum chemistry values of adult pregnant and newborn New Zealand rabbits (*Oryctolagus cuniculus*). *Laboratory Animal Science* 39:437–439.

Caisey, J. D., and D. J. King. 1980. Clinical chemistry values for some common laboratory animals. *Clinical Chemistry* 26:1877–1879.

Funakawa, S., T. Itoh, K. Miyata, Y. Tochino, and M. Nakamura. 1984. Sex difference of N-acetyl-D-glucosaminidase activity in the kidney, urine and plasma of mice. *Renal Physiology* 7:124–128.

Garattini, S. 1981. Toxic effects of chemicals: Difficulties in extrapolating data from animals to man. *CRC Critical Reviews in Toxicology* 16:1–29.

Hackbarth, H., E. Baunack, and M. Winn. 1981. Strain differences in kidney function of inbred rats: 1. Glomerular filtration rate and renal plasma flow. *Laboratory Animals* 15:125–128.

LaBorde, J. B., K. S. Wall, B. Bolon, T. S. Kumpe, R. Patton, Q. Zheng, R. Kodell, and J. F. Young. 1999. Hematology and serum chemistry parameters of the pregnant rat. *Laboratory Animals* 33:275–287.

Liberati, T. A., S. R. Sansone, and M. H. Feuston. 2004. Hematology and clinical chemistry values in pregnant Wistar Hanover rats compared with nonmated controls. *Veterinary Clinical Pathology* 33:68–73.

Loeb, W. F., and F. W. Quimby. 1999. *The clinical chemistry of laboratory animals*, 2nd ed. Boca Raton, FL: Taylor & Francis.

Matsuzawa, T., M. Nomura, and T. Unno. 1993. Clinical pathology reference ranges of laboratory animals. *Journal of Veterinary Medical Science* 55:351–62.

Maxwell, K. O., C. Wish, J. C. Murphy, and J. G. Fox. 1985. Serum chemistry references values in two strains of Syrian hamsters. *Laboratory Animal Science* 35:67–70.

Mitruka, B. M., and H. M. Rawnsley. 1977. *Clinical biochemical and hematological reference values in normal experimental animals.* New York: Masson Publishing USA Inc.

Myers, K. R., and K. M. Mackenzie. 1985. A comparison of 24-hour urine output in male and female mice and rats. *Laboratory Animal Science* 35:546–547.

Nachbaur, J., M. R. Clarke, J. P. Provost, and J. L. Dancla. 1977. Variations of sodium, potassium and chloride plasma levels in the rat with age and sex. *Laboratory Animal Science* 27:972–975.

Nakamura, M., T. ltoh, K. Miyata, N. Higashiyama, H. Takesue, and S. Nishiyama. 1983. Difference in urinary N-acetyl-p-D-glucosaminidase activity between male and female beagle dogs. *Renal Physiology (Basel)* 6:130–133.

Neuhaus, O. W., and W. Flory. 1978. Age-dependent changes in the excretion of urinary proteins by the rat. *Nephron* 22:570–576.

Palm, M. 1997. Clinical pathology values in pregnant and nonpregnant rabbits *Scandinavian Journal of Laboratory Animal Science* 24:177–183.

———. 1998. The incidence of chronic progressive nephrosis in young Sprague–Dawley rats for two different strains. *Laboratory Animals* 32:477–482.

Papworth, T. A., and S. K. Clubb. 1995. Clinical pathology in the female rat during the pre- and postnatal period. *Comparative Haematology International* 5:13–24.

Petterino, C., and A. Argentino-Storino. 2006. Clinical chemistry and hematology historical data in control Sprague–Dawley rats from preclinical toxicity studies. *Experimental and Toxicological Pathology* 57:213–219.

Pickrell, J. A., S. J. Schluter, J. J. Belasich, E. V. Stewart, J. Meyer, C. H. Hobbs, and R. K. Jones. 1974. Relationship of age of normal dogs to blood serum constituents and reliability of measured single values. *American Journal of Veterinary Research* 35:897–903.

Stoykova, S., C. Philippon, F. Labaille, D. Prevot, and Y. Manuel. 1983. Comparative study of alanine-amino-peptidase and gamma-glutamyl-transferase activity in normal Wistar rat urine. *Laboratory Animals* 17:246–251.

Uchiyama, T., K. Tokoi, and T. Deki. 1985. Successive changes in the blood composition of the experimental normal beagle dogs accompanied with age. *Experimental Animals* 34:367–377.

Vadiei, K., K. L. Berens, and D. R. Luke. 1990. Isolation-induced renal functional changes in rats from four breeders. *Laboratory Animal Science* 40:56–59.

Wolford, S. T., R. A. Schroer, F. X. Gohs, P. P. Gallo, M. Brodeck, H. B. Falk, and R. Ruhren. 1987. Age-related changes in serum chemistry and hematology values in normal Sprague–Dawley rats. *Fundamental and Applied Toxicology* 8:80–88.

Blood Volumes and Frequency

BVA/FRAME/RSPCA/UFAW Joint Working Group on Refinement. 1993. Removal of blood from laboratory mammals and birds. First report 1993. *Laboratory Animals* 27:1–22.

Diehl, K-H., R. Hull, D. Morton, R. Pfister, Y. Rabemampianina, D. Smith, J-M. Vidal, and C. van de Vorstenbosch. 2001. A good practice guide to the administration of substances and removal of blood including routes and volumes. *Journal of Applied Toxicology* 21:15–23.

Evans, G. O. 1994. Removal of blood from laboratory mammals and birds. *Laboratory Animals* 28:178–179.

Fowler, J. S. L. 1982. Animal clinical chemistry and haematology for the toxicologist. *Archives of Toxicology* 5 (Suppl.): 152–159.

McGuill, M. W., and A. N. Rowan. 1989. Biological effects of blood loss: Implications for sampling volumes and techniques. *ILAR News* 31:15–18.

Blood Collection Procedures for Rats and Mice

Archer, R. K., and J. Riley. 1981. Standardized method for bleeding rats. *Laboratory Animals* 14:25–28.

Bernardi, C., D. Moneta, M. Brughera, M. Di Salvo, D. Lamparelli, G. Mazué, and M. J. Iatropoulos. 1996. Hematology and clinical chemistry in rats: Comparison of different blood collection sites. *Comparative Hematology International* 6:160–166.

Cardy, R. H., and J. W. Warner. 1979. Effects of sequential bleeding on body weight gain in rats. *Laboratory Animal Science* 29:179–181.

Cochetto, D. M., and T. D. Bjornsson. 1983. Methods for vascular access and collection of body fluids from the laboratory rat. *Journal of Pharmaceutical Sciences* 72:465–492.

Conybeare, G., G. B. Leslie, K. Angles, R. J. Barrett, J. S. H. Luke, and D. R. Gask. 1988. An improved simple technique for the collection of blood samples from rats and mice. *Laboratory Animals* 22:177–182.

Dameron, G. W., K. W. Weingand, J. M. Duderstadt, L. W. Odioso, T. A. Dierckman, W. Schwecke, and K. Baran. 1992. Effects of bleeding site on clinical laboratory testing of rats: Orbital venous plexus versus posterior vena cava. *Laboratory Animal Science* 42:299–301.

Fowler, J. S. L., J. S. Brown, and E. W. Flower. 1980. Comparison between ether and carbon dioxide anaesthesia for removal of small blood samples from rats. *Laboratory Animals* 14:275–278.

Itumi, Y., F. Sugiyama, Y. Sugiyama, and K-I. Yagami. 1993. Comparison between the blood from orbital sinus and heart in analyzing plasma biochemical values—Increase of plasma enzymes in the blood from orbital sinus. *Experimental Animals* 42:99–102.

Landi, M. S., and J. T. Kissinger. 1994. The effects of four types of restraint on serum alanine aminotransferase and aspartate aminotransferase in *Macaca fascicularis*. In *Welfare and science, proceedings of the fifth FELASA symposium*, pp. 37–40. London: Royal Society of Medicine Press.

Mahl, A., P. Heining, P. Ulrich, J. Jakubowski, M. Bobadilla, W. Zeller, R. Bergmann, T. Singer, and L. Meister. 2000. Comparison of clinical pathology parameters with two different blood sampling techniques in rats: Retrobulbar plexus versus sublingual vein. *Laboratory Animals* 34:351–361.

Matsuzawa, T., H. Tabata, M. Sakazume, S. Yoshida, and S. Nakamura. 1994. A comparison of the effect of bleeding site on hematological and plasma chemistry values of F344 rats: The inferior vena cava, abdominal aorta, and orbital venous plexus. *Comparative Haematology International* 4:207–211.

Nahas, K., J-P. Provost, Ph. Baneux, and Y. Rabemampianina. 2000. Effects of acute blood removal via the sublingual vein on hematological and clinical parameters in Sprague–Dawley rats. *Laboratory Animals* 34:362–371.

Neptun, D. A., C. N. Smith, and R. D. Irons. 1985. Effect of sampling site and collection method on variations in baseline clinical pathology parameters in Fischer 344 rats. I. Clinical chemistry. *Fundamental and Applied Toxicology* 5:1180–1185.

Pearl, W., T. Balazs, and D. A. Buyske. 1966. The stress on serum transaminase activity in the rat. *Life Sciences* 5:67–74.

Riley, V. 1960. Adaptation of orbital bleeding technique to rapid serial blood studies. *Proceedings of the Society for Experimental Biology and Medicine* 104:751–754.

Sanchez, O., A. Arnau, M. Pareja, E. Poch, I. Ramirez, and M. Soley. 2002. Acute stress-induced tissue injury in mice: Differences between emotional and social stress. *Cellular Stress Chaperones* 7:36–46.

Schnell, M. S., C. Hardy, M. Hawley, K. J. Propert, and J. M. Wilson. 2002. Effect of blood collection technique in mice on clinical pathology parameters. *Human Gene Therapy* 13:155–162.

Suber, R. L., and R. L. Kodell. 1985. The effects of three phlebotomy techniques on hematological and clinical chemical evaluation in Sprague–Dawley rats. *Veterinary Clinical Pathology* 14:23–30.

Swaim, L. D., H. W. Taylor, and G. C. Jersey. 1985. The effect of handling techniques on serum ALT activity in mice. *Journal of Applied Toxicology* 5:160–162.

Upton, P. K., and D. J. Morgan. 1975. The effect of sampling technique on some blood parameters in the rat. *Laboratory Animals* 9:85–91.

Walter, G. L. 1999. Effects of carbon dioxide inhalation on hematology, coagulation and serum clinical chemistry values in rats. *Toxicologic Pathology* 27:217–225.

Blood Collection Procedures in Other Species

Bennett, J. S., K. A. Gossett, M. P. McCarthy, and E. D. Simpson. 1992. Effects of ketamine hydrochloride on serum biochemical and hematologic variables in Rhesus monkeys (*Macaca mulatta*). *Veterinary Clinical Pathology* 21:15–18.

Davy, C. W., P. N. Trennery, J. G. Edmunds, J. F. Altman, and D. A. Eichler. 1987. Local myotoxicity of ketamine hydrochloride in the marmoset. *Laboratory Animals* 21:60–67.

Fayoll, P., H. Lefebvre, and J. P. Braun. 1992. Effects of incorrect venepuncture on plasma creatine kinase activity in dog and horse. *British Veterinary Journal* 148:161–162.

Jensen, A. L., A. Wenck, and J. Koch. 1994. Comparison of results of hematological and clinical chemical analyses of blood samples obtained from the cephalic and external jugular veins in dogs. *Research in Veterinary Science* 56:24–29.

Effects of Intramuscular Toxicity

Gloor, H. O., C. Vorburger, and J. Schädelin. 1977. Intramusculäre injektionen und serumkreatinphosphokinase-aktivität. *Schweizerische Medizinische Wochenschrift* 107:948–952.

Meltzer, H. Y., S. Mrozak, and M. Boyer. 1970. Effects of intramuscular injections on serum creatine phosphokinase activity. *American Journal of Medical Science* 259:42–48.

Steiness, E., F. Rasmussen, O. Svendsen, and P. Nielsen. 1978. A comparative study of serum phosphokinase activity in rabbits, pigs and humans after intramuscular injections of local damaging drugs. *Acta Pharmacologica Toxicologica* 42:357–364.

Surber, C., and U. C. Dubach. 1989. Tests for local toxicity of intramuscular drug preparations. Comparison of in vivo and in vitro findings. *Arzeneimittel-Forschung* 39:1586–1589.

Plasma Protein Binding

Chou, R. C., and G. Levy. 1984. Comparative in vivo and in vitro studies of phenytoin protein binding and in vitro lipolysis in plasma of pregnant and nonpregnant rats. *Journal of Pharmaceutical Science* 73:1121–1124.

Hulse, M., S. Feldman, and J. V. Bruckner. 1981. Effect of blood sampling schedules on protein drug binding in the rat. *Journal of Pharmacology and Experimental Therapeutics* 218:416–420.

Proost, J. H., J. M. Wierda, and D. K. Meijer. 1996. An extended pharmacokinetic/pharmaco-dynamic model describing the quantitative influence of plasma protein binding, tissue binding and receptor binding on the potency and time course of action of drugs. *Journal of Pharmacokinetics and Biopharmaceutics* 24:45–77.

Tamura, A., K. Sugimoto, T. Sato, and T. Fujii. 1990. The effects of haematocrit, plasma protein concentration and temperature of drug-containing blood in vitro on the concentrations of the drug in the plasma. *Journal of Pharmacy and Pharmacology* 42:577–580.

Anticoagulants

Aktas, M., D. Auguste, P. Corcordet, P. Vinclair, H. Lefebvre, and P. L. Toutain. 1994. Creatine kinase in dog plasma: Preanalytical factors of variations, reference values and diagnostic significance. *Research in Veterinary Science* 56:30–36.

Ceron, J. J., A. S. Martínez-Subiela, C. Henneman, and F. Tecles. 2004. The effects of different anticoagulants on routine canine plasma biochemistry. *Veterinary Journal* 167:294–301.

Evans, G. O. 1985. Lactate dehydrogenase activity in platelets and plasma. *Clinical Chemistry* 31:165–166.

Friedel, R., and H. Mattenheimer. 1970. Release of metabolic enzymes from platelets during blood clotting of man, dog, rabbit and rat. *Clinica Chimica Acta* 30:37–46.

ICCLS. Clinical and Laboratory Standards Institute. 2003. *H01 tubes and additives for venous blood specimen collection,* 5th ed. Wayne, PA: Clinical Laboratory Standards Institute.

Korsrud, G. O., and K. D. Trick. 1973. Activities of several enzymes in serum and heparinized plasma from rats. *Clinica Chimica Acta* 48:311–315.

Miles, R. R., R. F. Roberts, A. R. Putman, and W. L. Roberts. 2004. Comparison of serum and heparinized plasma samples for measurement of chemistry analytes. *Clinica Chimica Acta* 50:1704–1705.

Reimann, K. A., G. G. Knowlen, and H. W. Tvedten. 1989. Factitious hyperkalemia in dogs with thrombocytosis. The effect of platelets on serum potassium. *Journal of Veterinary Internal Medicine* 3:47–52.

Shibata, S., and B. Kobayashi. 1978. Blood platelets as a possible source of creatine kinase in rat plasma and serum. *Thrombosis and Hemostasis (Stuttgart)* 39:701–706.

Zhang, D. J., R. K. Elswick, W. G. Miller, and J. L. Bailey. 1998. Effect of serum-clot contact time on clinical chemistry laboratory results. *Clinical Chemistry* 44:1325–1338.

Urine

Kurien, B. T., N. E. Everds, and R. H. Scofield. 2004. Experimental animal urine collection: A review. *Laboratory Animals* 38:333–351.

Obatomi, D. K., and D. T. Plummer. 1993. Influence of hydration states on the acute nephro-toxic effect of gentamicin. *Toxicology* 80:141–152.

————. 1997. Diuresis dependent excretion of enzymes in rat urine. *Biochemical Society Transactions* 25:67S.

Plummer, D. T., and P. J. Wright. 1970. The collection of rat urine free of fecal contamination. *Journal of Physiology* 209 (Suppl.): 16 pp.

Stokke, O. 1974. Preservation of gamma glutamyl transpeptidase in human urine. *Clinica Chimica Acta* 57:143–148.

Sample Storage

Berg, K. J., D. T. Kristofferson, O. Djøseland, A. Hartmann, E. Breistein, K. K. Lund, J. Narverud, J. Ø. Nossen, and J. Stenstrøm. 1998. Reference range of some enzymes and proteins in untimed overnight urine and their stability after freezing. *Clinica Chimica Acta* 272:225–230.

Falk, H. B., R. A. Schroer, J. J. Novak, and S. M. Heft. 1981. The effect of freezing on various serum chemistry parameters from common lab. animals. *Clinical Chemistry* 27:1039.

Hirata, M., G. Nomura, and Y. Tanimoto. 1979. Stability of serum components in monkey, dog and rat. *Experimental Animals* 28:401–404.

Ito, S., T. Matsuzawa, M. Saida, S. Izumisawa, and M. Iwasaki. 1998. Time and temperature effects on potassium concentration of stored whole blood from four mammalian species. *Comparative Hematology International* 8:77–81.

Matteuchi, E., G. Gregori, L. Pellegrini, R. Navalesi, and O. Giampietro. 1991. How can storage time and temperature affect enzymic activities in urines? *Enzyme* 45:116–120.

Pickrell, J. A., M. E. Light, J. L. Mauderley, P. B. Beckley, B. A. Muggenburg, and U. C. Luft. 1973. Certain effects of sampling and storage on canine blood of different oxygen tensions. *American Journal of Veterinary Research* 34:241–244.

Pickrell, J. A., J. L. Mauderley, B. A. Muggenburg, and U. C. Luft. 1973. Influence of fasting on blood gas tension, pH and related values in dogs. *American Journal of Veterinary Research* 34:805–808.

Szenci, O., E. Brydl, and C. A. Bajcsy. 1991. Effect of storage on measured ionized calcium and acid–base variables in equine, ovine, and canine venous blood. *Journal of the American Veterinary Medical Association* 199:1167–1169.

Hemolysis and Lipemia

Chin, B. H., T. R. Tipton, and S. J. Kozbelt. 1979. The interfering effects of hemolyzed blood rat serum chemistry. *Toxicologic Pathology* 7:19–22.

Coldman, M. F., and W. Good. 1967. The distribution of sodium, potassium and glucose in the blood of some mammals. *Comparative Biochemistry and Physiology* 21:201–206.

Coulter, D. B., and L. L. Small. 1971. Effects of hemolysis on plasma electrolyte concentrations of canine and porcine blood. *Cornell Veterinarian* 61:660–666.

Czerwek, B. H., and H. Bleuel. 1981. Normal values of alkaline phosphatase, glutamic oxaloacetate transaminase and glutamic pyruvic transaminase in the serum of experimental animals using optimized methods, and the effects of hemolysis on these values. *Experimental Pathology* 19:161–163.

Davy, C. W., M. R. Jackson, and J. M. Walker. 1984. The effect of hemolysis on some clinical chemistry parameters in the marmoset (*Callithrix jacchus*). *Laboratory Animals* 18:161–166.

Greenson, J. K., S. J. Farber, and S. B. Dubin. 1989. The effects of hemolysis on creatine kinase determination. *Archives of Pathology and Laboratory Medicine* 112:184–185.

Jacobs, R. M., J. H. Lumsden, and E. Grift. 1992. Effects of bilirubinemia, hemolysis and lipemia on clinical chemistry analytes in bovine, canine, equine and feline sera. *Canadian Veterinary Journal* 33:605–607.

Leard, B. L., R. D. Alsaker, W. P. Porter, and L. P. Sobel. 1990. The effect of hemolysis on certain canine serum chemistry parameters. *Laboratory Animals* 24:32–35.

O'Neill, S. L., and B. F. Feldman. 1989. Hemolysis as a factor in clinical chemistry and hematology of the dog. *Veterinary Clinical Pathology* 18:58–68.

Reimers, T. J., S. V. Lamb, S. A. Bartlett, R. A. Matamoros, R. G. Cowan, and J. S. Engle. 1991. Effects of hemolysis and storage on quantification of hormones in blood samples from dogs, cattle and horses. *American Journal of Veterinary Research* 52:1075–1079.

Sapin, R., J-C. Ongagna, F. Gasser, and D. Grucker. 1998. Insulin measurements in hemolyzed serum: Influence of insulinase inhibitors. *Clinica Chimica Acta* 274:111–117.

Environment, Transportation, and Stress

Bean-Knudsen, D. E., and J. E. Wagner. 1987. Effect of shipping stress on clinicopathologic indicators in F344/N rats. *American Journal of Veterinary Research* 48:306–308.

Bickhardt, K., D. Büttner, U. Muschen, and H. Plonait. 1983. Influence of bleeding procedure and some environmental conditions on stress-dependent blood constituents of laboratory rats. *Laboratory Animals* 17:161–165.

Dobrakovová, M., and J. Jurčovičová. 1984. Corticosterone and prolactin responses to repeated handling and transfer of male rats. *Experimental and Clinical Endocrinology* 83:21–27.

Drozdowicz, C. K., T. A. Bowman, M. L. Webb, and C. M. Lang. 1990. Effect of in-house transport on murine corticosterone concentration and blood lymphocyte populations. *American Journal of Veterinary Research* 51:1841–1846.

Eriksson, E., F. Royo, K. Lyberg, H. E. Carlsson, and J. Hau. 2004. Effect of metabolic cage housing on immunoglobulin A and corticosterone excretion in feces and urine of young male rats. *Experimental Physiology* 89:427–433.

Fouts, J. R. 1976. Overview of the field of environmental factors affecting chemicalor drug effects in animals. *Federal Proceedings* 35:1162–1165.

Garbus, J., B. Highman, and P. D. Atland. 1967. Alterations in serum enzymes and iosenzymes in various species induced by epinephrine. *Comparative Biochemistry and Physiology* 22:507–516.

Garnier, F., E. Benoit, M. Virat, R. Ochoa, and P. Delatour. 1990. Adrenal cortical response in clinically normal dogs before and after adaptation to a housing environment. *Laboratory Animals* 24:40–43.

Gärtner, K., D. Büttner, R. Döhler, R. Friedel, J. Lindena, and I. Trautschold. 1980. Stress response to handling and experimental procedures. *Laboratory Animals* 14:267–274.

Haemisch, A., G. Guerra, and J. Hurkert. 1999. Adaptation of corticosterone—but not β-endomorphin—secretion to repeated blood sampling in rats. *Laboratory Animals* 33:185–191.

Kuhn, G., and W. Hardegg. 1988. Effects of indoor and outdoor maintenance upon food intake, body weight and different blood parameters. *Zeitschrift für Versuchstierkunde* 31:205–214.

Kuhn, G., K. Lichtwald, W. Hardegg, and H. H. Abel. 1991. Reaktionen von corticoiden enzymaktivitaten und hamatologischen parametern auf transportstress bei hunden. *Journal of Experimental Animal Science* 34:99–104.

Peng, X., C. M. Lang, C. K. Drozdowicz, and B. M. Ohlsson-Wilhelm. 1989. Effect of cage density on plasma corticosterone and peripheral lymphocyte populations of laboratory mice. *Laboratory Animals* 23:302–306.

Pérez, C., J. R. Canal, E. Dominguez, J. E. Campillo, M. Gullén, and M. D. Torres. 1997. Individual housing influences certain biochemical parameters in the rat. *Laboratory Animals* 31:357–361.

Riley, V. 1981. Psychoneuroendocrine influence on immunocompetence and neoplasia. *Science* 212:1100–1109.

Rowan, A. N. 1990. Refinement of animal research technique and validity of research data. *Fundamental and Applied Toxicology* 15:25–32.

Royo, F., N. Björk, H-E. Carlsson, S. Mayo, and J. Hau. 2004. Impact of chronic catheterization and automated blood sampling (Accusampler) on serum corticosterone and fecal immunoreactive corticosterone metabolites and immunoglobulin A in male rats. *Journal of Endocrinology* 180:145–153.

Toth, L. A., and B. January. 1990. Physiological stabilization of rabbits after shipping. *Laboratory Animal Science* 40:384–387.

Tuli, J. S., J. A. Smith, and D. B. Morton. 1995. Stress measurements in mice after transportation. *Laboratory Animals* 29:132–138l.

Vadiei, K., K. L. Berens, and D. R. Luke. 1990. Isolation-induced renal functional changes in rats from four breeders. *Laboratory Animal Science* 40:56–59.

Vogel, W. H. 1987. Stress—the neglected variable in experimental pharmacology and toxicology. *Trends in Pharmacological Sciences* 8:35–38.

Whary, M., R. Peper, G. Borkowski, W. Lawrence, and F. Ferguson. 1993. The effects of group housing on the research use of the laboratory rabbit. *Laboratory Animals* 27:330–341.

Nutrition and Fluid Balance

Apostoulou, A., L. Saidt, and W. R. Brown. 1976. Effect of overnight fasting of young rats on water consumption, body weight, blood sampling and blood composition. *Laboratory Animal Science* 26:959–960.

Bertani, T., C. Zoja, M. Abbate, M. Rossini, and G. Remuzzi. 1989. Age-related nephropathy and proteinuria in rats with intact kidneys exposed to diets with different protein content. *Laboratory Investigation* 60:196–204.

Boemke, W., U. Palm, G. Kacmarczyk, and H. W. Reinhardt. 1990. Effect of high sodium and high water intake on 24-h potassium balance in dogs. *Zeitschrift für Versuchstierkunde* 33:79–85.

Boyd, J. W. 1981. The relationships between blood haemoglobin concentration packed cell volume and plasma protein concentration in dehydration. *British Veterinary Journal* 137:166–172.

Clausing, P., and M. Gottschalk. 1989. Effects of drinking water acidification, restriction of water supply and individual caging on parameters of toxicological studies in rats. *Z. Versuchstierkd* 32:129–134.

Cokelaere, M., E. Decuypere, G. Flo, V. M. Darras, and E. R. Kühn. 1996. Influence of feeding pattern on thyroid hormones. *Hormone and Metabolism Research* 28:315–318.

Dancla, J. L., and J. Nachbaur. 1981. The effect of diet on some clinical chemistry parameters in mice. *Journal of Clinical Chemistry and Clinical Biochemistry* 119:abstract.

Evans, G. O. 1987. Postprandial changes in canine plasma creatinine. *Journal of Small Animal Practice* 28:311–315.

Hammond, K. A., and D. N. Janes. 1998. The effects of increased protein intake on kidney size and function. *Journal of Experimental Biology* 201:2081–2090.

Hart, R. W., K. Keenan, A. Turturro, K. M. Abdo, J. Leakey, and B. Lyn-Cook. 1995. Calorie restriction and toxicity. *Fundamental and Applied Toxicology* 25:184–195.

Ingbar, D. H., and V. A. Galton. 1975. The effect of food deprivation on the peripheral metabolism of thyroxine in rats. *Endocrinology* 96:1525–1532.

Jenkins, F. P., and J. A. Robinson. 1975. Serum biochemical changes in rats deprived of food or water for 24 h. *Proceedings of the Nutrition Society* 34:37A.

Kast, A., and J. Nishikawa. 1981. The effect of fasting on acute oral toxicity of drugs in rats and mice. *Laboratory Animals* 15:359–364.

Kutscher, C. 1988. Plasma volume change during water deprivation in gerbils, hamsters, guinea pigs and rats. *Comparative Biochemistry and Physiology* 25:929–936.

Levin, S., D. Semler, and Z. Ruben. 1993. Effects of two week feed restriction on some toxicological parameters in Sprague–Dawley rats. *Toxicologic Pathology* 21:1–14.

Macconi, D., W. Laurens, S. Paris, C. Battaglia, T. Bertani, G. Remuzzi, and A. Remuzzi. 1997. Selective dietary restriction of protein and calorie intakes prevents spontaneous proteinuria in male MFW rats. *Experimental Nephrology* 5:404–413.

Maejima, K., and S. Nagase. 1991. Effect of starvation and refeeding on the circadian rhythm of hematological and clinico-biochemical values and water intake of rats. *Experimental Animals* 40:389–393.

Matsuzawa, T., and M. Sakaume. 1994. Effects of fasting on hematology and clinical chemistry values in the rat and dog. *Comparative Hematology International* 4:152–156.

Meijer, G. W., J. De Bruijne, and A. C. Beynen. 1987. Dietary cholesterol-fat type combinations and carbohydrate and lipid metabolism in rats and mice. *International Journal of Vitamin and Nutrition Research* 57:319–326.

Meyer, O. A., E. Kristiansen, and G. Wurtzen. 1989. Effects of dietary protein and butylated hydroxytoluene on the kidneys of rats. *Laboratory Animals* 23:175–179.

Oishi, S., H. Ishi, and K. Hiraga. 1979. The effect of food restriction for 4 weeks on common toxicity parameters in male rats. *Toxicology and Applied Pharmacology* 47:15–22.

Omaye, S. T. 1986. Effects of diet on toxicity testing. *Federal Proceedings* 45:133–135.

Pickering, R. G., and C. E. Pickering. 1984. The effects of reduced dietary intake upon the body and organ weights, and some clinical chemistry and hematological variates of the young Wistar rat. *Toxicology Letters* 21:271–277.

Schwartz, E., J. Tornaben, and G. C. Boxhill. 1973. The effects of food restriction on hematology, clinical chemistry and pathology in the albino rat. *Toxicology and Applied Pharmacology* 25:515–524.

Single, K. M., L. L. Reed, D. L. Bove, and J. A. Dill. 1998. Effects of water dilution, housing, and food on rat urine collected from the metabolism cage. *Laboratory Animal Science* 48:520–525.

Slaughter, H. S., H. S. Gorko, M. A. Wilkinson, and E. L. Car. 1998. Clinical pathology ranges for diet restricted Crl:CD and reg (SD)IGS BR rats: A comparison to diet restricted Crl:CD and reg (SD)BR rats. *Clinical Chemistry* 44:A109.

Stonard, M. D., D. M. Samuels, and E. A. Lock. 1984. The pathogenesis of nephrocalcinosis induced by different diets in female rats, and the effect on renal function. *Food and Chemical Toxicology* 22:139–146.

Street, A. E., H. Chesterman, G. K. Smith, and R. M. Quinton. 1968. The effect of diet on blood urea levels in the beagle. *Journal of Pharmacy and Pharmacology* 20:325–326.

Waner, T., and A. Nyska. 1994. The influence of fasting on blood glucose, triglycerides, cholesterol and alkaline phosphatase in rats. *Veterinary Clinical Pathology* 23:78–80.

Watson, A. D., D. B. Church, and A. J. Fairburn. 1981. Postprandial changes in plasm aurea and creatinine concentration in dogs. *American Journal of Veterinary Research* 42:1878–1880.

Yoshida, T., K. Ohtoh, H. Narita, F. Ohkubo, F. Cho, and Y. Yoshikawa. 1994. Feeding experiment on laboratory-bred male cynomolgus monkeys. II. Hematological and serum biochemical studies. *Experimental Animals* 43:199–207.

Chronobiochemical Rhythms

Arendt, J. 1998. Biological rhythms: The science of chronobiology. *Journal of the Royal College of Physicians, London* 32:27–35.

Batalla, A., M. F. Malmary, J. Cambar, C. Labat, and J. Oustrin. 1994. Dosing time-dependent nephrotoxicity of cyclosporine A during 21-day administration to Wistar rats. *Chronobiology International* 3:187–195.

Cal, J. C., F. Lemoigne, R. Crockett, and J. Cambar. 1987. Circadian rhythm in gamma glutamyltranspeptidase and leucine aminopetidase urinary activity in rats. *Chronobiology International* 4:153–160.

Cambar, J., C. Dorian, and J. C. Cal. 1987. Chronobiochemistry and renal physiopathology. *Pathologie Biologie* 35:977–984.

Do, T. X., P. Boignard, A. Girault, P. Planchenault, R. Breget, and M. Prelot. 1992. Etude experimentale des variations diurnes et nocturnes de quelques activites enzymatiques renales de rats Sprague Dawley. *Science et Techniques de l'Animal de Laboratoire* 17:207–211.

Fukuda, S., H. Nagashima, K. Morioka, and J. Aoki. 1988. Fluctuations in peripheral serum testosterone levels within a day, with age and by sexual stimulation in male beagle dogs bred indoors. *Jikken Dobutsu* 37:381–386.

Grotsch, H., M. Hropot, E. Klaus, V. Malerczyk, and H. Mattenheimer. 1985. Enzymuria of the rat: Biorhythms and sex differences. *Journal of Clinical Chemistry and Clinical Biochemistry* 23:343–347.

Kempainnen, R. J., and J. L. Sartin. 1984. Evidence for episodic but not circadian activity in plasma concentrations of adrenocorticotrophin, cortisol and thyroxine in dogs. *Endocrinology* 103:219–226.

LeBrun, M., L. Grenier, M. G. Bergeron, L. Tibault, G. Labrecque, and D. Beauchamp. 1999. Effects of fasting on temporal variation in the nephrotoxicity of amphotericin B in rats. *Antimicrobial Agents and Chemotherapy* 43:520–524.

Moore-Ede, M. C., and F. M. Sulzman. 1981. Internal temporal order. In *Handbook of behavioral neurobiology, biological rhythms,* vol. 4, ed. J. Aschoff, pp. 215–241. New York: Plenum Press.

Murphy, P. J., and S. S. Campbell. 1996. Physiology of the circadian system in animals and humans. *Journal of Clinical Neurophysiology* 13:2–16.

Nigi, H., and R. Torii. 1991. Periovulatory time courses of serum LH in the Japanese monkey (*Macaco fuscata*). *Experimental Animals* 40:401–405.

Orth, D. N., M. E. Peterson, and W. D. Drucker. 1988. Plasma immunoreactive propiomelanocortin peptides and cortisol in normal dogs and dogs with Cushing's syndrome: Diurnal rhythm and responses to various stimuli. *Endocrinology* 122:1250–1262.

Pariat, C. I., P. Ingrand, J. Cambar, E. de Lemos, A. Piriou, and P. T. Courtois. 1990. Seasonal effects on the daily variations of gentamicin-induced nephrotoxicity. *Archives of Toxicology* 64:205–209.

Torii, R., and H. Nigi. 1994. Hypothalamo–pituitary testicular function in male Japanese monkeys (*Macaco fuscata*) in nonmating season. *Experimental Animals* 43:381–387.

Wong, C-C., K-D. Dohler, H. Geerlings, and A. von zur Muhlen. 1983. Influence of age, strain and season on circadian periodicity, gonadal and adrenal hormones in the serum of male laboratory rats. *Hormone Research* 17:202–215.

Yamauchi, H., E. Kobayashi, K. I. Sugimoto, S. Tsuruoka, M. Ybana, M. Ishii, and A. Fujimura. 1998. Time dependent cyclosporine A-induced nephrotoxicity in rats. *Clinical Experiments in Pharmacology and Physiology* 25:435–440.

13 Analytical Variables and Biosafety

13.1 INTRODUCTION

In this chapter, some of the analytical variables that need to be considered when performing studies and interpreting data are discussed, including analytical interferences due to xenobiotics. Analytical variations in biochemical measurements usually are much less than variations due to preanalytical factors (i.e., the biological components discussed in the previous chapter). The factors governing analytical procedures can be divided into the six "M" factors: (1M) manpower or analysts; (2M) methods or analytical procedures; (3M) machines or analytical equipment and reagents; (4M) materials (samples, reference materials, standards, or calibrants); (5M) manipulation of data for the calculation of results, reformatting of reported data, and data transmission to host computers; and (6M) method interferents. Good laboratory practice (GLP) demands attention to all of these M factors and includes the more basic tasks (e.g., reagent preparation, labeling, and assignment of expiry dates).

The availability and suitability of automated biochemistry analyzers for most of the core tests have improved over the last decade, with reductions of test sample volumes; this now allows a greater number of tests to be performed with the samples obtained from laboratory animals. Alongside the commercial development of analytical capabilities, the incorporation of software into analyzers enables "real-time monitoring" of the quality of data, data manipulation, and calculation of results. For many analyzers, the manufacturers supply locked-in reagents and methods that help to provide procedures for maintaining good laboratory practice (e.g., reagents with bar-coded expiry dates). In the last decade, a larger number of immunoassays for animal hormones and proteins have been made commercially available, as well as multiplexing assays that allow the simultaneous measurements of several analytes (e.g., cytokines with immunobeads or electroluminescent detection with patterned arrays).

Not all of the analytical equipment and reagents used in human medicine are appropriate for use with animal species, and they may have some limitations when used with laboratory animal samples. Many gaps remain in the commercial development of assays suitable for laboratory animals and niche products, partly because the diagnostic market is driven by the needs of human medical practice. In this discussion, some of the following terms may be regarded as interchangeable because, despite the available guidelines, common practice and publications continue to use and interchange these terms (e.g., *assay*—measurement procedure; *sample*—specimen; *analyte*—measurand, test, parameter; *interfering substance*—interferent, influence quantity).

13.2   ANALYZERS AND METHODOLOGY

When an analyzer is acquired, there should be an installation qualification (IQ) and an operational qualification (OQ). The supplier will normally carry out installation procedures and ensure the analyzer is properly installed (IQ), and this requires documentation for GLP purposes (CLSI/GP31-P). For operational qualification, a number of analytical issues must be addressed by the users to ensure the performance of the analyzer and that the methods to be utilized are characterized and documented. There are several international guidelines for analyzer evaluations and laboratory practice; some of them, provided by the Clinical Laboratory and Standards Institute (CLSI), are referenced at the end of this chapter

As a "golden rule," analyzer software should only be accessed by the supplier and no attempt should be made to modify the software other than those programs where the user has been given access (e.g., test parameters, control ranges). The manufacturer's software development should be confidentially documented by the manufacturer as intellectual property, and the installation of all software updates subsequent to installation should be recorded. Requests for remote access to analyzers are increasing as suppliers try to troubleshoot analyzer malfunctions and reduce the number of site maintenance visits. These remote access requests should be carefully controlled when experimental data are stored in the analyzer memory (CLSI: GP31-P, GP19-A2, and AUTO11-A). Some aspects of operational qualification should include measures of imprecision, accuracy, linearity, and carryover between samples.

Imprecision of a method (more widely described as precision) is described by a numerical value (often expressed as standard deviation—SD—or coefficient of variation—CV%) obtained from a series of replicate measurements; it is a measure of the closeness of agreement between independent test/measurement results obtained under stipulated conditions (CLSI: EP05-A2; EP13-R).

For each method, the laboratory should establish data that reflect the relative precision (or imprecision). Within-run (or batch) precision is the variability found when the same material is analyzed repetitively in the same analytical run or, alternatively, when duplicate analyses are made within an analytical batch. This can be extended to within-day precision and then further to day-to-day or between-day (or both/between batches) precision measurement when the variability found is for the same material analyzed on different days.

With current instrumentation and reagents, the intrabatch analytical coefficient of variation values of less than 5% are achievable for most of the common tests. It is usually a little higher for immunoassays, tests where sample volumes have been scaled below that recommended, and manual tests. Thus, as a general rule, analytical variance is a smaller component than the biological variance in the total variance, and general targets for analytical goals in human medicine are given in a number of publications (WASP 1979; Petersen et al. 1994, 2000; Fraser 2004).

Accuracy (or *inaccuracy* or the less frequently referred-to *trueness*) describes the numerical value of the difference between the means of series of replicate values or a single measurement and the true value of the analyte or measurand. Sometimes this difference is referred to as bias or systematic error (CLSI: EP15-A2). Inaccuracy remains a major challenge for biochemical measurements with laboratory animal samples in the absence of any or very few primary reference materials with accepted known and accurate values for individual species (CLSI: EP09-A2).

Tietz (1994) has drawn attention to the need to return to the concept of accuracy in laboratory tests in human medicine, and this remains a constant challenge for laboratories involved in animal studies, where the lack of primary species-specific standards and methods remains. Laboratories have become increasingly dependent on commercially available multianalyte calibration materials and their assigned values. Sometimes when species-specific reference standards are lacking, it is necessary to use methodology that can distinguish effects between control and treatment groups but where there is an element of inaccuracy in the test (e.g., in some endocrine and specific protein assays). Comparison to other previous technologies and manual methods helps in determining relative inaccuracy or bias of a new method compared to a previous method—with the knowledge that manual methods are less precise and that there is no absolute certainty that previous methods are accurate.

Analytical specificity relates to accuracy and the ability to determine the analyte exclusively without being affected by other substances. *Analytical sensitivity* is described by the slope of the calibration curve and the ability of an analytical procedure to produce a signal for a defined change of unit. The terms *sensitivity* and *specificity* for analytical procedures have different definitions when applied to diagnostic procedures (see Chapter 14), and they should not be confused.

Linearity of a method should be established or a series of standards selected for use with non-linear-method calibration. This can be checked by preparing and analyzing serial dilutions of aqueous reference standard solutions, quality control materials, enzyme solutions, or commercially available materials for demonstrating linearity (again, these are designed for use in human medicine) and comparing the determined values with the theoretical values calculated for the dilutions. The serial dilutions used for linearity checks can also help establish the analytical sensitivity when defined as the minimal detectable change from one concentration to another.

The *limit of detection* is defined as the smallest concentration or quantity of analyte that can be detected with reasonable certainty for a given analytic procedure (CLSI: EP06-A; Linnet and Kondratovich 2004). *Carryover* between samples can be checked by analyzing samples with low and high values to determine if there is an effect between samples. Typically, this can be done by analyzing samples in a pattern of three low values, followed by three high values, and then followed by the further three of the low value samples. The carryover between samples is minimal with most current analyzers using small sample volumes.

Enzyme-linked immunosorbent assays (ELISA) are being used increasingly, although these assays are often less precise than some routine clinical chemistry methods. Additional imprecision may be caused by incomplete washing and aspiration of the wells, inadequate mixing of reagents within the wells, pipetting errors and contamination during the washing procedures, and incorrect timings for the various steps involving reagent additions, washing, and incubation. In addition to these problems, the measuring range may be inappropriate for the species, or immunospecificity may be lacking.

Most manufacturers provide some indication of the performance of their analyzers with preferred reagents in terms of imprecision, linearity, and reportable ranges. All analytical methods should be assessed by the user for imprecision, accuracy, linearity, limits of detection, and carryover between samples.

Although the lower volumes required per test are advantageous, they are accompanied by a higher risk of sample evaporation, and this can markedly affect results (Burtis, Begovitch, and Watson 1975; Salzmann and Male 1993). Wherever possible, analytical methods should not be changed during a study (although this is sometimes a problem with studies of 2 years' duration). By ensuring that calibration and quality control procedures are followed, relative inaccuracy within a study and between studies for an assay should be maintained and minimized.

13.3   ANALYZER MAINTENANCE

Based on manufacturers' recommendations and experience, laboratories perform regular preventative maintenance procedures on the analyzers, with some additional maintenance procedures initiated in response to internal quality control performance or analyzer malfunctions. Calibration and quality control performances should always be checked after maintenance visits because replacement parts and disturbances of the optical and hydraulic systems sometimes adversely affect subsequent analyzer performance (sometimes called PMT—postmaintenance visit trauma). These procedures form part of good laboratory practice.

13.4   CALIBRATION, QUALITY CONTROL MATERIALS, AND PROCEDURES

All automated analyzers should be calibrated according to the manufacturer's recommended methods and performed according to the manufacturer's specifications. The calibration and quality control materials are often of animal or human origin, but they are not currently from the laboratory animal species relevant for toxicology except for some hormones and proteins. Occasionally, some problems arise because of inaccurately calibrant values assigned by the manufacturer. Troponin I assays are an example: values were assigned by the various manufacturers (Tate et al. 1999) and the values for calibrant and quality control materials were found to differ markedly between manufacturers.

Many biochemical analyzers rely on single-point calibration at values that are normal for humans but differ from those of laboratory animals; such reliance requires the analyzer to be linear over a range that includes normal and extremely abnormal values as far as practicable. To ensure correct calibration and consistent analyzer performance, quality control materials should be used for every batch of analyses performed. Many laboratories use trilevel materials similar in properties to the calibration materials and with quoted assay values that are relative to low, normal, and high human blood samples. It is good practice to cross-reference new batches of quality control materials with previous batches because there may be slight differences that are sometimes unacceptable and due to shipment and delivery problems.

Most of the current major analyzers or host computers have all of the common tools used for quality control procedures where out of range values can be flagged and trends plotted (e.g., Levey–Jenning plots, Cusum charts, application of Westgard rules; Westgard and Groth 1981; Hinckley 1997). Monitoring of internal quality control materials aids the recognition of drifts in accuracy, poor precision, and analyzer malfunctions. Even the best quality control procedures will not detect random errors that may occur due to poor sampling or reagent problems. Gross errors, unfortunately, do occur in even the best managed laboratories; examples include wrongly identifying samples at the time of collection and analysis, and these errors are often difficult to detect.

To aid control procedures, many laboratories participate in external quality assessment schemes (also termed external proficiency testing). In these assessment schemes, the pools of material may be human or animal in origin and are distributed to a number of participating laboratories for comparative purposes. Given the various analyzer technologies, it is perhaps not surprising that results obtained by various analyzers differ to some extent and these proficiency schemes do alert laboratories to poor performance.

13.5 ANALYTICAL DIFFERENCES ASSOCIATED WITH METHODOLOGIES

From external proficiency schemes and other published comparisons, it is recognized that different analyzers and reagents produce slightly different results. Even two analyzers from the same manufacturer with the same reagents and in the same laboratory may produce slightly different results. Certain test methodologies are known to give differing results with some laboratory animals; these commonly used tests include some enzymes, albumin, and creatinine. Test differences were also indicated in a survey using a rat serum by a number of Japanese laboratories (Matsuzawa et al. 1997). Variations in analytical methodologies and units often can lead to problems when data are compared for the same test compound in different toxicological studies and obtained from several laboratories. In these situations, it is useful to know the analytical bias that may have been introduced by such methodological changes and to take these factors into account when interpreting data.

13.5.1 ENZYMES

Reagents for enzyme measurement are known not to be optimal for the different species (e.g., the substrate concentrations required for the measurement of plasma aspartate aminotransferase [AST/GOT] in rats, dogs, and monkeys differed from the concentrations used for these human plasma enzymes (Dooley 1979). However, there remains a lack of data on the optimal conditions—in terms of buffer, substrate concentration, reaction times, etc.—required for the different species. There are no nationally or internationally agreed-upon recommendations for laboratory animal samples, so most analysts use reagents formulated for human enzymes. Temperature has an effect on enzyme measurements, and most laboratories have now adopted 37°C as the measurement temperature.

Some examples of methodological effects on enzymes include alkaline phosphatase, gamma glutamyltransferase, aminotransferases, and cholinesterases (see Chapter 2). The majority of methods for alkaline phosphatase employ 4-nitrophenylphosphate as the substrate, but the two main alternative buffers—diethanolamine and 2-aminopropanol—give interspecies differences (Masson and Holmgren 1992). Using the two different substrates (gamma-glutamyl-4-nitroanilide and gamma-glutamyl-3-carboxy-4-nitroanilide) gave different results following cholestasis induced by the oral administration of alpha-napthylisothiocyanate to rats (Evans 1986a). In most rats, plasma GGT activity is low (usually less than 3 IU/L). This is at the very low end of the measuring ranges designed for humans; thus, with small changes in absorbance, plasma GGT may change from 1 to 3 IU/L. This might be statistically significant but must be interpreted knowing the imprecision of the method in this range.

Pyridoxal phosphate is a cofactor for both of the aspartate and alanine aminotransferases (AST: ALT) and is often supplied as a separate component of reagent assay kits. The inclusion of pyridoxal phosphate can increase the measured activities of both aminotransferases' activity by a small percentage (Stokol and Erb 1998), but this also can alter statistical differences observed between treatment groups in rat studies (Evans and Whitehorn 1995).

13.5.2   CREATININE

Plasma and urinary creatinine are commonly measured by the colorimetric alkaline picrate method of Jaffé, but there are alternative methods that are enzymatic or use high-performance liquid chromatography. The enzymatic methods use creatinine amidohydrolase or creatinine iminohydrolase and are more specific for creatinine. The measurement of plasma creatinine may be affected by endogenous noncreatinine chromogens (e.g., bilirubin and ketones); this can overestimate plasma creatinine in dogs by up to 45% and to an even greater extent in rats and mice (Meyer et al. 1985; Evans 1986b; Jung et al. 1987; Braun, Lefebvre, and Watson 2004; Yuen et al. 2004; Palm and Lundblad 2005).

13.5.3   ALBUMIN AND OTHER PLASMA PROTEINS

Variations of dye-binding with albumin from different species have been described. The commonest dye-binding method for plasma albumin uses bromcresol green (or BCG) dye, and it is essential to make absorbance measurements within 60 s if overestimation of albumin resulting from other reactions with alpha-1-globulin fractions is to be avoided (Gustafsson 1976). Some investigators have reported problems when using BCG to measure rabbit albumin, but others have not confirmed this finding (Fox 1989; Hall 1992; Evans 1994). Other albumin binding dyes including bromcresol purple are not suitable for many species (Witiak and Whitehouse 1969; Metz and Schutze 1975; Evans and Parsons 1988).

Some other methodological issues relate to calibration and separation techniques. Very few specific proteins for the laboratory animals are available and of sufficient purity to be used as primary calibrants. Alterations of electrophoretic apparatus, support media, and buffers will alter the apparent number of protein fractions obtained on separation. The different dyes used for staining the protein fractions vary in their dye-binding capacity and thus can cause the albumin electrophoretic values to differ from those obtained with BCG dye.

13.6 INTERFERENCE WITH ASSAYS

When data from toxicological studies are examined, differences are sometimes found for clinical chemistry data that cannot be explained simply on the grounds of observed toxicity, histopathological findings, clinical observations, statistical analyses, or pre-analytical variables. In these cases, it is worth considering whether the differences are due to analytical interference caused by the test compound and/or its metabolites on the assay in question. This general consideration of effects due to metabolites applies throughout the following sections, where only the xenobiotic/test compound may be mentioned. The analytical interferences may be exaggerated in toxicology studies where the concentrations of the test compound may be several multiples of the therapeutic dosages, and there may be evidence of a relationship to dose levels. Early recognition of potential interference in plasma or urine chemistry measurements during the preclinical or development phase of a test compound can assist in identifying and prevent misleading interpretations made during later stages of compound development.

Xenobiotics may interfere with analytical methods in several different ways, and these may have a negative or positive effect on the analytical result. The effect may be caused directly by the xenobiotic (or metabolite) or through its influence as an accelerator or inhibitor of the chemical reactions used to measure the analyte. Potentially interfering substances may originate from either endogenous or exogenous sources, and the interference may be analytical, physical, chemical, or biological. Methodological interferences are more likely to occur in analytical procedures that use nonspecific reactions. The extent of the interference will depend on the level of interferent in the test samples, and the degree of interference may vary for the same analyte when different analytical methods and/or analyzers are employed. (A xenobiotic that causes interference is sometimes called an interferent.)

Physical interferences often arise when the test compound or metabolite has the same color as the endpoint color of the reaction used to measure the analyte. Any compound that imparts an unusual color to blood or urine may cause interference, depending on the analytical technology (e.g., disulphine blue) (Halloran and Torrens 1983). Some analyzers have programs that assess the degrees of hemolysis and lipemia in the samples, but these are designed for use with human samples (Vermeer, Thomassen, and de Jonge 2005) and some dyes (e.g., Patent Blue V. can interfere with these serum indices but not the analytical methods; Darby and Broomhead 2008). Some xenobiotics may interfere due to their fluorescent properties.

13.6.1 HEMOLYSIS AND LIPEMIA

These are examples of endogenous causes of interference in some plasma measurements. The presence of hemolysis can affect colorimetric methods using absorbance

reading at 540–580 nm, where hemoglobin shows a spectral peak; effects of hemolysis have been reported in several species (Chin, Tyler, and Kozbelt 1979; Davy,
Jackson, and Walker 1984; Sonntag 1986; O'Neill and Feldman 1989; Leard et al.
1990; Reimers et al. 1991; Jacobs, Lumsden, and Grift 1992). Some blood substitutes may cause effects due to their color or by interference with light measurements
(Chang 1997; Sakai et al. 2003).

Lipemia may interfere with some measurements through turbidity (Hortin and
Goolsby 1997) or by alterations to the plasma volume (McGowan, Artiss, and Zak
1984) (e.g., plasma displacement effects causing pseudohyponatremia; Weisberg
1989). The turbidity due to lipemia may be reduced by ultracentrifugation or precipitation techniques, but these procedures may alter apparent analyte concentrations (Thompson and Kunze 1984). Synthetic lipid emulsions are often used to test
for effects caused by lipemia, but these emulsions do not always mimic the physicochemical effects of hyperlipemia caused by perturbations of lipid metabolism
(Bornhorst, Roberts, and Roberts 2004).

13.6.2 INTERFERENCES WITH URINARY GLUCOSE AND ENZYMES—ENDOGENOUS INHIBITORS

Two examples of endogenous effects on urinary measurements are ascorbate and
glucose and urinary enzyme inhibitors. When present in high concentrations, *urinary ascorbate* can lead to false negative test strip reaction when testing for glucose
in mice and dogs because the ascorbate interferes with the glucose oxidase/peroxi-
dase detection system (Watts 1968; Taylor and Neal 1982; Berg 1986; Rotblatt and
Koda-Kimble 1987). Rats can excrete more ascorbate in some cases of hepatotoxicity (Poon et al. 1994), thus potentially affecting test strip results.

Some *urinary enzymes* are inhibited by low molecular weight endogenous molecules in the urine, and these inhibitors require removal by gel filtration, dialysis,
or ultrafiltration prior to analysis (Amador, Zimmerman, and Wacker 1963; Werner,
Maruhn, and Atoba 1969; Raab 1972; Werner and Gabrielson 1977; Berscheid et al.
1983; Kumar et al. 1987). The inhibitory effects on some of these enzymes are less
than in the original methods due to lower sample volumes in proportion to the total
reaction volumes and improved methods.

13.6.3 INTERFERENCES WITH SERUM SEPARATING GELS

Some laboratories use one of the several serum separating gel materials to separate
serum. These polymeric materials have a density between that of serum and the
blood cells and thus form a layer on top of the packed cells during centrifugation.
Although some effects are of a preanalytical nature (e.g., lower potassium values
for several species; Caisey and King 1980), some effects, such as increased CRP
(C-reactive protein) (Chang et al. 2003) and increased progesterone (Ferry, Collins,
and Sykes 1999), appear to affect the test measurement. Other investigators (Sunaga
et al. 1992) have reported no marked differences for several analytes using three
different separators with several species. Some evidence suggests that some of these

serum separators may have a potential to interact with therapeutic drugs in human serum (Landt, Smith, and Hortin 1993; Dasgupta et al. 1994).

13.6.4 INTERFERENCE IN PEROXIDASE CASCADE METHODS

Interference in peroxidase cascade methods is an example of exogenous interference caused by xenobiotics. In several methods, the analyte is measured by a series of reactions that generate hydrogen peroxide, which in the presence of peroxidase reagent leads to the oxidation of a final product chromophore. Examples of these methods using 4-aminophenazone and phenol to yield quinnoneimine as chromogen (Trinder 1969; Fossati, Principe, and Berti 1980) after peroxidase reactions include glucose, cholesterol, triglycerides, urate, and creatinine. In these methods, relatively specific enzyme-mediated reactions occur in the first-stage reactions, but the subsequent stages are subject to interference from a variety of compounds (Kaufmann-Raab et al. 1976; Weber and van Zanten 1991; Karon, Daly, and Scott 1998).

13.6.5 SOME OTHER ANALYTICAL EFFECTS

These include plasma protein binding with xenobiotics (see Chapter 8) and the differing properties of enzyme reagents to hydrolyze plasma cholesterol esters and triglycerides (see Chapter 9). Some compounds cause a false positive protein reaction with test strips and quantitative total proteins (e.g., some aminoglycosides; Yosselson-Superstine and Sinai 1986; Marshall and Williams 2003). False positive reactions may be checked by using alternative methods such as electrophoresis, immunoassays for specific urinary proteins, or in vitro testing (Appel, Hubbuch, and Koler 1991).

13.7 INTERFERENCE TESTING

Various guidelines have been proposed for testing drug interference in clinical chemistry measurements, and some suggest performing in vitro studies (Powers et al. 1986; Malya et al. 1988; Kallner and Tryding 1989; Kroll and Elin 1994; Breuer 1996; CLSI EP 7 2005). Currently, it is recommended that drugs be tested at therapeutic and above therapeutic concentrations (Sonntag and Scholer 2001; CLSI EP 7 2005; Brambila et al. 2008).

Although manufacturers of in vitro diagnostic (IVD) analytical systems should include an evaluation of effects due to potentially interfering substances in their risk analyses at the design stage, this requirement cannot cover the many novel compounds being tested in toxicology studies. Proposals for in vitro interference testing are not always practicable (particularly when the interference effect is due to a metabolite), although in vitro studies can be useful when testing series of compounds similar in chemical structure and/or therapeutic target and where there has been some association with marked interference effects. When an interference effect is suspected, it is useful to perform the analysis using a method with a different principle (e.g., enzymatic method for creatinine vs. alkaline picrate method).

Some of the problems of testing for interferences are illustrated by studies with several cephalosporins, which interfere with creatinine measurements. With alkaline picrate reagents, cephalosporins can interfere either positively or negatively with serum creatinine measurements depending on the instrumentation and reaction conditions (Kirby et al. 1982; Baer et al. 1983; Kroll et al. 1985; Letellier and Desjarlais 1985a; Okudo, Ito, and Nishida 1984; Brambila et al. 2008). By altering the timing of the blood sample in relation to dosing with cefoxitin, the interference was reduced as the plasma drug levels fell (Durham, Bignell, and Wise 1979). From a study of 20 drugs with seven different instruments, Letellier and Desjarlais (1985b) concluded that interferences changed in magnitude and direction, depending on the instrumentation and reaction conditions.

Given the variety of available analytical methods and analyzers, it is not possible to test every combination of analyzers and reagents, and it is important to recognize that these factors change with time as analytical technology develops (Evans 1985). Some proposals for defining clinically significant interference as compared to significant effects on the analyte have been made (Fuentes-Arderiu and Fraser 1991; Castano-Vidriales 1994).

13.8   DATA BANKS

Several literature surveys of the effects of drugs and other substances have been published (Caraway 1962; Wirth and Thompson 1965; Elking and Kabat 1968; Lubran 1969; van Peenen and Files 1969; Christian 1970; Sher 1982; Salway 1990; Tryding, Tufvesson, and Sonntag 1996), and a very large database is now available online that includes effects due to "natural" products (Young 2008). Although these databases are primarily designed to help in human medicine, they can be used as an aid in identifying possible mechanisms for interferences due to test compounds.

13.9   BIOHAZARDS AND CHEMICAL SAFETY

When transporting, receiving, or analyzing diverse blood samples, every effort should be made to reduce the chemical and biohazards for laboratory staff (Truchaud et al. 1994; WHO 2004; Green and Hunt 2006). Suitable containers and bags should be used to transport samples from the animal care buildings to the laboratory. Allergies to laboratory animals remain a risk for laboratory workers, and efforts should be made to minimize exposure to animal dander, etc. Although most laboratories use purpose-bred animals, occasionally bacteria, parasites, and yeasts may be found in blood (Owen 1992). When immunosuppressants or immunostimulants are being tested, this may increase the risks of viral infections and potential viral transmission. When wild-caught nonhuman primates or other species are being studied (e.g., in Third World countries), the risks from viral infections must be considered. Guidance for periodic cleaning and disinfection of analyzers is usually provided by manufacturers, but more frequent measures may be required following analysis of infectious materials.

Local safety procedures should be written to address and avoid potential risks to the analyst. During the analytical preparation stages, several risks for accidents should be minimized; these include aerosols produced in breakages by centrifugation, metal foil caps, moving mechanical parts, and electrical safety—particularly following liquid spillages. Adequate warnings are usually provided by analyzer manufacturers on electrical and laser beam hazards, and chemical hazards are usually indicated by the reagent manufacturers. Samples from some studies may contain radioactivity, and these should be treated according to local rules pertaining to radiation safety.

REFERENCES

Analysis

Burtis, C. A., J. M. Begovitch, and J. S. Watson. 1975. Factors influencing evaporation from sample cups and assessment of their effect on analytical error. *Clinical Chemistry* 21:1907–1917.

Fraser, C. G. 2004. Test result variation and the quality of evidence-based clinical guidelines. *Clinica Chimica Acta* 346:19–24.

Hinckley, M. C. 1997. Defining the best quality-control systems by design and inspection. *Clinical Chemistry* 4:873–879.

Linnet, K., and M. Kondratovich. 2004. Partly nonparametric approach for determining the limit of detection. *Clinical Chemistry* 50:632–640.

Petersen, P. H., C. G. Fraser, H. Baadenhuijsen, J. C. Libeer, and C. Ricos. 1994. Analytical quality specifications in clinical chemistry. *Clinical Chemistry* 40:670–671.

Petersen, P. H., S. Sandberg, C. G. Fraser, and H. Goldschmidt. 2000. A model for setting analytical quality specifications and design of control for measurements on the ordinal scale. *Clinical Chemistry and Laboratory Medicine* 38:545–551.

Salzmann, M. B., and I. A. Male. 1993. Keep the lid on it: Artifactual hypernatremia in samples from pediatric patients. *Annals of Clinical Biochemistry* 30:211–212.

Tate, J. R., D. Heathcote, J. Rayfield, and P. E. Hickman. 1999. The lack of standardization of cardiac troponin I assay systems. *Clinica Chimica Acta* 284:141–149.

Tietz, N. W. 1994. Accuracy in clinical chemistry—Does anybody care? *Clinical Chemistry* 40:859–861.

WASP. 1979. Analytical goals in clinical chemistry: Their relationship to medical care. Proceedings of the subcommittee on analytical goals in clinical chemistry World Association of Societies of Pathology. *American Journal of Clinical Pathology* 71:624–630.

Westgard, J. O., and T. Groth. 1981. Design and evaluation of statistical control processes: Application of a computer "quality control simulator" program. *Clinical Chemistry* 27:1536–1547.

Analytical Differences Associated with Methodologies

Braun, J. P., H. P. Lefebvre, and A. D. Watson. 2004. Creatinine in the dog: A review. *Veterinary Clinical Pathology* 32:162–179.

Dooley, J. F. 1979. The role of clinical chemistry in chemical and drug safety evaluation by use of laboratory animals. *Clinical Chemistry* 25:345–347.

Evans, G. O. 1986a. Further observations on plasma γ-glutamyltransferase activity after oral administration of α-napthylisothiocyanate. *Human Toxicology* 5:120–121.

———. 1986b. The use of an enzymatic kit to measure plasma creatinine in the mouse and three other species. *Comparative Biochemistry and Physiology* 85B:193–195.

———. 1994. Plasma albumin measurement in New Zealand White rabbits. *World Rabbit Science* 1:25–27.

Evans, G. O., and C. E. Parsons. 1988. A comparison of two dye binding methods for the determination of dog, rat and human plasma albumin. *Journal of Comparative Pathology* 98:453–460.

Evans, G. O., and L. C. Whitehorn. 1995. Effects of pyridoxal 5'-phosphate on plasma alanine aminotransferase determinations in toxicological studies. *Toxicology Letters* 80:34–37.

Fox, R. R. 1989. The rabbit. In *The clinical chemistry of laboratory animals,* ed. W. F. Loeb and F. W. Quimby, pp. 45–46. New York: Pergamon Press.

Gustafsson, J. E. 1976. Improved specificity of serum albumin determination and estimation of "acute phase reactants" by use of the bromcresol green reaction. *Clinical Chemistry* 22:616–622.

Hall, R. E. 1992. Clinical pathology of laboratory animals. In *Animal models of toxicology,* ed. S. C. Gad and C. P. Chengelis. New York: Marcel Dekker.

Jung, K., C. Wesslau, F. Priem, G. Schreiber, and A. Zubek. 1987. Specific creatinine determination in laboratory animals using the enzymatic test kit "Creatinine–PAP." *Journal of Clinical Chemistry and Clinical Biochemistry* 25:357–361.

Masson, P., and J. Holmgren. 1992. Comparative study of alkaline phosphatase in human and animal samples using methods based on AMP and DEA buffers: Effect on quality control. *Scandinavian Journal of Clinical and Laboratory Investigation* 52:773–775.

Matsuzawa, T. et al. 1997. A survey of the values of clinical chemistry parameters obtained for a common rat blood sample in ninety-eight Japanese laboratories. *Journal of Toxicological Sciences* 22:25–45.

Metz, A., and A. Schuzte. 1975. Vergleichende untersuchungen zur bestimmung von gesamt-protein und albumin im serum von mensch, affe, hund and ratte. *Zeitschrift für Klinische Chemie und Klinische Biochemie* 13:423–426.

Meyer, M. H., R. A. Meyer, R. W. Gray, and R. L. Irwin. 1985. Picric acid methods greatly overestimate serum creatinine in mice: More accurate results with high performance liquid chromatography. *Analytical Biochemistry* 144:285–290.

Palm, M., and A. Lundblad. 2005. Creatinine concentration in plasma from dog, rat and mouse: A comparison of 3 different methods. *Veterinary Clinical Pathology* 34:232–236.

Stokol, T., and H. Erb. 1998. The apo-enzyme content of aminotransferases in healthy and diseased domestic animals. *Veterinary Clinical Pathology* 27:71–78.

Witiak, D.T., and M. W. Whitehouse. 1969. Species differences in the albumin binding of 2,4,6,-trinitrobezaldehyde, chlorophenoxyacetic acids, 2-(4'-hydroxybenzeneazo) benzoic acid and some other acidic drugs—The unique behavior of rat plasma albumin. *Biochemical Pharmacology* 18:971–977.

Yuen, P. S., S. R. Dunn, T. Miyalji, H. Yasuda, K. Sharma, and R. A. Star. 2004. A simplified method for HPLC determination of creatinine in mouse serum. *American Journal of Physiology and Renal Physiology* 286:F1116–1119.

Hemolysis, Lipemia, and Dyes

Bornhorst, J. A., R. F. Roberts, and W. L. Roberts. 2004. Assay specific differences in lipemic interferences in native and Intralipid-supplemented samples. *Clinical Chemistry* 50:2197–2201.

Chang, T. M. S., ed. 1997. *Blood substitutes: Principles, methods, products and clinical trials,* vols. 1 and 2. Basel, Switzerland: Karger AB.

Chin, B. H., T. R. Tyler, and S. J. Kozbelt. 1979. The interfering effects of hemolyzed blood on rat serum chemistry. *Toxicologic Pathology* 7:19–21.

Darby, D., and C. Broomhead. 2008. Interferences with serum indices measurement, but not chemical analysis on the Roche Modular by Patent Blue V. *Annals of Clinical Biochemistry* 45:289–292.

Davy, C. W., M. R. Jackson, and J. M. Walker. 1984. The effect of hemolysis on some clinical chemistry parameters in the marmoset (*Callithrix jacchus*). *Laboratory Animals* 18:161–168.

Halloran, S. P., and D. J. Torrens. 1983. Effects of the drug disulphine blue on routine biochemical investigations. *Annals of Clinical Biochemistry* 20:317–320.

Hortin, G. L., and K. Goolsby. 1997. Lipemia interference with a rate-blanked creatinine method. *Clinical Chemistry* 43:408–410.

Jacobs, R. M., J. H. Lumsden, and E. Grift. 1992. Effects of bilirubinemia, hemolysis and lipemia on clinical chemistry analytes in bovine, canine, equine and feline sera. *Canadian Veterinary Journal* 33:605–607.

Leard, B. L., R. D. Alsaker, W. P. Porter, and L. P. Sobel. 1990. The effect of hemolysis on certain canine serum chemistry parameters. *Laboratory Animals* 24:32–35.

McGowan, M. W., J. D. Artiss, and B. Zak. 1984. Description of analytical problems arising from elevated serum lipids. *Analytical Biochemistry* 142:239–251.

O'Neill, S. L., and B. F. Feldman. 1989. Hemolysis as a factor in clinical chemistry and hematology of the dog. *Veterinary Clinical Pathology* 18:58–68.

Reimers, T. J., S. V. Lamb, S. A. Bartlett, R. A. Matamoros, R. G. Cowan, and J. S. Engle. 1991. Effects of hemolysis and storage on quantification of hormones in blood samples from dogs, cattle and horses. *American Journal of Veterinary Research* 52:1075–1079.

Sakai, H., K. Tomiyama, Y. Masada, S. Takeoka, H. Horinouchi, and K. Kobayashi. 2003. Pretreatment of serum containing hemoglobin vesicles (oxygen carriers) to prevent their interference in laboratory tests. *Clinical Chemistry and Laboratory Medicine* 41:22–31.

Sonntag, O. 1986. Hemolysis as an interference factor in clinical chemistry. *Journal of Clinical Chemistry and Clinical Biochemistry* 24:127–139.

Thompson, M. B., and D. J. Kunze. 1984. Polyethylene glycol-6000 as a clearing agent for lipemic serum samples from dogs and the effects on 13 serum assays. *American Journal of Veterinary Research* 45:2154–2157.

Vermeer, H. J., E. Thomassen, and N. de Jonge. 2005. Automated processing of serum indices used for interference detection by the laboratory information system. *Clinical Chemistry* 51:244–247.

Weisberg, L. S. 1989. Pseudohyponatremia: A reappraisal. *American Journal of Medicine* 86:315–318.

Interferences with Urinary Glucose and Enzymes

Amador, E., T. S. Zimmerman, and W. E. Wacker. 1963. Urinary alkaline phosphatase activity. II. An analytical validation of the assay method. *Journal of the American Medical Association* 185:953–957.

Berg, B. 1986. Ascorbate interference in the estimation of urinary glucose by test strips. *Journal of Clinical Chemistry and Clinical Biochemistry* 24:89–96.

Berscheid, G., H. Grotsch, M. Hropot, E. Klaus, and H. Mattenheimer. 1983. Enzymuria in the rat: The preparation of urine for enzyme analysis. *Journal of Clinical Chemistry and Clinical Biochemistry* 21:799–804.

Kumar, A., H. N. Pandey, G. Harma, D. N. Pandley, and B. K. Sur. 1987. Urinary aspartate transaminase (AST) activity and detection of inhibitors in normal urine. *Industrial Journal of Physiology and Pharmacology* 31:12–18.

Poon, R., I. Chu, P. Lecavalier, A. Bergman, and D. C. Villeneuve. 1994. Urinary ascorbic acid—HPLC determination and application as a noninvasive marker of hepatic response. *Journal of Biochemical Toxicology* 9:297–304.

Raab, W. P. 1972. Diagnostic value of urinary enzyme determinations. *Clinical Chemistry* 18:5–25.

Rotblatt, M. D., and M. A. Koda-Kimble. 1987. Review of drug interference with urine glucose tests. *Diabetes Care* 10:103–110.

Taylor, D. M., and D. L. Neal. 1982. False negative hyperglucosuria test-strip reactions in laboratory mice. *Laboratory Animals* 116:192–197.

Watts, C. 1968. Failure of an impregnated cellulose strip as a test for glucose in urine. *Veterinary Record* 82:48–52.

Werner, M., and D. Gabrielson. 1977. Ultrafiltration for improved assay of urinary enzymes. *Clinical Chemistry* 23:700–704.

Werner, M., D. Maruhn, and M. Atoba. 1969. Use of gel filtration in the assay of urinary enzymes. *Journal of Chromatography* 40:254–263.

Separator Gels

Caisey, J. D., and D. J. King. 1980. Clinical chemistry values for some common laboratory animals. *Clinical Chemistry* 26:1877–1879.

Chang, C-Y., J-Y. Lu, T-I. Chien, J-T. Kao, M-C. Lin, P-C. Shih, and S-N. Yan. 2003. Interference caused by the contents of serum separator tubes in the Vitros CRP assay. *Annals of Clinical Biochemistry* 40:249–251.

Dasgupta, A., R. Dean, S. Saldana, G. Kinnaman, and R. W. McLawhon. 1994. Absorption of therapeutic drugs by barrier gels in serum separator blood collection tubes. *American Journal of Clinical Pathology* 101:456–461.

Ferry, J. D., S. Collins, and E. Sykes. 1999. Effect of serum volume and time of exposure to gel barrier tubes on results for progesterone by Roche Diagnostics Elecsys 2010. *Clinical Chemistry* 45:1574–1575.

Landt, M., C. H. Smith, and G. L. Hortin. 1993. Evaluation of evacuated blood collection tubes: Effects of three types of polymeric separators on therapeutic drug monitoring specimens. *Clinical Chemistry* 39:1712–1717.

Sunaga, T., M. Hirata, K. Ichinohe, E. Saito, S. Suzuki, and Y. Tanimoto. 1992. The influence of serum separators on biochemical values in experimental animals. *Jikken Dobutso* 41:533–536.

Interference in Peroxidase Cascade Methods

Fossati, P., L. Principe, and G. Berti. 1980. Use of 3,5,dichoro-2-hydroxybenzene sulphonic acid-4 aminophenazone chromogenic system in direct assay of uric acid in serum and urine. *Clinical Chemistry* 26:227–231.

Karon, B. S., T. M. Daly, and M. G. Scott. 1998. Mechanisms of dopamine and dobutamine interference in biochemical tests that use peroxide and peroxidase to generate chromophore. *Clinical Chemistry* 44:55–60.

Kaufmann-Raab, I., H. G. Jonen, E. Jahnchen, G. F. Kahl, and U. Groth. 1976. Interference by acetaminophen in the glucose oxidase-peroxidase method for blood glucose determination. *Clinical Chemistry* 22:1729–1731.

Trinder, P. 1969. Determination of glucose in blood using glucose oxidase alternative oxygen acceptor. *Annals of Clinical Biochemistry* 24:24–27.

Weber, J. A., and A. P. van Zanten. 1991. Interferences in current methods for creatinine. *Clinical Chemistry* 37:695–700.

Other Analytical Effects

Appel, W., A. Hubbuch, and P. U. Koler. 1991. In vitro testing for interference by drugs in quantitative urine analysis. Results of an expert discussion and initial experience gained with the new testing list. *Laboratory Medicine* 15:399–403.

Marshall, T., and K. M. Williams. 2003. Aminoglycoside interference in the pyrogallol red-molybdate protein assay is increased by the addition of sodium dodecyl sulphate to the dye reagent. *Clinical Chemistry* 49:2111–2113.

Yosselson-Superstine, S., and Sinai, Y. 1986. Urine protein interference. *Journal of Clinical Chemistry and Clinical Biochemistry* 24:103–106.

Interference Testing

Baer, D. M., R. N. Jones, J. P. Mullooly, and W. Horner. 1983. Protocol for the study of drug interference in laboratory tests: Cefotaxime intereference in 24 clinical tests. *Clinical Chemistry* 29:1736–1740.

Brambila, S., A. Valaperta, C. Filippi, E. Baldassarre, S. Magnini, F. Rossi, and A. Montanelli. 2008. *Clinical Chemistry* 54 (Suppl.): A221.

Breuer, J. 1996. Report on symposium "Drug effects in clinical chemistry methods." *European Journal of Clinical Chemistry and Clinical Biochemistry* 34:385–386.

Castano-Vidriales, J. L. 1994. Interferences in clinical chemistry. *Journal of the International Federation of Clinical Chemistry* 6:10–14.

Durham, S. R., A. H. Bignell, and R. Wise. 1979. Interference of cefoxitin in the creatinine estimation and its clinical relevance. *Journal of Clinical Pathology* 32:1148–1151.

Evans, G. O. 1985. Changes of methodology and their potential effects on data banks for drug effects on clinical laboratory tests. *Annals of Clinical Biochemistry* 22:397–401.

Fuentes-Arderiu, X., and C. G. Fraser. 1991. Analytical gels for interference. *Annals of Clinical Biochemistry* 28:393–395.

Kallner, A., and N. Tryding. 1989. IFCC guidelines to the evaluation of drug effects in clinical chemistry. *Scandinavian Journal of Clinical and Laboratory Investigation* 49:1–29.

Kirby, M. G., P. Gal, H. W. Baird, and B. Roberts. 1982. Cefoxitin interference with serum creatinine measurement varies with the assay system. *Clinical Chemistry* 28:1981.

Kroll, M. H., and R. J. Elin. 1994. Interference with clinical laboratory analyses. *Clinical Chemistry* 40:1996–2005.

Kroll, M. H., L. Nealon, M. A. Vogel, and R. J. Elin. 1985. How certain drugs interfere negatively with the Jaffe reaction for creatinine. *Clinical Chemistry* 31:306–308.

Letellier G. and Desjarlais F. 1985a. Analytical interference of drugs in clinical chemistry: 1. Study of twenty drugs on seven different instruments. *Clinical Biochemistry* 18:345–351.

———. 1985b. Analytical interference of drugs in clinical chemistry: II. The interference of cephalosporins with the determination of serum creatinine concentration by the reaction. *Clinical Biochemistry* 18:352–356.

Malya, P. A., J. Nachbaur, J. P. Dooley, J. Breur, M. M. Galteau, G. Siest, and N. Tryding. 1988. International Federation of Clinical Chemistry Scientific Committee: Drug interferences and drug effects in clinical chemistry. Part 4. Clinical laboratory tests on laboratory animals during toxicity studies. *Journal of Clinical Chemistry and Clinical Biochemistry* 26:175–179.

Okudo, T., J. Ito, and M. Nishida. 1984. "Interferovalue" indicates the interference of substances with creatinine determination. *Clinical Chemistry* 30:1888–1889.

Powers, D. M., J. C. Boyd, M. R. Glick, M. L. Kotschi, G. Letellier, W. G. Miller, D. A. Nealon, and A. E. Hartmann. 1986. *Interference testing in clinical chemistry: Proposed guidelines.* N.C.C.L.S. EP7/P. Villanova, PA: National Committee for Clinical Laboratory Standards.

Sonntag, O., and A. Scholer. 2001. Drug interference in clinical chemistry: Recommendation of drugs and their concentrations to be used in drug interference studies. *Annals of Clinical Biochemistry* 38:376–385.

Databases

Caraway, W. T. 1962. Chemical and diagnostic specificity of laboratory tests. *American Journal of Clinical Pathology* 37:1453–1458.

Christian, D. G. 1970. Drug interference with laboratory blood chemistry determinations. *American Journal of Clinical Pathology* 54:118–142.

Elking, P., and H. F. Kabat. 1968. Drug induced modifications of laboratory test values. *American Journal of Hospital Pharmacy* 25:485–519.

Lubran, M. 1969. The effects of drugs on laboratory values. *Medical Clinics of North America* 53:211–222.

Salway, J. G. 1990. *Drug test interactions handbook.* London: Chapman & Hall.

Sher, P. P. 1982. Drug interferences with clinical laboratory tests. *Drugs* 24:24–63.

Tryding, N., C. Tufvesson, and O. Sonntag. 1996. *Drug effects in clinical chemistry,* 7th ed. Stockholm: Apoteksbolaget AB.

van Peenen, H. J., and J. Files. 1969. The effect of medication on laboratory test results. *American Journal of Clinical Pathology* 52:666–670.

Wirth, W. A., and R. L. Thompson. 1965. The effect of various conditions and substances on the result of laboratory procedures. *American Journal of Clinical Pathology* 43:579–590.

Young, D. 2008. *Young's effects.* Online http://www.fxol.org

Biohazards and Chemical Safety

Green, D. O., and D. L. Hunt. 2006. *Biological safety: Principles and practice,* 4th ed. Washington, D.C.: American Society for Microbiology Press.

Owen, D. G. 1992. *Parasites of laboratory animals. Laboratory animal handbook,* vol. 12. London: Royal Society of Medicine Press.

Truchaud, A., P. Schnipelsky, H. L. Pardue, J. Place, and K. Ozawa. 1994. Increasing the biosafety of analytical systems in the clinical laboratory. *Clinica Chimica Acta* 226: S5–S13.

World Health Organization. 2004. *WHO laboratory biosafety manual,* 3rd ed. Geneva: World Health Organization.

Clinical and Laboratory Standards Institute Guidelines (http://www.clsi.org/)

C24-A3. 2006. *Statistical quality control for quantitative measurements: Principles and definitions,* 2nd ed. Approved guideline.

C28-A2. 2008. *How to define and determine reference intervals in the clinical laboratory,* 2nd ed. Approved guideline.

EP05-A2. 2004. *Evaluation of precision performance of quantitative measurement methods,* 2nd ed. Approved guideline.

EP06-A. 2003. *Evaluation of linearity of quantitative measurement procedures: A statistical approach,* 1st ed. Approved guideline.

EP07-A2. 2005. *Interference testing in clinical chemistry,* 2nd ed. Approved guideline.

EP09-A2. 2002. *Method comparison and bias estimation using patient samples,* 2nd ed. Approved guideline.

EP13-R. 1995. *Laboratory statistics—Standard deviation,* 1st ed. A report.

EP14-A2. 2005. *Evaluation of matrix effects,* 2nd ed. Approved guideline.

EP15-A2. 2006. *User verification of performance for precision and trueness,* 2nd ed. Approved guideline.

EP17-A. 2004. *Protocols for determination of limits of detection and limits of quantitation,* 1st ed. Approved guideline.

EP21-A. 2003. *Estimation of total analytical error for clinical laboratory methods,* 1st ed. Approved guideline.

GP17-A2. 2004. *Clinical laboratory safety,* 2nd ed. Approved guideline.

GP19-A2. 2003. *Laboratory instruments and data management systems: Design of software user interfaces and end-user software systems validation, operation and monitoring,* 2nd ed. Approved guideline.

GP29-A. 2002. *Assessment of laboratory tests when proficiency testing is not available,* 1st ed. Approved guideline.

GP31-P. 2007. *Laboratory instrument implementation, verification, and maintenance.* Proposed guideline.

HO1-A5. 2003. *Tubes and additives for venous blood specimen collection,* 5th ed. Approved guideline.

LA1-A2. 2004. *Assessing the quality of radioimmunoassay systems,* 2nd ed.

ILA21-A2. 2008. *Clinical evaluation of immunoassays,* 2nd ed. Approved guideline.

ILA-23A. 2004. *Immunoassay systems: Radioimmunoassays and enzyme, fluorescence and luminescence immunoassays,* 1st ed. Approved guideline.

ILA-30A. 2008. *Immunoassay interference by endogenous antibodies,* 1st ed. Approved guideline.

MP29-A3. 2005. *Protection of laboratory workers from occupationally acquired infections,* 3rd ed. Approved guideline.

AUTO11-A. 2006. *IT security of in vitro diagnostic instruments and software systems,* 1st ed. Approved standard.

14 Data Processing and Interpretation

14.1 INTRODUCTION

After the data have been produced, the next steps are to analyze them and to summarize the observed effects using experience and statistical analyses, if appropriate. In the two previous chapters, some of the preanalytical and analytical variables affecting animal laboratory data have been discussed. Some of this information will be relevant to the interpretation of effects observed in a study.

14.2 DATA DEFINITION AND SECURITY

Laboratory data produced for a toxicology study may be voluminous, particularly for a rodent study, where more than 5,000 clinical chemistry values may be generated; the majority of these data are obtained using automated biochemical analyzers. These analyzers have proprietary software with some selectable options for the user, details of which should be retained for reference and in the event of analyzer software crashes. The analyzers may be connected to a laboratory information management system (LIMS), and the access to both the analyzer software and LIMS must be controlled by the local operating procedures and IT/IS policies (also see OECD 1995; FDA 2003). Manufacturers are increasing their requests for remote access in attempts to "troubleshoot" analyzer problems and to reduce the number of site maintenance visits. However, this access should be controlled as part of data security procedures. When analyzers are not connected to a LIMS or data are generated by manual methods, data can be entered manually into the LIMS or the data processing package. "Double entry" procedures reduce the number of errors generated in manual data entries. Some of the relevant guidelines from the Clinical and Laboratory Standards Institute are referenced at the end of this chapter.

In generating analytical results, analyzers make several readings over the measuring time period (e.g., enzyme activities may be monitored by more than 30 absorbance readings from which data are selected for calculating results). With some analyzers, these data can be viewed and accessed; other analyzers are limited to showing only the results (e.g., for urine test strips). Options exist to store both the calculated result and the data used to calculate the result, so it is important to define the constitution of the raw data because these data must be retained and eventually archived for regulated studies. The definitions of electronic raw data were outlined by a U.S. Food and Drug Administration (FDA) guidance document, which was subsequently reviewed (FDA 2003). The standard operating procedures of the laboratory should ensure that data in paper or electronic format are stored securely. Editing of data must be properly tracked with reasons for changes and identity of the person making changes, while ensuring that this person is authorized to make such changes.

Each regulatory study design, protocol, or plan defines the tests required, and any additional tests must be approved by formal approved amendments to the study plan or protocol. With some analyzers, it is possible to select "reflex" testing, which automatically initiates follow-up testing when certain test results are obtained on the first analysis requests. The use of reflex tests is best avoided, but if they are used, the reasons should be well documented.

14.3 REPEATED ANALYSES ON THE SAME SAMPLE

Unlike toxicokinetics, where samples may be analyzed in triplicate or quadruplicate, most clinical chemistry samples for core tests are analyzed once due to the small sample volumes available. Trained analysts will invariably spot aberrant sample values, which have been affected by poor sample aspiration leading to "short" samples (i.e., insufficient sample volume used for the test, small clots, or analyzer flags for insufficient sample). Other results may look suspect (e.g., a very high potassium value with low calcium, suggesting the incorrect use of anticoagulants). The natural responses to such findings are to repeat the analysis for confirmation when the sample is sufficient. If a value is outside the flagged reference ranges preselected on the analyzer, why repeat one sample if all the surrounding sample values appear to be within these ranges? After the analysis is repeated, is the first or second result correct? The laboratory should examine the reasons for repeating sample analysis and why certain results are accepted or rejected. If the number of replicate measurements varies between individual animals, then the inclusion of all data can be statistically complex. Whatever the final decision as to the validity of results, the laboratory should ensure that the standard operating procedures provide sufficient and adequate guidance for repeating analyses.

14.4 SIMPLE DATA TERMINOLOGY

Some commonly used terminology includes:

n or N represents the number of samples included in a study group or used in a single group for method comparisons.

Standard deviation (S.D.) is the square root of the variance that is a measure of the scatter of values about the mean value; the smaller the value is, the more indicative of the tighter clustering of data about the mean. By calculating the mean and S.D. for a reference population, ±1 S.D. will contain 68% of all values, ±2 S.D. will contain 95.5% of all values, and ±3 S.D. will contain 99.7% of all values.

Standard error of the mean (S.E.M. or S.E): the magnitude of S.E.M. values is dependent on the S.D. and number of results within the group. Although S.E.M. values appear smaller than S.D. values, there is doubtful value in expressing the results as S.E.M, and results should be expressed as S.D. in preference wherever possible.

Confidence limits relate to a normal distribution, and commonly the limits applied are 95% or mean ± 2 S.D.

Transformation of data: for distributions that are not parametric, data can be converted to $\log_{10}$ or $\log_e$ values to obtain a log-normal distribution prior to applying a parametric method of comparison such as t-test or ANOVA.

Power relates to the probability of a statistical test rejecting the null hypothesis when it is false.

Probability values (p or P) are usually presented as $p < 0.001$ (***), $p < 0.01$ (**), or $p < 0.05$ (*) (Jones 1988; Romano 1988).

To interpret clinical chemistry measurements, we need to consider some of the variables in toxicological experiments.

14.5   INTRA- AND INTERINDIVIDUAL VARIATIONS

Biological variations occur both intra- (within) and inter- (between) animal. The animals used in toxicity studies are purposely bred with known genetic backgrounds, using a carefully controlled environment with special reference to pathogens and adequate diet. The exceptions are some nonhuman primates in which the genetic backgrounds and refinements are less well known in the captive bred populations. In some countries, the supply and control of laboratory animal breeding are less consistent. More recently, a countering debate has suggested that the use of less well controlled genetic populations would aid the detection of idiosyncratic adverse reactions. In Chapter 12, several preanalytical biological variations were discussed, and these variations are higher than those found in humans because many more of these preanalytical variables cannot be well controlled with animals. These inter- and intra-animal variances can be expected to be higher, with increasing toxicity associated with escalating doses.

A simple procedure to obtain an estimate of biological variation can be used in some larger species for example dogs, where values for an individual animal can be compared for pretreatment and serial samples to obtain an indication of the intra- and interanimal variations. In larger laboratory animals, when blood volumes permit, it is useful to take two pretreatment values. This has several advantages in that it gives a stronger indication of the intra- and interanimal variations in studies where the group sizes are usually small as well as allowing some confirmation of any outlying values particular to an individual animal. This may enable the animal to be excluded from the study or reassigned to a different treatment group where the outlying values are unlikely to affect the overall conclusions of the study. It is more difficult to obtain estimates of the biological variation for the smaller laboratory animals such as rats because the volumes of blood required for repetitive analysis result in changes including hematological and body fluid balance perturbations. In many of the shorter toxicology studies, samples are only taken at a single time point toward the end of a study.

In general, the variations due to analytical components in clinical chemistry measurements usually are much less than variations due to the preanalytical factors. The contributions of both analytical and biological variation to a measurement may be expressed by the formula:

$$\text{Standard deviation } ab = \text{square root of } (\text{S.D.}^2a + \text{S.D.}^2b)$$

where

S.D. a is the analytical variation and

S.D. b is the biological variation.

A similar formula can be used when the corresponding coefficients of variations are substituted to obtain a measure of imprecision. The probability that the difference between test values from the same animal is significant at the 95% level (i.e., this difference occurs by chance at fewer than 1 in 20 occasions) can be expressed by the formula $2.8 \times \text{SD } ab$ and is known as a *critical difference*. The critical difference may also be calculated by the formula:

$$1.96 \times \text{the square root of } 2 \times (\text{biological coefficient of variation}^2 \text{ for intraindividual} + \text{analytical coefficient of variation}^2)$$

In some reported canine studies, 1.96 is replaced by 2 (Fraser 2001, 2004; Martinez-Subiela, Tecles, and Cerón 2003; Jensen and Aaes 1992).

Some measurements of the biological variation that occur for both intra- and inter-individual animals have been made in rat studies (Lindena, Büttner, and Trautschold 1984; Carakostas and Banerjee 1990) and dog studies (Leissing, Izzo, and Sargent 1985). Other studies have reported on examples for both intra- and inter-individual variations for canine thyroid function (Jensen and Høier 1996), glomerular filtration rate (Kampa et al. 2002), and urine osmolality (van Vonderen, Kooistra, and Rijnberk 1997). Some data have been published for biological variations and critical difference calculations for dogs (e.g., fructosamine [Jensen and Aaes 1992] and acute phase proteins [Martinez-Subiela et al. 2003]) and for rabbits [Jensen, Wedø, and Bantz 1992].

The biological variations are usually greater for rodents compared to dogs, with plasma enzymes showing greater biological variations compared to total protein, sodium, and calcium in most species. Plasma total bilirubin and GGT show wide coefficients of variations in rodents due to the analytical variations associated with their measurements at low values. The analytical variations for hormones are greater than for core plasma measurements, and the hormonal biological variations are much greater for rodents. In studies where toxic effects are observed, the biological variations for some tests will increase—not necessarily due to toxicity.

14.6   REFERENCE VALUES

Despite numerous attempts to direct investigators away from using the terminology, the term *normal ranges* still is frequently used instead of *reference ranges*. Reference or test values are determined for samples collected from healthy animals (reference individuals with described procedures for sample collections, sample processing, analytical methodology, etc.) (IFCC 1987; Kley et al. 2004). A number of animals must be used to determine the reference range; this number should exceed 40 and ideally be at least more than 100 animals. When more than 120 animals are sampled to establish the reference values, there seems to be a diminishing improvement or alteration in the ranges obtained when compared to ranges using up to 120 animals. For fewer than 40 animals, the lowest and highest observed values provide a reasonable estimate of the central 95% reference interval. Reference ranges should be based on the literature or determined in house and qualified by:

strain, age, and gender;
dosing regime—oral, intravenous, or inhalation;
animal supplier;
sample collection method;
analytical methods;
exclusion criteria;
number of animals; and
period of data collection.

A 10-year period database has limited use if the items listed above are not logged because many of these parameters will have changed during the 10 years. Data obtained by new methodology (e.g., following introduction of a new biochemical analyzer) should be compared with current methodology to detect possible changes to existing reference ranges.

Although several laboratories use historical reference ranges based on the mean ±2 S.D. values of data collected over a number of studies (JPMA 1993), many of the test values do not follow a normal (or Gaussian) distribution with peaks in the middle of the distribution and with a perfectly symmetrical or bell-shaped distribution. Parametric testing assumes that the data are normally distributed, the distributions are similar in the groups being compared, and there are no extreme or outlying values. In some cases, modest departures from these assumptions will allow satisfactory parametric analysis of the data, and this parametric analysis may lead to the detection of smaller differences between the populations. The data distributions may be skewed to the left (negative in direction) or leptokuric (showing positive kurtosis). Nonparametric analyses should be used to estimate the 2.5–97.5 percentiles to define a 95% reference interval for non-Gaussian distributions. Transformation of non-Gaussian distribution data (e.g., by log transformation) may help in establishing the reference intervals and in dealing with some study data sets.

Some investigators rely heavily on reference ranges to identify outlying values, but accumulation of such data without cognizance of the influence of preanalytical and analytical factors can lead to misleading interpretations. Literature values for reference ranges that do not specify the methods used to obtain the ranges should be treated with caution. Reference ranges should not be used to dismiss values outside the range as being of little or no consequence; conversely, values may change within the reference range and may be important. Reference ranges are a guide, and these comments emphasize the need for concurrent control animal data in each study.

14.7   CONTROL GROUPS

Control groups should always be included in study designs, and they should be matched by gender and sex. Even if the compound is designed for use with one sex (e.g., female hormone therapy), male animals should be studied to identify toxicities unrelated to the pharmacological actions of the test compound. If the vehicle for the test article is novel, then an additional control group should be included in the study design. For inhalation studies, it is useful to include an "air"-only control group in addition to the vehicle control group. Animals should be randomized when assigned to groups and for sampling procedures.

For both rodents and nonrodents, clinical pathology testing should be performed on the same animals as those examined for histopathological findings. It is also recommended that blood samples from recovery or withdrawal satellite groups should be analyzed at study termination.

Usually, a study design will include a control group, which provides a picture of test result variations that occur in the absence of the test compound. It is important to recognize that even within this control group, one or more individuals may have some data that can be ascribed as abnormal or outside an expected reference range for healthy animals. In studies of dogs and nonhuman primates where the animal numbers may be fewer than five per group, it is useful to take at least two samples prior to the commencement of the studies, about 1 week apart. This brings the benefits of having some indication of intra- and interanimal variation, and these results may affect the allocation of animals to groups; this also introduces naïve animals to the local blood collection procedures and animal care staff.

Several reports have drawn attention to the variations observed in distributions for the same analyte in control groups between differing studies of rats in the same laboratory (Weil 1982; Gaylor et al. 1987; Waner 1991; Kobashyi 2005). It must not be assumed that data are always distributed in the same way for each analyte in every study.

14.8   STUDY SIZE

The size of a study should be determined by using power analysis to avoid excessively large studies and to minimize the number of animals in a study. (Unfortunately, this is not always the case because study designs tend to follow traditional in-house designs.) The number of animals in each treatment group is usually larger in rodent studies compared to the group numbers for other species; this tends to produce more uniform results in rodent studies, but even here group sizes may be no more than 25 animals per group per sex in longer-term studies. In dog and nonhuman primate studies, the group size may often be fewer than five per group, and in preliminary studies the group sizes of rodent studies may also be small. The studies are often underpowered in the number of animals within a study, but there is increasing pressure to minimize the number of animals in studies. When studies are designed, some restrictions may apply—for example, on the amount of blood to be taken at necropsy or during a study when other demands may require taking samples primarily for pharmacokinetics. This problem may be obviated by using separate groups for pharmacokinetics in rodent studies; however, this increases the number of animals required.

14.9   STATISTICAL PROCEDURES

The quotation attributed to Benjamin Disraeli, "There are three kinds of lies: lies, damned lies and statistics," is unfortunately often quoted to dismiss statistical findings. And perhaps an opposite view is "like dreams, statistics are a form of wish fulfillment." ~ J. Baudrillard

There are numerous statistical methods for parametric and nonparametric analyses, and the choice is often made locally (Table 14.1; also see the reference section). Waner (1992) surveyed a number of laboratories and reported that a variety of statistical methods was being used to analyze toxicology studies. A recent study performed by

TABLE 14.1

Some Statistical Tests Applied in Toxicology Studies

Tests for Non-Normality

Chi-square
Kolmgorov–Smirnov
Shapiro–Wilk

Tests for Homogeneity of Variance

Bartlett's test
Levene's test

Tests for Normally Distributed Data

Analysis of variance (ANOVA)
Analysis of covariance (ANCOVA)
Duncan's multiple test range
Dunnett's test
Fisher's least significant difference (LSD) test
Linear regression to test for dose–effect trends
Pairwise comparison
Pearson's correlation coefficient
Student's t-test
Williams's t-test

Tests for Nonparametric Distributed Data

Dunn's test
Jonckheere's test
Kendall's coeffcient of rank correlation
Kruskal–Wallis ANOVA
Mann–Whitney U test (similar to t-test)
Shirley's test
Wilcoxon signed rank test (paired or matched pairs)

13 laboratories (as part of an evaluation of a proposed regulatory guideline) showed a similar variety of statistical methods (OECD 2006), even though all of the laboratories were supposedly using the same study design. When different statistical methods are used, there may be subtle differences in the statistical sensitivity; some procedures may yield statistical significances and others might not produce statistical significances.

Some laboratories use decision trees in applying several of these statistical procedures; these procedures usually include an examination of data distributions, application of favored parametric and nonparametric tests, and a test for dose–response relationships (Gad and Weil 1989; Dickens and Robinson 1996). Nonparametric tests can be applied for group comparisons with the assumption that similarly shaped distributions are being compared, but the group sizes, which were the same at the start of a study, may change at the time of sampling due to interim deaths or difficulties with sampling procedures. The use of inappropriate statistical methods should be avoided, and it is of limited use when the group sizes are small (e.g., in dog and nonhuman primate studies).

Many LIMSs capture the study data and contain simple programs that calculate group mean and standard deviation (or standard mean error) values—sometimes termed descriptive statistical data. The user should recognize that these statistical programs work with the assumptions that the groups are adequately sized and all distributions are Gaussian. These assumptions may be incorrect and thus all individual data should be examined.

In small groups of fewer than 12 animals, there may be individual outlying values (termed *outliers*) that may have a considerable effect on the calculated group mean and standard deviation values, and it is important to identify these individual animals. Due to the relatively small sample volumes available, it often is not possible to confirm outlying values by repeat analysis. In dog and nonhuman primate studies where the group sizes are often fewer than five animals per group, the standard deviation values are of little value and the individual values should receive greater examination.

Given the small group sizes, statistically significant differences are often found in the clinical chemistry data sets. For example, in a study of four dose groups per sex and 20 biochemical measurements, it is not uncommon to find at least one or two statistical differences between groups. These differences are highlighted by probability values (*, **, ***) and this sometimes leads to "star gazing," where every attempt is made to give biological significance to a statistical probability value, although some of these differences are due to chance. There is common ground between biological and statistical significances where both show effects or both show no effects. It is more difficult when there is a biological significance or statistical significance not supported by the other; these differences can sometimes lead to data torture—"If you torture your data long enough, they will tell you what you want to hear" (Mills 1993).

Although multivariate analysis or principal component analysis procedures could be employed to explore relationships among a number of biochemical variables, this technique appears to be rarely used in toxicology except in metabonomics. However, it may have application when linking the results of new and rarer tests with the core tests.

Small changes are often observed, with study data showing apparently random changes in individual groups. Glocklin (1983) suggested that "frequently, statistically significant group differences in hematology or serum chemistry have no relevance unless certain of these changes correlate directly with each other or with some pathological lesion." This assumes that the statistical methods chosen to analyze the data are appropriate, but it fails to recognize that plasma or urine biochemistry may be a more sensitive indicator of early toxicity, or that the timing of sampling in relation to exposure and necropsy is critical.

14.10 DATA INTERPRETATION

In some studies, by comparing groups or with baseline/predosing data for larger animals, there will be clear evidence of effects and dose relationships due to the test compound; in other studies, there may be "random" changes between and within dosed groups. Data should be examined for dose relationships and possible expected relationships among several parameters (e.g., increases of plasma enzymes and total bilirubin). Usually, an alteration of test results will be supported by other evidence gathered mainly from hematology, histopathology, and clinical observations, which allow confirmation of a biochemical finding and a decision as to whether an effect is due to toxicology or pharmacology, or is a biological variation. However, some studies comparing histopathological evidence of liver injury with various plasma tests for hepatotoxicity show that we should not expect total agreement between the clinical chemistry and pathology findings (Carakostas et al. 1986; Travlos et al. 1996; Fujii 1997). Sometimes, the changes appear to be minor and are dismissed due to a lack of corroborating evidence, but it is important to reflect on these findings in subsequent studies with the same test compound to see if a consistent pattern emerges.

If collected over a number of days or weeks, data should be inspected for any interbatch variations that may affect the final interpretation and processing. Any apparent outliers should be examined for any obvious confounding factors (e.g., extreme difficulties in obtaining blood sample or evidence of gross hemolysis, which would lead to exclusion of data items) and for any trends toward similar extreme values. Although it is always the outliers that catch the reader's eye, it must always be remembered that animals with values within the reference range may be or are undergoing a reaction to the test compound. Samples taken from animals in extremis often are widely divergent from reference and control group values.

In longer-term rodent studies, data interpretation can be more problematic after the animals have reached the age of 18 months because of the onset and progression of age-associated disease. As these animals approach the end of their life spans, rodents tend to display patterns of declining organ functions, increased incidence of tumors, and hormonal perturbations (e.g., thyroids and reproductive organs). These changes may result in the intergroup relationships showing different statistical relationships during a 2-year study, although the toxic effects are continuing in similar proportionality.

In earlier chapters, the diagnostic values, organ and tissue specificity, and limitations of some tests have been discussed, and this knowledge should be applied when interpreting data. A test value change due to cellular injury should be distinguished from a change due to an adaptive response. Variations in the rates for analyte production and clearance must be considered, and the binding of an analyte can complicate this interpretation if the free concentration is more relevant than the total concentration. Two examples of adaptive change have been mentioned in previous chapters: plasma aminotransferase values are increased without evidence of hepatotoxicity (Chapter 3) and increased proteinuria occurs due to competitive binding for renal transport systems (Chapter 4). The timing of sampling procedures in relationship to the timing of the dose and duration of exposure also plays an important part in data interpretation because plasma chemistry and urine measurements may reflect transient or reversible changes (e.g., plasma troponins in cardiotoxicity and urine enzymes in renal toxicity). Some of the changes observed in toxicity studies may be due to exaggerated or unexpected pharmacodynamic effects.

The findings of biochemical effects in preclinical toxicology studies are relatively common; Heywood (1981, 1983) found more than 30% of a mixture of tested compounds affected blood chemistry measurements in rats, dogs, and monkeys; there were species differences, and these findings were less common in monkeys. In 61 subchronic rat studies conducted by the U.S. National Toxicology Program, liver and kidney lesions were reported in 31 and 41% of the studies, respectively (Travlos et al. 1996), but the incidence of these findings will depend on the discovery and development interests of the particular organization.

14.10.1 SUMMARY QUESTIONS FOR INTERPRETING DATA

Is the effect on a biochemical measurement

    due to pharmacological action;
    normal or exaggerated;
    desirable or adverse;
    dose related or a hormetic response;
    due to toxicity;
    due to test compound (or enantiomer);
    due to metabolite;
    due to prodrug component rather than drug itself;
    due to vehicle or excipient;
    due to preanalytical factor;
    due to interference with analytical methodology;
    greater than inter- and intra-animal variation;
    greater than analytical variation;
    a change that occurs over time and, if so, in what sequence;
    related to other clinical chemistry measurements;
    an occurrence in one or more species;
    an adaptive response; or
    due to a combination of any of these factors?

14.11   PREDICTIVE VALUES

As new biomarkers are developed for application in toxicology, some of the procedures used in similar situations with evidence-based human medicine should be considered. These procedures include the concepts of sensitivity/specificity and receiver operator characteristics (ROCs).

14.11.1   SENSITIVITY AND SPECIFICITY

Sometimes the question asked about a new test is how predictive or how sensitive it is. (Sensitivity of a test can have a very different meaning to an analyst looking for the lowest level of quantification.) The concepts of sensitivity and specificity are applied to assays used for disease diagnosis. The sensitivity of an assay is the fraction of those with a specific disease that the assay correctly predicts, and the specificity is the fraction of those without the disease that the assay correctly predicts; these can be expressed in formulae where

TP = true positive: number of affected individuals correctly classified by the test;
FP = false positive: number of nonaffected individuals misclassified by the test;
FN = false negative: number of individuals misclassified by the test; and
TN = true negative: number of nonaffected individuals correctly classified by the test.

Then, sensitivity is expressed by

$$\frac{TP}{TP + FN} \times 100$$

and specificity is expressed by (Griner et al. 1981)

$$\frac{TN}{FP + TN} \times 100$$

If a test has a high sensitivity with a value of 0.9999, then there is a 99.99% chance of the test's being positive; conversely, if a test has a high specificity of 0.9999, then there is a 99.99% chance of the test's being negative. If these values are applied to a population of 10,000 subjects, where there is a 1.5% incidence rate of the condition being tested for, there will be 151 positive results in which 1 result is false, and the chances of the test's being truly positive are 150 out of 151 (i.e., the test is highly predictive). However, if the incidence rate of the condition is 1 in 10,000, then one true false negative but two positive results—one truly positive and one falsely positive—can be expected (i.e., there is a 50–50 chance of the positive results' being true). These expressions for sensitivity and specificity can be used to assess the diagnostic value of a particular test and to assess the predictive values when extrapolating from animals to humans.

14.11.2 RECEIVER OPERATING CHARACTERISTIC (OR RELATIVE OPERATING CHARACTERISTIC: ROC)

Sensitivity versus specificity can be plotted when the data are initially classified as individuals with or without the feature of interest (i.e., the toxic effect under investigation) and using differing cut-off limits to define those values that are positive (Jensen and Poulsen 1992; Jensen, Thofner, and Iverasen 1996; Jensen 2000: Gardner and Greiner 2006). These ROC plots, which may produce four variants according to the way data are projected on the axis, can then be used to compare two tests to determine which test gives the better discrimination where specificity is superior at any level of sensitivity. Furthermore, the areas under the ROC curves can be calculated and tested by statistical techniques for significant difference between the two ROC curves.

14.12 EXTRAPOLATION OF ANIMAL DATA TO HUMANS

To estimate the predictive value of animal studies, the concepts of sensitivity and specificity were applied to data from dog and monkey studies with anticancer drugs and the observed human toxicities (Schein et al. 1970; Schein and Anderson 1973) and for hepatotoxicity (Thomann, Achermann, and Ziel 1981). In several retrospective studies of new drugs, it has been shown that some animal studies have been predictive for adverse events in humans; some animal studies predict toxicities that are not observed in humans, while other studies have failed to detect adverse effects and predict toxicity in humans (Litchfield 1962; Fletcher 1978; Heywood 1990; Olsen et al. 2000). What these and other published studies fail to show is the large number of unpublished studies that have prevented compounds from being given to humans because of the adverse results obtained from animal toxicity studies. Alternatively, the presence of adverse signals from animal studies has not prevented the administration of compounds to humans, and this has led to a questioning about the significance of these animal data and how they are reviewed. These comparative prediction studies often lack relevant exposure data to the test compound, which limits extrapolation between species so that the predictive values of the animals can be more effectively tested. The failure of predictions could be related to differing metabolism between species.

A preclinical toxicology study should be designed to determine the range of toxicities in the selected animal species, enable extrapolation to other species including humans, and determine safe levels of exposure (Garratini 1985; Zbinden 1991). In addition, the animal studies should help to determine the risks of adverse toxic effects, which may result from exposure to chemicals or biologicals, and to minimize or prevent adverse health effects.

In establishing safety margins, consideration must be given to the relationships among the no observed effect level (NOEL), no observed adverse effect level (NOAEL), and the exposure levels expected in humans (Lewis et al. 2002). By their very nature, the detection of idiosyncratic adverse effects, where maybe only one in a million subjects suffers an adverse effect, remains a challenge. Unfortunately, there are several examples where preclinical testing has failed to ensure human safety.

Animal studies will continue to have a major part to play in assessing exposures to xenobiotics in human and animals until we find suitable replacements.

As pathology began as a science of observation, so did clinical pathology begin as measurements of chemicals in blood, urine, and other body fluids and making associations between the measurements and diseases. Biochemical analyses are an important, key part in the safety assessment of pharmaceuticals and chemicals, helping to identify target organs and adverse effects. The same biochemical measurements often act as a bridge between animal studies and human exposures and risk. In addition, some of the measurements indicate the efficacy of the therapeutic properties suggested by the development of novel pharmaceuticals and their successful use for both human and animal medicines. Clinical chemistry is a key gatekeeper in preclinical safety assessment of xenobiotics.

REFERENCES

FDA. 2003. *Guidance for industry. Part 11. Electronic records; electronic signatures—Scope and application.* Washington, D.C.: U.S. Food and Drug Administration.

OECD. 1995. No. 10: *The application of the principles of GLP to computerized systems.* Paris: Organization for Economic Co-operation and Development.

Clinical and Laboratory Standards Institute Guidelines (http://www.clsi.org/)

AUTO08-A. 2006. *Managing and validating laboratory information systems.* Approved guideline.

AUTO09-A. 2006. *Remote access to clinical laboratory diagnostic devices via the Internet.* Approved standard.

AUTO11-A. 2006. *IT security of in vitro diagnostic instruments and software systems.* Approved standard.

CP28-P3. 2008. *Defining, establishing and verifying reference intervals in the clinical laboratory,* 3rd ed. Proposed guideline.

GP02-A5. 2006. *Laboratory documents; development and control,* 5th ed. Approved guideline.

GP19-A2. 2003. *Laboratory instruments and data management systems: Design of software user interfaces and end-user software systems validation, operation and monitoring,* 2nd ed. Approved guideline.

Intra- and Interindividual Variations, Critical Differences, and Reference Ranges

Carakostas, M. C., and A. K. Banerjee. 1990. Interpreting rodent clinical laboratory data in safety assessment studies: Biological and analytical components of variation. *Fundamental and Applied Toxicology* 15:744–753.

Fraser, C. G. 2001. *Biological variation: From principles to practice.* Washington, D.C.: AACC Press.

———. 2004. Inherent biological variation and reference values. *Clinical Chemistry and Laboratory Medicine* 42:758–764.

Gaylor, D. W., R. L. Suber, G. L. Wolff, and J. A. Crowell. 1987. Statistical variation of selected clinical pathological and biochemical measurements in rodents. *Proceedings of the Society for Experimental Biology and Medicine* 185:361–367.

IFCC. 1987. Approved recommendation (1987) on the theory of reference values. Part 5. Statistical treatment of collected reference values. Determination of reference limits. *Clinica Chimica Acta* 170:S13–32.

Jensen, A. L., and H. Aaes. 1992. Reference interval and critical difference for canine fructosamine concentration. *Veterinary Research Communications* 16:317–325.

Jensen, A. L., and R. Høier. 1996. Evaluation of thyroid function in dogs by hormone analysis: Effects on data of biological variation. *Veterinary Clinical Pathology* 25:130–134.

Jensen, A. L., E. Wedø, and M. Bantz. 1992. Critical differences of clinical chemistry components in blood from laboratory rabbits. *Scandinavian Journal of Laboratory Animal Science* 19:179–184.

Jones, P. K. 1988. R. A. Fisher and the 0.05 level of significance in medical studies. *Journal of Laboratory and Clinical Medicine* 111:491–492.

JPMA. 1993. Issues associated with laboratory tests in toxicology studies for 1991–1992, pp. 44–46. Japan Pharmaceutical Manufacturers Association. Drug Evaluation Committee, Basic Research Group.

Kampa, N., I. Boström, P. Lord, U. Wennstrom, P. Öhagen, and E. Maripuu. 2002. Day-to-day variability in glomerular filtration rate in normal dogs by scintographic technique. *Journal of Veterinary Pathology* A50:37–41.

Kley, S., P. Tshudi, A. Busato, and F. Gaschen. 2004. Establishing canine clinical chemistry references values for the Hitachi 912 using the International Federation of Clinical Chemistry (IFCC) recommendations. *Comparative Clinical Pathology* 12:106–112.

Kobashyi, K. 2005. Analysis of quantitative data obtained from toxicity studies showing non-normal distribution. *Journal of Toxicological Sciences* 30:127–134.

Leissing, N., R. Izzo, and H. Sargent. 1985. Variance estimates and individuality ratios of 25 serum constituents in beagles. *Clinical Chemistry* 31:83–86.

Lindena, J., D. Büttner, and I. Trautschold. 1984. Biological, analytical and experimental components of variance in a long-term study of plasma constituents in the rat. *Journal of Clinical Chemistry and Clinical Biochemistry* 22:97–104.

Martinez-Subiela, S., F. Tecles, and J. J. Cerón. 2003. Critical differences of acute phase proteins in canine serum samples. *Veterinary Journal* 166:233–237.

Romano, P. E. 1988. The insignificance of a probability value of $p < 0.05$ in the evaluation of medical scientific studies. *Journal of Laboratory and Clinical Medicine* 111:501–503.

van Vonderen, I. K., H. S. Kooistra, and A. Rijnberk. 1997. Intra- and interindividual variation in urine osmolality and urine specific gravity in healthy pet dogs of various ages. *Journal of Veterinary Internal Medicine* 11:30–35.

Waner, T. 1991. Population distribution profiles of the activities of blood alanine and aspartate aminotransferase in the normal F344 inbred rat by age and sex. *Laboratory Animals* 25:263–271.

Weil, S. W. 1982. Statistical analysis and normality of selected hematologic and clinical chemistry measurements used in toxicologic studies. *Archives of Toxicology* 5 (Suppl.): 237–253.

Statistical Procedures

Baudrillard, J. 1966. In: *The Colombia world of quotations*, eds. Andrews, R., M. Biggs, and M. Seidel. New York: Columbia University Press.

Dickens, A., and J. Robinson. 1996. Statistical approaches. In *Animal clinical chemistry: A primer for toxicologists,* ed. G. O. Evans. London: Taylor & Francis Ltd.

Gad, S. C., and C. S. Weil. 1989. Statistics for toxicologists. In *Principles and methods of toxicology,* 2nd ed., ed. A. W. Hayes, pp. 435–483. New York: Raven Press.

Glocklin, V. C. 1983. The role of data organization in the evaluation of toxicology studies in drug application. *Drug Information Journal* 17:139–151.

Mills, J. L. 1993. Data torturing. *New England Journal of Medicine* 329:1196–1199.

OECD. 2006. Series on testing and assessment, no. 59. Report of validation of the updated guideline 407: Repeat dose 28-day oral toxicity in laboratory rats. Paris: Organization for Economic Cooperation and Development.

Waner, T. 1992. Current statistical approaches to clinical pathological data from toxicological studies. *Toxicologic Pathology* 20:477–479.

Some Statistical Tests Mentioned in Table 14.1

Armitage, P., and G. Berry. 2001. *Statistical methods in medical research,* 2nd ed. Oxford, England: Blackwell Scientific Publications.

Dunnett, C. W. 1955. A multiple comparison procedure for comparing several treatments with a control. *Journal of the American Statistical Association* 50:1096–1121.

———. 1964. New table for multiple comparisons with a control. *Biometrics* 20:482–491.

Jonckheere, A. R. 1954. A distribution-free *k*-sample test against ordered alternatives. *Biometrika* 41:13–45.

Levene, H. 1960. *Contributions to probability and statistics.* Stanford, CA: Stanford University Press.

Shirley, E. 1977. A nonparametric equivalent of Williams' test for contrasting increasing dose levels of a treatment. *Biometrics* 33:386–389.

Snedcor, G. W., and W. G. Cochran. 1980. *Statistical methods,* 7th ed. Ames: Iowa State University Press.

Williams, D. A. 1972. The comparison of several dose levels with a zero dose control. *Biometrics* 28:519–531.

Data Interpretation

Carakostas, M. C., K. A. Gossett, G. E. Church, and B. L. Cleghorn. 1986. Evaluating toxin-induced hepatic injury in rats by laboratory results and discriminant analysis. *Veterinary Pathology* 23:264–269.

Fujii, T. 1997. Toxicological correlation between changes in blood biochemical parameters and liver histopathological findings. *Journal of Toxicological Sciences* 22:161–183.

Heywood. R. 1981. Target organ toxicity. *Toxicology Letters* 8:349–358.

———. 1983. Target organ toxicity II. *Toxicology Letters* 18:83–88.

Travlos, G. S., R. W. Morris, M. R. Elwell, A. Duke, S. Rosenblum, and M. B. Thompson. 1996. Frequency and relationships of clinical chemistry and liver and kidney histopathology in 13-week toxicity studies in rats. *Toxicology* 107:17–29.

Predictive Values and Receiver Operating Characteristics

Gardner, I. A., and M. Greiner. 2006. Receiver–operator characteristic curves and likelihood ratios: Improvements over traditional methods for the evaluation and application of veterinary clinical pathology tests. *Veterinary Clinical Pathology* 35:8–17.

Griner, P. F., R. J. Mayewski, A. I. Mushlin, and P. Greenland. 1981. Selection and interpretation of diagnostic tests and procedures. *Annals of Internal Medicine* 94:553–600.

Jensen, A. L. 2000. Alternative ways of evaluating test results. *Revue Médecine Vétérinaire* 151:593–599.

Jensen, A. L., and J. S. Poulsen. 1992. Evaluation of diagnostic tests using relative operating characteristic (ROC) curves and the differential positive rate. An example using total serum bile acid concentration and the alanine aminotransferase activity in the diagnosis of canine hepatobiliary diseases. *Zentralblatt für Veterinarmedizin. Reihe A* 39:656–658.

Jensen, A. L., M. T. Thofner, and L. Iverasen. 1996. Application of receiver operating characteristic (ROC) curves to veterinary clinical pathology. *Comparative Hematology International* 6:176–181.

Extrapolation

Fletcher, A. P. 1978. Drug safety tests and subsequent clinical experience. *Journal of the Royal Society of Medicine* 71:693–696.

Garratini, S. 1985. Toxic effects of chemicals: Difficulties in extrapolating data from animals to man. *CRC Critical Reviews in Toxicology* 16:1–29.

Heywood, R. 1990. Clinical toxicity—Could it have been predicted? In *Animal toxicity studies: Their relevance for man,* ed. C. E. Lumley and S. W. Walker, pp. 57–67. CMR Workshop series. Lancaster, England: Quay Publishing.

Lewis, R. W., R. Billington, E. Debryune, A. Gamner, B. Lang, and F. Carpanini. 2002. Recognition of adverse and nonadverse effects in toxicology studies. *Toxicologic Pathology* 30:66–74.

Litchfield, J. T. 1962. Evaluation of the safety of new drugs by means of tests in animals. *Clinical Pharmacology and Therapeutics* 3:665–672.

Olson, H. et al. 2000. Concordance of the toxicity of pharmaceuticals in humans and in animals. *Regulatory Toxicology and Pharmacology* 32:56–67.

Schein, P. S., and T. Anderson. 1973. The efficacy of animal studies in predicting clinical toxicity of cancer chemotherapeutic drugs. *International Journal of Clinical Pharmacology* 8:22–38.

Schein, P. S., R. D. Davis, S. Carter, J. Newman, D. R. Schein, and D. P. Rall. 1970. The evaluation of cancer drugs in dogs and monkeys for the prediction of qualitative toxicities in man. *Clinical Pharmacology and Therapeutics* 11:3–40.

Thomann, P., H. R. Achermann, and R. Ziel. 1981. Standard animal models of hepatotoxicity—Species differences and relevance for man. In *Drug reactions and the liver,* ed. M. Davis, J. M. Tredger, and R. Williams, pp. 321–327. London: Pitman Medical.

Zbinden, G. 1991. Predictive values of animal studies in toxicology. *Regulatory Toxicology and Pharmacology* 14:167–177.

Appendix A
References for Laboratory
Animal Clinical Chemistry Data

For general information on laboratory animals, the Laboratory Animal Pocket Reference Series published by the CRC Press provides information on biological data, husbandry, management, veterinary care, experimental methodology, and resources. The series includes *The Laboratory Rat, The Laboratory Non-human Primate, The Laboratory Rabbit, The Laboratory Hamster and Gerbil, The Laboratory Mouse, The Laboratory Guinea Pig,* and *The Laboratory Swine.*

REFERENCE VALUES

Throughout this book, attention has been drawn to the variables that affect the reference data ranges for laboratory animals. Some references—general and for some species— are given here, and some additional references are provided at the end of each chapter.

GENERAL

Kaneko, J. J., J. W. Harvey, and M. L. Bruss, eds. 1997. *Clinical biochemistry of domestic animals,* 5th ed. San Diego, CA: Academic Press.

Laird, C. W. 1974. Clinical pathology: Blood chemistry. In *Handbook of laboratory animal science,* vol. 2, ed. E. C. Melby and N. H. Altman, pp. 347–436. Cleveland, OH: CRC Press.

Levine, B. S. 1995. Animal clinical pathology. In *CRC Handbook of Toxicology,* ed. M. J. Derelanko and M. A. Hollinger, pp. 518–535. Boca Raton, FL: CRC Press.

Loeb, W. F., and F. W. Quimby, eds. 1999. *The clinical chemistry of laboratory animals,* 2nd ed. Boca Raton, FL: CRC Press.

Matsuzawa, T., M. Nomura, and T. Unno. 1993. Clinical pathology reference ranges of laboratory animals. *Journal of Veterinary Medical Science* 55:351–362.

Mitruka, B. M., and H. M. Rawnsley. 1977. *Clinical biochemical and hematological reference values in normal experimental animals.* New York: Masson Publishing Inc.

Wolford, S. T., R. A. Schroer, F. X. Gohs, P. P. Gallo, M. Brodeck, H. B. Falk, and R. Ruhren. 1986. Reference range data base for serum chemistry and hematology values in laboratory animals. *Journal of Toxicology and Environmental Health* 8:161–188.

SPECIES

Dog, *Canis familiaris*

Andersen, A. C., and O. W. Schalm. 1970. Hematology. In *The beagle as an experimental dog,* ed. Andersen, A. C., and L. S. Good, pp. 261–281. Ames: The Iowa State University Press.

Fukuda, S., N. Kawashima, H. Iida, J. Aoki, and K. Tokita. 1989. Age dependency of hematological values and concentrations of serum constituents in normal beagles from 1 to 14
years of age. *Nippon Juigaku Zasshi* 51:636–641.

Ikeuchi, J., T. Yoshizaki, and M. Hiarat. 1991. Plasma biochemistry values of young beagle
dogs. *Journal of Toxicological Sciences* 16:49–59.

Kaspar, L. V., and W. P. Norris. 1977. Serum chemistry values of normal dogs (beagles):
Associations with age, sex and family line. *Laboratory Animal Science* 27: 980–985.

Kraft, W., K. Hartmann, and R. Dereser. 1996. Altersabhängigkeiten von laborwerten bei hund
und katze. Teil III. Bilirubin, kreatinin und protein im blutserum. *Tierarztliche Praxis
Suppl.* 24:610–615.

Lane, I. F., D. H. Shaw, S. A. Burton, and A. W. Donald. 2000. Quantitative analysis in healthy
beagle puppies from 9 to 27 weeks of age. *American Journal of Veterinary Research*
61:577–581.

Lulich, J. P., C. A. Osborne, D. J. Polzin, S. D. Johnston, and M. L. Parker. 1991. Urine metabolite values in fed and nonfed clinically normal beagles. *American Journal of Veterinary
Research* 52:1573–1578.

Michaelson, S. M., K. Scheer, and S. Gilt. 1966. The blood of the normal beagle. *Journal of
the American Veterinary Medical Association* 148:532–534.

Passing, H., and R. Brunk. 1981. Statistische Untersuchungen auf alters-und geschlechtsspezi-
fische Unterschiede von Blutparametern an englischen Beagle-Hunden. II. Klinische
Chemie. *Berliner und Munchener Tierarztliche Wochenschrift* 94:432–436.

Uchiyama, T., K. Tokoi, and T. Deki. 1985. Successive changes in the blood composition
of the experimental normal beagle dogs accompanied with age. *Experimental Animals*
34:367–377.

Wolford, S. T., R. A. Schroer, F. X. Gohs, P. P. Gallo, H. B. Falk, and A. R. Dente. 1988. Effect
of age on serum chemistry profile, electrophoresis and thyroid hormones in beagle dogs
two weeks to one year of age. *Veterinary Clinical Pathology* 17:35–42.

Ferret, *Mustela putorius furo*

Esteves, M. I., R. P. Marini, E. B. Ryden, J. C. Murphy, and J. G. Fox. 1994. Estimation of
glomerular filtration rate and evaluation of renal function in ferrets (*Mustela putorius
furo*). *American Journal of Veterinary Research* 55:166–172.

Fox, J. G. 1998. Normal clinical and biologic parameters. In *Biology and diseases of the ferret*,
ed. J. G. Fox, pp. 183–210. Oxford, England: Blackwell Publishing.

Fox, J. G., B. P. Hotaling, B. P. Ackerman, and K. Hewes. 1986. Serum chemistry and hematology
reference values in the ferret (*Mustela putorius furo*). *Laboratory Animal Science* 36:583.

Lee, E. J., W. E. Moore, H. C. Fryer, and H. C. Minocha. 1982. Hematological and serum
chemistry profiles of ferrets (*Mustela putorius furo*). *Laboratory Animals* 16:133–137.

Ohwada, K., and K. Kathira. 1993. Reference values for organ weight, hematology and serum
chemistry in the female ferret (*Mustela putrius furo*). *Jikken Dobutsu* 42:135–142.

Thornton, P. C., P. A. Wright, P. J Sacra, and T. E. W. Goodier. 1979. The ferret. *Mustela putorius furo* as a new species in toxicology. *Laboratory Animals* 13:119–124.

Gerbil, *Meriones unguiculatus*

Mays, A. 1969. Baseline hematological and blood biochemical parameters of the Mongolian
gerbil (*Meriones unguiculatus*). *Laboratory Animal Care* 19:383–342.

Guinea Pig, *Cavia porcellus*

Kitagaki, M., M. Yamaguchi, M. Nakamura, K. Sakurada, T. Suwa, and H. Sasa. 2005. Age-
related changes in hematology and serum chemistry of Weiser–Maples guinea pigs
(*Cavia porcellus*). *Laboratory Animals* 39:321–330.

Sisk, D. B. 1976. Physiology. In *The biology of the guinea pig,* ed. J. E. Wagner and P. J. Manner, pp. 64–74. New York: Academic Press Inc.

Waner, T., Y. Avidar, H. C. Peh, R. Zass, and E. Bogin. 1996. Hematology and clinical blood chemistry and hematology values of normal and euthymic hairless Dunkin–Hartley guinea pigs (*Cavia porcellus*). *Veterinary Clinical Pathology* 25:61–64.

Yoshihara, K., A. Wanatabe, T. Inaba, M. Kuramoto, and K. Shiratori. 1995. A biological study of inbred Weiser–Maples guinea pigs—Urinalysis, hematological and blood chemical values and organ weights. *Experimental Animals* 43:737–745.

Hamster, *Mesocricetus auratus* (Syrian Hamster); *Cricetulus griseus* (Chinese Hamster)

Bannon, P. D., and G. H. Friedell. 1966. Values for plasma constituents in normal and tumor bearing golden hamsters. *Laboratory Animal Care* 16:417–420.

Dent, N. J. 1977. The use of the Syrian hamster to establish its clinical chemistry and hematology profile. In *Clinical toxicology,* vol. XVIII, ed. W. A. Duncan and B. J. Leonard, pp. 321–323. Amsterdam: Excerpta Medica.

Dontenwill, W., H-J. Chevalier, H-P. Harke, U. Lafrenz, G. Reckzeh, and F. Leuschner. 1974. Biochemical and hematological investigations in Syrian golden hamsters after cigarette smoke inhalation. *Laboratory Animals* 8:217–235.

Maxwell, K. O., C. Wish, J. C. Murphy, and J. G. Fox. 1985. Serum chemistry reference values in two strains of Syrian hamster. *Laboratory Animal Science* 35:67–70.

Tomson, F. N., and K. J. Wardrop. 1987. Clinical chemistry and hematology. In *Laboratory hamsters,* ed. G. L. van Hoosier and C. W. McPherson, pp. 43–59. Orlando, FL: Academic Press Inc.

Trautwein, E. A., J. Liang, and K. C. Hayes. 1993. Plasma lipoproteins, biliary lipids and bile acid profiles differ in various strains of Syrian hamsters, *Mesocritus auratus*. *Comparative Biochemistry and Physiology* 104A:829–835.

Marmoset, *Callithrix jacchus*

Davy, C. W., M. R. Jackson, and J. Walker. 1984. Reference intervals for some clinical chemistry parameters in the marmoset (*Callithrix jacchus*): Effect of age and sex. *Laboratory Animals* 18:135–142.

———. 1984. The effect of hemolysis on some clinical chemistry parameters in the marmoset. *Laboratory Animals* 18:161–168.

Holmes, A. W., M. Passovoy, and R. B. Capps. 1967. Marmosets as laboratory animals. III. Blood chemistry of laboratory-kept marmosets with particular attention to liver function and structure. *Laboratory Animal Care* 17:41–47.

McNees, D. W., R. W. Lewis, B. J. Ponzio, R. F. Sis, and F. J. Stein. 1983. Blood chemistry of the common marmoset (*Callithrix jacchus*) maintained in an indoor–outdoor environment: Primate comparisons. *Primates* 25:103–109.

Yarbrough, L. W., J. L. Tollett, R. D. Montrey, and R. J. Beattie. 1984. Serum biochemical, hematological and body measurement data for common marmosets (*Callithrix jacchus jacchus*). *Laboratory Animal Science* 34:276–280.

Micropigs

Ellegaard, L., S. Damm-Jorgensen, S. Klastrup, A. Kornerup-Hansen, and O. Svendsen. 1995. Hematological and clinical chemistry values in 3- and 6-months-old Göttingen minipigs. *Scandinavian Journal of Laboratory and Clinical Animal Science* 22:239–248.

Parsons, A. H., and R. E. Wells. 1986. Serum biochemistry of healthy Yucatan miniature pigs. *Laboratory Animal Science* 36:428–430.

Radin, M. J., M. G. Weiser, and M. J. Fettman. 1986. Hematologic and serum biochemical values for Yucatan miniature swine. *Laboratory Animal Science* 36:425–427.

Rispat, G., M. Slaoui, D. Weber, P. Salemink, C. Berthoux, and R. Shrivastava. 1993. Hematological and plasma biochemical values for healthy Yucatan micropigs. *Laboratory Animals* 27:368–373.

Tsutsumi, H., K. Katagiri, M. Morimoto, T. Nasu, M. Tanigawa, and K. Mamba. 2004. Diurnal variation and age-related changes of bone turnover markers in female Göttingen minipigs. *Laboratory Animals* 38:439–446.

Mouse, *Mus*

Boehm, O., B. Zur, A. Koch, N. Tran, R. Freyenhagen, M. Hartmann, and K. Zacharowski. 2007. Clinical chemistry reference database for Wistar rats and C57/BL6 mice. *Biological Chemistry* 388:547–554.

Camus, M-C., M. J. Chapman, P. Forgez, and P. M. Lapaud. 1983. Distribution and characterization of the serum lipoproteins and apoproteins in the mouse, *Mus musculus. Journal of Lipid Research* 24:1210–1299.

Cotchin, E., and F. J. C. Roe. 1967. *Pathology of laboratory rats and mice.* Oxford, England: Blackwell Scientific Publications.

Everett, R. M., and S. D. Harrison. 1983. Clinical biochemistry. In *The mouse in biomedical research,* ed. H. L. Foster, J. D. Small, and J. G. Fox, pp. 313–326. New York: Academic Press.

Frith, C. H., R. L. Suber, and R. Umholtz. 1980. Hematologic and clinical chemistry findings in control BALB/c and C57BL/6 mice. *Laboratory Animal Science* 30: 835–840.

Schneck, K., M. Washington, D. Holder, K. Lodge, and S. Motzel. 2000. Hematological and serum reference values in nontransgenic FVB mice. *Comparative Medicine* 50:32–35.

Nonhuman Primate, *Macaca fascicularis* (Cynomolgus); *Macaca artoides* (Stump Tailed Monkey)

Buchl, S. J., and B. Howard. 1997. Hematologic and serum biochemical and electrolyte values in clinically normal domestically bred Rhesus monkeys (*Macaca mulatta*) according to age sex and gravidity. *Laboratory Animal Science* 47:528–533.

de Neef, K. J., K. Nieuwenhuijsen, A. J. J. C. Lammers, A. J. M. Degen, and F. Verbon. 1987. Blood variables in adult stumptail macques (*Macaca artoides*) living in a captive group: Annual variability. *Journal of Medical Primatology* 16:237–247.

Fuchs, E., J. Hensel, M. Böer, and M. H. Weber. 1989. Urinproteine bei primaten. *Klinische Wochenschrift* 67 (Suppl. XV11): 19–22.

Matsumoto, K., H. Akagi, T. Ochiai, K. Hagino, K. Sekita, Y. Kawasaki, M. A. Matin, and T. Furuya. 1980. Comparative blood values of *Macaca mulatta* and *Macaca fascicularis. Experimental Animals* 29:335–340.

Matsuzawa, T., and Y. Nagia. 1994. Comparative hematological and plasma chemistry values in purpose-bred squirrel, cynomolgus and Rhesus monkeys. *Comparative Hematology International* 4:43–48.

Schuurman, H-J., and H. T. Smith. 2005. Reference values for clinical chemistry and clinical hematology parameters in cynomolgus monkeys. *Xenotransplantation* 12:72–75.

Verlangieri, A. J., J. C. DePriest, and J. C. Kapeghian. 1985. Normal serum biochemical, hematological and EKG parameters in anesthetized adult male *Macaca fascicularis* and *Macaca artoides. Laboratory Animal Science* 35:63–66.

Rabbit, *Oryctolagus cuniculus*

Bortolotti, A., D. Castelli, and M. Bonati. 1989. Hematology and serum chemistry values of adult, pregnant and newborn New Zealand rabbits (*Oryctolagus cuniculus*). *Laboratory Animal Science* 39:437–439.

Evans, G. O. 1994. Plasma albumin measurements in New Zealand white rabbits. *World Rabbit Science* 2:25–27.

Hewitt, C. D., D. J. Innes, J. Savory, and M. R. Wills. 1989. Normal biochemical and hematological values in New Zealand white rabbits. *Clinical Chemistry* 35:1777–1779.

Kozma, C., W. Macklin, L. M. Cummins, and R. Mauer. 1974. Anatomy, physiology and biochemistry of the rabbit. In *The biology of the laboratory rabbit,* ed. S. H. Weisbroth, R. E. Flatt, and A. L. Kraus, pp. 50–72. New York: Academic Press Inc.

McLaughlin, R. M., and R. E. Fish. 1994. Clinical chemistry and hematology. In *The biology of the laboratory rabbit,* 2nd ed., ed. P. J. Manning, D. H. Ringler, and C. E. Newcomer, pp. 111–124. San Diego, CA: Academic Press Inc.

Rat, *Rattus norvegicus*

Boehm, O., B. Zur, A. Koch, N. Tran, R. Freyenhagen, M. Hartmann, and K. Zacharowski. 2007. Clinical chemistry reference database for Wistar rats and C57/BL6 mice. *Biological Chemistry* 388:547–554.

Car, B. D., V. M. Eng, N. E. Everds, and D. I. Bounous. 2005. Clinical pathology. In *The laboratory rat,* 2nd ed., ed. M. A. Suckow, S. H. Weisbroth, and C. L. Franklin, pp. 127–147. New York: Academic Press.

Cotchin, E., and J. C. Roe. 1967. *Pathology of laboratory rats and mice.* Oxford, England: Blackwell Scientific Publications.

Kozma, C. K., S. H. Weisbroth, S. L. Stratman, and M. Conejeros. 1969. Normal biological values for Long–Evans rats. *Laboratory Animal Care* 19:747–755.

Lewi, P. J., and R. P. Marsbloom. 1981. *Toxicology reference data—Wistar rat.* Amsterdam: Elsevier/North–Holland Biomedical Press.

Libertati, T. A., S. R. Sansone, and M. H. Feuston. 2004. Hematology and clinical chemistry values in pregnant Wistar Hannover rats compared with nonmated controls. *Veterinary Clinical Pathology* 33:68–73.

Lillie, L., N. J. Temple, and L. Z. Florence. 1996. Reference values for young normal Sprague–Dawley rats: Weight gain, hematology and clinical chemistry. *Human and Experimental Toxicology* 15:612–616.

Loeb, W. F., and M. C. Carakostas. 1992. Changes in serum biochemistry. In *Pathobiology of the aging rat,* ed. U. Mohr, D. L. Dungworth, and C. C. Capen, pp. 7–13. Washington, D.C.: ILSI Press.

Neptun, D. A., C. A. Smith, and R. D. Irons. 1985. Effect of sampling site and collection method on variations in baseline clinical pathology parameters in Fischer-344 rats. 1. Clinical chemistry. *Fundamental and Applied Toxicology* 5:1180–1185.

Papworth, T. A., and S. K. Clubb. 1995. Clinical pathology in the neonatal rat. *Comparative Haematology International* 5:237–250.

Pettersen, J. C., R. L. Morrissey, D. R. Saunders, K. L. Pavkov, L. G. Luempert, J. C. Turnier, D. W. Matheson, and D. R. Schwarzt. 1996. A 2-year comparison study of Crl: CD BR and Hsd: Sprague–Dawley SD rats. *Fundamental and Applied Toxicology* 33:196–211.

Ringler, D. H., and L. Dabich. 1979. Hematology and clinical biochemistry. In *The laboratory rat,* vol. 1, ed. H. J. Baker, J. R. Lindsey, and S. H. Weisbroth, pp. 105–121. Orlando, FL: Academic Press Inc.

Shevlock, P. N., S. R. Khan, and R. L. Hackett. 1993. Urinary chemistry of the normal Sprague–Dawley rat. *Urological Research* 21:309–312.

Trevisan, A., M. Giraldo, M. Borella, and S. Maso. 2001. Historical control data on urinary and renal tissue biomarkers in naive Wistar rats. *Journal of Applied Toxicology* 21:409–413.

Waner, T., A. Nyska, and R. Chen. 1991. Population distribution profiles of the activities of blood alanine and aspartate aminotransferases in the normal F344 inbred rat by age and sex. *Laboratory Animals* 25:263–271.

Wolford, S. T., R. A. Schroer, P. P. Gallo, F. X. Gohs, M. Brodeck, H. B. Falk, and R. Ruhren. 1987. Age-related changes in serum chemistry and hematology values in normal Sprague–Dawley rats. *Fundamental and Applied Toxicology* 8:80–88.

Appendix B
SI Unitage and Conversions

The International System of Units (Systeme International: SI) was adopted in 1960 by the General Conference of Weights and Measures as a coherent system based on seven basic units: the meter, kilogram, second, ampere, kelvin, candela, and mole. In human medicine, the system has not been adopted universally.

Some of the common clinical chemistry units are provided here with factors to convert from the traditional non-SI units to SI unitage in plasma or serum.

REFERENCES

Baron, D. N., P. M. G. Broughton, M. Cohen, T. S. Lansley, S. M. Lewis, and N. K. Shinton. 1974. The use of SI units in reporting results obtained in hospital laboratories. *Journal of Clinical Pathology* 27:590–597.

Dykbaer, R. 1979. International Union of Pure and Applied Chemistry and International Federation of Clinical Chemistry. IUPAC section on clinical chemistry: Commission on Quantities and Units in Clinical Chemistry and IFCC Committee on Standards Expert Panel on Quantities and Units approved recommendation (1978). List of quantities in clinical chemistry. IUPAC and IFCC. *Clinica Chimica Acta* 96:185–204F.

Editorial. 1986. Now read this: The SI units are here. *Journal of the American Medical Association* 255:2329–2339.

Laposata, M. 1992. *SI unit conversion guide.* Waltham, MA: Massachusetts Medical Society (New England Journal of Medicine).

Olesen, H. 1996. Properties and units in the clinical laboratory science 1. Syntax and semantic rules, IUPAC-IFCC recommendations 1995. *Clinica Chimica Acta* 245:S5–22.

UNITS FOR VOLUMES, MASSES, AND MOLES

fl or fL = femtoliter (10^{-15}/L)	fg = femtogram	fmol = femtomole
pl or pL = picoliter (10^{-12}/L)	pg = picogram	pmol = picomole
nl or nL = nanoliter (10^{-9}/L)	ng = nanogram	pmol = picomole
μl or μL = microliter (10^{-6}/L)	μg = microgram	μmol = micromole
mL = milliliter (10^{-3}/L)	mg = milligram	mmol = millimole
dl or dL = deciliter (10^{-1}/L)		
kDa = kilodalton		

MOLARITY AND MOLALITY

The mole is a unit of mass and is expressed as the molecular weight of substance in grams (g). A molar solution will contain one mole solute per liter of solution. A molal solution contains one mole solute per 1000 g of solvent.

TABLE B.1
SI Units and Conversion Factors

Analyte	SI Unit	Traditional Unit	Conversion Factor to SI
Albumin	g/L	g/dL	10
	μmol /L	g/dL	149
Bicarbonate	mmol/L	meq/L	1
Total bilirubin	μmol/L	mg/dL	17.1
Calcium	mmol/L	mg/dL	0.25
		meq/L	0.5
Chloride	mmol/L	mg/dL	1
Cholesterol	mmol/L	mg/dL	0.0259
Cortisol	nmol/L	μg/dl	27.6
Creatinine	μmol/L	mg/dL	88.4
Ferritin	ng/mL	μg/L	1
Fibrinogen	g/L	mg/dl	0.01
Folate	nmol/L	μg/L	2.27
Globulin	g/L	g/dL	10
Glucose	mmol/L	mg/dL	0.0555
	mmol/L	g/dL	55.5
Haptoglobin	mg/L	mg/dl	10
Inorganic phosphate	mmol/L	mg/dL	0.323
Iron	μmol/L	μg/dL	0.179
Magnesium	mmol/L	mg/dL	0.411
		meq/L	0.5
Potassium	mmol/L	meq/L	1
Sodium	mmol/L	meq/L	1
Thyroxine	nmol/L	μg/dL	12.9
Total protein	g/L	mg/dL	10
Tri-iodothyronine	nmol/L	ng/dL	0.015
Triglycerides	mmol/L	mg/dL	0.0113
Urate (uric acid)	μmol/l	mg/dL	59.48
Urea	mmol/L	mg/dL	0.166

Note: For some substances, a different factor will need to be used (e.g., for urinary creatinine, a factor of 8.84 will convert grams per liter to millimoles per liter).

OTHER NOTES

1. **pH/Hydrogen ion**

   The recommended SI unit is nmol/L. This relationship is expressed by the formula:

   $pH = -\log_{10}[H^+]$, where $[H^+]$ is expressed in mol/L.

2. **Blood urea nitrogen**

   To convert mg/dL to mmol/L, multiply by 0.357.

   To convert urea nitrogen values to mg/dL, multiply by 2.14 to obtain urea mg/dL values.

3. **Osmolarity and osmolality**

   Osmolarity refers to the molar concentration (mol/L), whereas osmolality refers to molal concentrations and is usually expressed as moOsmol/kg body water.

4. **Enzymes**

   Enzyme values vary considerably between laboratories, and these values are dependent on measurement temperature, substrate concentration, pH, buffer, activators, and other methodological variations. Enzyme activities may be expressed by various units; these units include:

   International unit—defined as the enzyme activity that will convert one micromole of substrate per minute under defined conditions. It may be expressed as IU/L, or sometimes as U/L or mIU/mL. One IU/L corresponds to 16.67 nanokatals per liter.

   Katal—defined as the catalytic activity that will convert one mole of substrate per second under defined conditions. One nanokatal (nKat) equals 109 mol/s or 0.06 IU/L.

If the reaction conditions vary (e.g., using different substrates for the same enzyme), then using these conversion factors may be inappropriate for comparison. Even for common enzymes such as the aminotransferases, there are several different national and international recommended methods for use with human sera or plasma, and these yield differing values despite conformity in units. There are no internationally recommended conditions for samples obtained from laboratory animals.

Appendix C
"Expectable" Ranges for Plasma/Serum

Investigators coming into the field of laboratory animal plasma/serum chemistry sometimes ask the question: "What values might I expect to encounter in healthy animals?" From the information provided in Chapters 12, 13, and 14, the reader will understand that these ranges can be affected by many pre-analytical and analytical variables on the measurements, and it must be emphasized that the local laboratory should be asked to comment on its own ranges and experience. Many data from older published studies have limited value for comparative purposes because the changes in animal breeding, genetic characterization, animal care, sample collection procedures, and improved analytical methods over time have altered the ranges obtained for healthy animals. The compendium of data provided by Loeb and Quimby (1999; see Appendix A, General References) is comprehensive, but these data illustrate the wide variations in published data for laboratory animals.

The following tables are provided to indicate the ranges of values that might be obtained for several species of laboratory animals. These ranges are based on published and unpublished data sources, and they should be treated as a guide. These "expectable ranges" and the references provided in Appendix A can be used for comparison when establishing locally determined ranges.

The values are provided in both SI and non-SI unitage (see Appendix B for conversion factors). The values for sodium, potassium, and chloride ranges are expressed as millimoles per liter, and these values are the same in milliequivalents per liter. Enzyme activities are expressed as measured at 37°C.

The abbreviations used are:

ALT: alanine aminotranferase;
AST: aspartate aminotransferase;
ALP: alkaline phosphatase;
CK: creatine kinase;
GGT: gamma glutamyl transferase;
LDH: lactate dehydrogenase; and
BUN: blood urea nitrogen.

Ranges for Dogs (Beagles Aged 8–12 Months)

Test	SI Unit	Range in SI Units	Non-SI Unit	Range in Non-SI Units
Bilirubin, total	μmol/L	2–14	mg/dL	0.1–0.80
Albumin	g/L	27–37	g/dL	2.7–3.7
Calcium	mmol/L	2.40–3.00	mg/dL	9.6–12.0
Chloride	mmol/L	105–118	mequiv/L	105–118
Cholesterol, total	mmol/L	2.59– 5.18	mg/dL	100–200
Creatinine	μmol/l	44–97	mg/dL	0.5–1.1
Glucose	mmol/L	3.33–6.66	mg/dL	60–120
Inorganic phosphate	mmol/L	1.29–2.91	mg/dL	4.0–9.0
Potassium	mmol/L	4.2–5.3	mequiv/L	4.2–5.3
Total protein	g/L	48–64	g/dL	4.8–6.4
Triglycerides	mmol/L	0.22–1.13	mg/dL	20–100
Sodium	mmol/L	140–154	mequiv/L	140–154
Urea	mmol/L	2.14–7.50	mg/dL; BUN	6–21

Enzymes

Test	SI Unit	Range in SI Units
ALT	IU/L	10–70
AST	IU/L	5–50
ALP	IU/L	30–180
CK	IU/L	30–260
GGT	IU/L	0–7
LDH	IU/L	20–250

Ranges for Ferrets

Test	SI Unit	Range in SI Units	Non-SI Unit	Range in Non-SI Units
Bilirubin, total	μmol/L	1–7	mg/dL	0–0.4
Albumin	g/L	26–40	g/dL	2.6–4.0
Calcium	mmol/L	2.10–2.70	mg/dL	8.4–10.8
Chloride	mmol/L	105–120	mequiv/L	105–120
Cholesterol, total	mmol/L	2.59–6.48	mg/dL	100–250
Creatinine	μmol/l	18–60	mg/dL	0.2–0.8
Glucose	mmol/L	4.40–8.80	mg/dL	80–160
Inorganic phosphate	mmol/L	1.60–2.91	mg/dL	5.0–9.0
Potassium	mmol/L	4.0–5.5	mequiv/L	4.0–5.5
Total protein	g/L	51–74	g/dL	5.1–7.4
Triglycerides	mmol/L	0.11–0.57	mg/dL	10–50
Sodium	mmol/L	148–154	mequiv/L	148–154
Urea	mmol/L	2.86–12.50	mg/dL; BUN	8–35

Enzymes				
ALT	IU/L	15–170		
AST	IU/L	20–100		
ALP	IU/L	200–350		
LDH	IU/L	250–1000		

Ranges for Guinea Pigs

Test	SI Unit	Range in SI Units	Non-SI Unit	Range in Non-SI Units
Bilirubin, total	μmol/L	0–5	mg/dL	0–0.3
Albumin	g/L	25–40	g/dL	2.5–4.0
Calcium	mmol/L	2.30–2.85	mg/dL	9.2–11.4
Chloride	mmol/L	100–112	mequiv/L	100–112
Cholesterol, total	mmol/L	0.65–2.07	mg/dL	25–80
Creatinine	μmol/l	35–106	mg/dL	0.4–1.2
Glucose	mmol/L	4.16–7.22	mg/dL	75–130
Inorganic phosphate	mmol/L	1.29–2.58	mg/dL; mequiv/L	4.0–8.0
Potassium	mmol/L	4.0–6.0	mequiv/L	4.0–6.0
Total protein	g/L	45–63	g/dL	4.5–6.3
Triglycerides	mmol/L	0.11–0.79	mg/dL	10–70
Sodium	mmol/L	133–142	mequiv/L	133–142
Urea	mmol/L	5.36–10.71	mg/dL; BUN	15–30

Enzymes

ALT	IU/L	10–90		
AST	IU/L	10–90		
ALP	IU/L	80–350		
CK	IU/L	50–150		
GGT	IU/L	1–12		
LDH	IU/L	20–120		

Ranges for Hamsters (Syrian)

Test	SI Unit	Range in SI Units	Non-SI Unit	Range in Non-SI Units
Bilirubin, total	μmol/L	2–12	mg/dL	0.1–0.7
Albumin	g/L	35–45	g/dL	3.5–4.5
Calcium	mmol/L	2.40–3.10	mg/dL	9.6–12.4
Chloride	mmol/L	98–110	mequiv/L	98–110
Cholesterol, total	mmol/L	1.81–5.18	mg/dL	70–200
Creatinine	μmol/l	26–79	mg/dl	0.3–0.9
Glucose	mmol/L	3.30–8.25	mg/dL	60–150
Inorganic phosphate	mmol/L	1.42–2.71	mg/dL	4.4–8.4
Potassium	mmol/l	4.0–6.0	mequiv/L	4.0–6.0
Total protein	g/L	54–70	g/dL	5.4–7.0
Triglycerides	mmol/L	2.26–3.96	mg/dL	200–350
Sodium	mmol/L	137–150	mequiv/L	137–150
Urea	mmol/L	4.28–10.71	mg/dL; BUN	12–30

Enzymes				
ALT	IU/L	20–50		
AST	IU/L	20–150		
ALP	IU/L	50–170		
LDH	IU/L	100–300		

Ranges for Marmoset *(Callithrix jacchus)*

Test	SI Unit	Range in SI Units	Non SI Unit	Range in Non-SI Units
Bilirubin, total	μmol/L	0–5	mg/dL	0–0.3
Albumin	g/L	36–52	g/dL	3.6–5.2
Calcium	mmol/L	2.70–3.10	mg/dL	10.8–12.4
Chloride	mmol/L	100–115	mequiv/L	100–115
Cholesterol, total	mmol/L	2.59–6.22	mg/dL	100–240
Creatinine	μmol/l	18–70	mg/dL	0.2–0.8
Glucose	mmol/L	4.40–15.54	mg/dL	80–280
Inorganic phosphate	mmol/L	0.81–2.58	mg/dL	2.5–8.0
Potassium	mmol/L	3.0–5.0	mequiv/L	3.0–5.0
Total protein	g/L	60–90	g/dL	6.0–9.0
Triglycerides	mmol/L	0.23–2.26	mg/dL	20–200
Sodium	mmol/L	145–160	mequiv/L	145–160
Urea	mmol/L	2.86–6.4	mg/dL; BUN	8–18

Enzymes

ALT	IU/L	2–30		
AST	IU/L	60–180		
ALP	IU/L	130–300		
CK	IU/L	100–650		
GGT	IU/L	0–15		
LDH	IU/L	150–700		

Ranges for Mice (CD1)

Test	SI Unit	Range in SI Units	Non-SI Unit	Range in Non-SI Units
Bilirubin, total	µmol/L	0–17	mg/dL	0–1.0
Albumin	g/L	28–40	g/dL	2.8–4.0
Calcium	mmol/L	2.00–3.00	mg/dL	8.0–12.0
Chloride	mmol/L	110–125	mequiv/L	110–125
Cholesterol, total	mmol/L	1.04–4.14	mg/dL	40–160
Creatinine	µmol/l	26–97	mg/dL	0.3–1.1
Glucose	mmol/L	1.67–13.90	mg/dL	30–250
Inorganic phosphate	mmol/L	1.94–3.88	mg/dL	6–12
Potassium	mmol/L	5.0–8.5	mequiv/L	5.0–8.5
Total protein	g/L	40–60	g/dL	4.0–6.0
Triglycerides	mmol/L	0.23–1.13	mg/dL	20–100
Sodium	mmol/L	146–170	mequiv/L	146–170
Urea	mmol/L	3.57–17.85	mg/dL; BUN	10–50
Enzymes				
ALT	IU/L	40–140		
AST	IU/L	50–250		
ALP	IU/L	20–100		

Ranges for Micropigs (Yucatan)

Test	SI unit	Range in SI Units	Non-SI Unit	Range in Non-SI Units
Bilirubin, total	μmol/L	0–12	mg/dL	0–0.7
Albumin	g/L	35–55	g/dL	3.5–5.5
Calcium	mmol/L	2.25–2.85	mg/dL	9.0–11.4
Chloride	mmol/L	98–110	mequiv/L	98–110
Cholesterol, total	mmol/L	1.55–3.62	mg/dL	60–140
Creatinine	μmol/l	53–106	mg/dL	0.6–1.2
Glucose	mmol/L	2.22–6.66	mg/dL	40–120
Inorganic phosphate	mmol/L	1.55–2.58	mg/dL	4.8–8.0
Potassium	mmol/L	3.5–5.5	mequiv/L	3.5–5.5
Total protein	g/L	63–83	g/dL	6.3–8.3
Triglycerides	mmol/L	0.11–0.62	mg/dL	10–55
Sodium	mmol/L	135–150	mequiv/L	135–150
Urea	mmol/L	4.28–8.57	mg/dL; BUN	12–24

Enzymes		
ALT	IU/L	20–80
AST	IU/L	10–80
ALP	IU/L	20–130
CK	IU/L	100–1500
LDH	IU/L	300–1000

Ranges for Monkeys (*Cynomolgus*)

Test	SI Unit	Range in SI Units	Non-SI Unit	Range in Non-SI Units
Bilirubin, total	μmol/L	2–15	mg/dL	0.1–0.9
Albumin	g/L	35–50	g/dL	3.5–5.0
Calcium	mmol/L	2.25–2.75	mg/dL	9.0–11.0
Chloride	mmol/L	100–115	mequiv/L	100–115
Cholesterol, total	mmol/L	2.33–4.92	mg/dL	90–190
Creatinine	μmol/l	44–114	mg/dL	0.5–1.3
Glucose	mmol/L	2.78–7.22	mg/dL	50–130
Inorganic phosphate	mmol/L	1.25–1.94	mg/dL	3.5–6.0
Potassium	mmol/L	3.5–6.0	mequiv/L	3.5–6.0
Total protein	g/L	70–90	g/dL	7.0–9.0
Triglycerides	mmol/L	0.26–1.02	g/dL	20–90
Sodium	mmol/L	142–152	mequiv/L	142–152
Urea	mmol/L	3.57–10.71	mg/dL; BUN	10–30

Enzymes				
ALT	IU/L	10–80		
AST	IU/L	10–80		
ALP	IU/L	30–360		
CK	IU/L	50–600		
LDH	IU/L	300–600		

Ranges for Rabbits (New Zealand White)

Test	SI Unit	Range in SI Units	Non-SI Unit	Range in Non-SI Units
Bilirubin, total	µmol/L	0–14	mg/dL	0.1–0.8
Albumin	g/L	29–42	g/dL	2.9–4.2
Calcium	mmol/L	3.00–4.25	mg/dL	12–17.0
Chloride	mmol/L	108–120	mequiv/L	108–120
Cholesterol, total	mmol/L	0.9–1.7	mg/dL	5–80
Creatinine	µmol/l	70–132	mg/dL	0.8–1.5
Glucose	mmol/L	5.56–8.88	mg/dL	100–160
Inorganic phosphate	mmol/L	0.85–2.27	mg/dL	2.5–7.0
Potassium	mmol/L	4.0–6.0	mequiv/L	4.0–6.0
Total protein	g/L	52–69	g/dL	5.2–6.9
Triglycerides	mmol/L	0.17–1.81	mg/dL	15–160
Sodium	mmol/L	138–158	mequiv/L	138–158
Urea	mmol/L	3.57–10.71	mg/dL; BUN	10–30

Enzymes

Test	SI Unit	Range in SI Units
ALT	IU/L	10–70
AST	IU/L	10–80
ALP	IU/L	40–140
CK	IU/L	150–1000
LDH	IU/L	30–140

Ranges for Rats (Wistar Aged 6–12 Weeks)

Test	SI Unit	Range in SI Units	Non-SI Unit	Range in Non-SI Units
Bilirubin, total	μmol/L	0–8.5	mg/dL	0–0.5
Albumin	g/L	30–50	g/dL	3.0–5.0
Calcium	mmol/L	2.25–4.00	mg/dL	9.0–12.0
Chloride	mmol/L	98–112	mequiv/L	98–112
Cholesterol, total	mmol/L	0.51–2.85	mg/dL	20–110
Creatinine	μmol/l	9–70	mg/dL	0.1–0.8
Glucose	mmol/L	7.77–12.21	mg/dL	140–220
Inorganic phosphate	mmol/L	1.29–2.58	mg/dL	4.0–8.0
Potassium	mmol/L	4.0–6.0	mequiv/L	4.0–6.0
Total protein	g/L	50–80	g/dL	5.0–8.0
Triglycerides	mmol/L	0.56–2.23	mg/dL	50–200
Sodium	mmol/L	138–152	mequiv/L	138–152
Urea	mmol/L	4.28–8.57	mg/dL	12–24
Enzymes				
ALT	IU/L	10–80		
AST	IU/L	20–100		
ALP	IU/L	70–450		
CK	IU/L	50–650		
GGT	IU/L	0–4		
LDH	IU/L	50–700		

Appendix D
General Abbreviations

This list includes some of the common acronyms used in toxicology and drug development, but every organization invents its own alphabet soup of acronyms, so beware!

AACC: American Association of Clinical Chemistry
ABPI: Association of British Pharmaceutical Industry
ADME: Absorption, distribution, metabolism and excretion
ADR: Adverse drug reaction
ANOVA: Analysis of variance
ANSI: American National Standards Institute
AUC: Area under the curve: plasma concentration-time curve
BP or Bp: Blood pressure
CAS: Chemical Abstract Service
CDC: Centers for Disease Control, United States
CFR: Code of Federal Regulation, United States
CFSAN: Center for Food Safety and Applied Nutrition, United States
CHIPS: Chemical hazards information, packaging, and supply
CL: Confidence limits
CNS: Central nervous system
CPMP: Committee for Proprietary Medicinal Products (EEC)
CRO: Contract research organization
CTC: Clinical trials certificate
CTM: Clinical trials material
CV: Coefficient of variation
CVS: Cardiovascular system
DACC: Division of Animal Clinical Chemistry, AACC
ECCP: European Comparative Clinical Pathology
ECG: Electrocardiogram
EDI: Estimated daily intake
EEC: European Economic Community
ELISA: Enzyme Linked Immunoabsorbent Assay
EMA: European Medicines Agency
EMEA: European Medicines Evaluation Agency
EPA: Environmental Protection Agency, United States
EQAS: External Quality Assessment Scheme
EU: European Union
FAO: Food and Agricultural Organization of the United Nations
FASEB: Federation of American Societies for Experimental Biology
FDA: Food and Drug Administration, United States

FD&C: Food, Drug and Cosmetic Act, United States

FIFRA: Federal Insecticide Fungicide and Rodenticide Act, United States

FOB: Functional observational battery

GCP: Good clinical practice

GI: Gastrointestinal

GIT: Gastrointestinal tract

GLP: Good laboratory practice

GMP: Good manufacturing practice

HPLC: High-performance liquid chromatography

HSE: Health and Safety Executive, United Kingdom

IARC: International Agency for Research on Cancer

IC: Incapacitating concentration

IC 50: Concentration causing (or calculated to cause) 50% incapacitation of the population studied (e.g., cells)

ICH: International Committee on Harmonization of technical requirements of pharmaceuticals for human use

ID 50: Dose causing 50% inhibition in the population studied

IM: Intramuscular

IND: Investigational new drug

IP: Intraperitoneal

IPCS: International Program on Chemical Safety, World Health Organization

IQ: Installation qualification

IRIS: Integrated risk information system

ISO: International Standards Organization

IV: Intravenous

JPMA: Japan Pharmaceutical Manufacturers Association

LAA: Laboratory animal allergy

LOAEL: Lowest observed adverse effect level

LOD: Limit of detection

LOEL: Lowest observed effect level

LOQ: Limit of quantification

MAA: Marketing authorization authority

MCA: Medicines Control Agency, United Kingdom; now MHRA

MDD: Maximum daily dose

MHRA: Medicines and Healthcare Products Regulatory Agency, United Kingdom

MHW: Ministry of Health and Welfare, Japan

MOA: Mode of action

MRC: Medical Research Council, United Kingdom

MSDS: Material safety data sheet

MTD: Maximum tolerated dose

MW: Molecular weight

NCE: New chemical entity

NICE: National Institute for Clinical Excellence, United Kingdom

NIEHS: National Institute of Environmental Health and Safety, United States

NIOSH: National Institute of Occupational Safety and Health, United States

NOAEL: No observable adverse effect level

NOEL: No observed effect level
NONS: Notification of new substances
NTP: National Toxicology Program, United States
OECD: Organization for Economic Cooperation and Development
OEL: Occupational exposure limit
OSHA: Occupational Safety and Health Administration
OTC: Over-the-counter (sale)
PC: Percutaneous
PCD: Programmed cell death
PEL: Permissible or permitted exposure level
PMA: Pharmaceutical Manufacturers Association, United States
PMDA: Pharmaceutical and Medical Devices Agency, Japan
PMN: Premanufacturing notification
PMS: Postmarketing surveillance
PO: Per oral
QA: Quality assurance
QC: Quality control
QSAR: Quantitative structure and activity relationship
RTECS: Registry of toxic effects of chemical substances
SAR: Structure activity relationship
SC: Subcutaneous
SD: Standard deviation
SE: Standard error
SEM: Standard error of the mean
SOP: Standard operating procedure
TDI: Total dietary intake
TLV: Threshold limit value
TSCA: Toxic Substances Control Act, United States
USDA: United States Department of Agriculture
US EPA: United States Environmental Protection Agency
USP: United States Pharmacopeia
VMD: Veterinary Medicine Directorate, United Kingdom
WHO: World Health Organization

Appendix E
Some Common Biochemical Abbreviations

ADP: Adenosine diphosphate
ATP: Adenosine triphosphate
CBP: Cortisol binding protein
CRF: Corticotrophin releasing factor
Da: Dalton, unit of mass
DNA: Deoxyribose nucleic acid
DPG: Diphosphoglycerate or diphosphoglyceric acid
EDTA: Ethylenediaminetetra-acetic acid
ELISA: Enzyme linked immunosorbent assay
EM pathway: Emden Meyerhof pathway
EPO: Erythropoietin
ESF: Erythropoietin stimulating factor
F6P: Fructose 6 phosphate
FSH: Foliotrophin (follicle stimulating hormone)
G6PD: Glucose 6 phosphate dehydrogenase
GH: Somatotrophin (growth hormone)
GHRH: Growth hormone releasing hormone
GnRF: Gonadotropin releasing factor
GSH: Reduced glutathione
GSSG: Oxidized glutathione
HMGCoA: 3-hydroxy-3-methyl-glutaryl-coenzyme A
IG or Ig: Immunoglobulin
IL: Interleukin
LCAT: Phosphatidylcholine sterol acyltransferase
LDH: Lactic dehydrogenase
LH: Luteotrophin (lutrophin; luteinizing hormone)
LPS: Lipopolysaccharide
NAD: Nicotinamide adenine dinucleotide
NADH: Reduced nicotinamide adenine dinucleotide
NADPH: Reduced nicotinamide adenine dinucleotide phosphate
PPAR: Peroxisome proliferator-activated receptor
PTH: Parathyrin (parathyroid hormone)
RT-PCR: Real-time polymerase chain reaction
T3: Triiodothyronine
T4: Thyroxine
TBG: Thyroxine binding globulin

Tg: Thyroglobulin
TH: Thyroid hormone
TRH: Thyrotropin-releasing hormone
TSH: Thyroid stimulating hormone (thyrotropin)
TTR: Transthyretin

Index